FIRST EXPOSURE TO

NEUROLOGY

FIRST EXPOSURE TO

NEUROLOGY

Howard S. Kirshner, MD

Professor and Vice Chairman
Department of Neurology
Director, Vanderbilt Stroke Center
Vanderbilt University Medical Center
Nashville, Tennessee

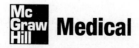 Medical

New York / Chicago / San Francisco / Lisbon / London / Madrid / Mexico City
Milan / New Delhi / San Juan / Seoul / Singapore / Sydney / Toronto

First Exposure to Neurology

1 2 3 4 5 6 7 8 9 0   DOC/DOC   0 9 8 7

ISBN-13: 978-0-07-145819-1
ISBN-10: 0-07-145819-0

This book was set in Palatino by International Typesetting and Composition.
The editors of this book were Jason Malley, Karen Edmonson, and Lester A. Sheinis.
The production supervisor was Sherri Souffrance.
Project management was handled by International Typesetting and Composition.
The cover designer was Janice Bielawa.
The indexer was Robert Swanson.
RR Donnelley was printer and binder.

This book is printed on acid-free paper.

Cataloging-in-publication data are on file at the Library of Congress

INTERNATIONAL EDITION ISBN 10:0-07-110490-9; ISBN 13:978-0-07-11490-6
Copyright © 2007. Exclusive rights by The McGraw-Hill Companies, Inc., for manufacture and export. This book cannot be reexported from the country to which it is consigned by McGraw-Hill. The International Edition is not available in North America.

CONTENTS

Bassel Abou-Khalil, MD
Professor of Neurology
Director, Epilepsy Division
Vanderbilt University School
 of Medicine
Nashville, Tennessee

Michael Edgeworth, MD
Assistant Professor
 of Neurology
Vanderbilt University School
 of Medicine
Nashville, Tennessee

Gerald M. Fenichel, MD
Professor, Chair Emeritus
Director, Child Neurology
Department of Neurology
Vanderbilt University School
 of Medicine
Nashville, Tennessee

Kimberly N. Hutchison, MD
Assistant Professor
 of Neurology
Vanderbilt University School
 of Medicine
Nashville, Tennessee

Howard S. Kirshner, MD
Professor and Vice Chairman
Department of Neurology
Director, Vanderbilt Stroke Center
Vanderbilt University School
 of Medicine
Nashville, Tennessee

Robert L. Macdonald, MD, PhD
Professor and Chairman
Department of Neurology
Vanderbilt University School
 of Medicine
Nashville, Tennessee

Karl E. Misulis, MD, PhD
Clinical Professor of Neurology
Vanderbilt University School
 of Medicine
Semmes-Murphey Clinic
Nashville, Tennessee

Paul L. Moots, MD
Associate Professor of Neurology
Director, Neurooncology Division
Vanderbilt University School
 of Medicine
Nashville, Tennessee

PREFACE

When I was approached by editors at McGraw-Hill to write a textbook of neurology for the medical student clerkship, my initial reaction was that there is already a wealth, almost a plethora, of textbooks on neurology. Some of these books are for general audiences, some for house officers, some for psychiatrists, some for practicing neurologists, but precious few are intended for medical students. Medical students on a required neurology clerkship represent a special audience. Students rotate on neurology for four weeks at most U.S. medical schools, even two weeks at some. As a course director at Vanderbilt for 23 years, I found myself in a quandary regarding what text to recommend, let alone require; most of the major texts are too long and too expensive for medical students to make the learning of the specialty more enjoyable and also to ensure that essential topics are covered.

With regard to the required topics a medical student in neurology should read, I had the privilege to serve on a small committee, chaired by Dr. Doug Gelb of the University of Michigan, to outline the minimum list of topics that every Neurology clerkship should include. In preparing this book, I have tried to adhere to the outline prepared by this committee and published in Neurology.[1] I hereby acknowledge my debt to Dr. Gelb and the other members of the committee, Dr. Gunderson, Dr. Henry, and Dr. Jozefowicz.

In preparing for the neurology clerkship, students do very well to review first the basics of neuroanatomy and second the neurological examination. This volume will provide only an outline and abbreviated discussion of these two topics. We shall then proceed directly to the subject matter of neurology, first the symptoms and signs and then the specific neurological disorders.

I wish to thank McGraw-Hill for giving me the opportunity to write this text. I sincerely hope that it will help the medical students, who have made my career so enjoyable. I have endeavored to make the book, like this preface, as succinct as possible. I also want to thank my editor, Jason Malley, and my current and past chairs of neurology at Vanderbilt University, Dr. Robert Macdonald and Dr. Gerald Fenichel, who helped the book along. Drs. Bassel Abou-Khalil, Mike Edgeworth, Gerald Fenichel, Kim Hutchison, Karl Misulis, and Paul Moots wrote chapters and Drs. Patrick Lavin, Adrian Jarquin-Valdivia and Tom Davis reviewed my attempts at chapters in their areas of expertise. I also acknowledge the invaluable help of my wife, Carol, and our children, Josh and Jodie, for always affording me the time to work on projects

---

[1] Gelb DJ, Gunderson CH, Henry KA, Kirshner HS, Jozefowicz RF. The neurology clerkship core curriculum. *Neurology* 2002;58:849–852.

like this, to the generations of medical students who have made my life more interesting, and to the patients—the patient sufferers of neurological disease, who have provided me the opportunity to pursue this wonderful and rewarding specialty.

Howard S. Kirshner

FIRST EXPOSURE TO

NEUROLOGY

APPROACHES TO THE NEUROLOGICAL PATIENT

THE NEUROLOGICAL

EXAMINATION

HOW TO TAKE A NEUROLOGICAL HISTORY

The first task of the student is the clinical history, or interview of the patient. Neurology differs from most specialties of medicine in the importance of localization of symptoms to a specific area of the nervous system. Most of our objective information for localizing a lesion comes from the neurological examination. Often, the history provides additional clues to localization. For example, in a seizure, onset with head turning to the right, followed by jerking of the R arm, would indicate a left hemisphere seizure focus, near the motor cortex. The patient might have a completely normal neurological examination, and in this case all of the localizing information would come from the history. More often, the examination provides the localizing information, but the history provides information about the etiology of the lesion, or the diagnosis. In other words, the examination tells us where the lesion is, but the history tells us what it is. This concept is critical to the understanding of the methodology of neurological diagnosis.

In neurology perhaps more than any other specialty of medicine, the precise time course in which symptoms develop often leads to the specific etiologic diagnosis. Brain tumors produce symptoms in an insidious, slowly developing fashion, whereas strokes occur more suddenly. A brain tumor patient and a stroke patient may have nearly identical examinations, such as right hemiparesis and aphasia; it is the history that distinguishes the two diagnoses. Specification of the precise temporal profile of the symptoms helps immensely in neurological diagnosis. In this context, the medical student can often contribute to patient care by calling family members or witnesses at the workplace and obtaining their descriptions of what went on with the patient. It is important in history taking to identify sources of information and to specify whether the information comes from direct observation or second-hand reports, and these descriptions should be taken as statements from the patient or observer rather than as objective facts. Sometimes patients relate more about what other doctors have diagnosed, rather than what symptoms they experienced. The student or physician must redirect the patient to describe his or her symptoms. In addition, patients often use vague terms to describe their symptoms, and the examiner must be sure that he or she understands what the patient means. For example, patients use the word "weakness" at times when they mean numbness. A host of symptoms can be encoded in the term *dizzy*, and the examiner should try to discern whether the patient is experiencing lightheadedness or presyncopal sensations, an abnormal sensation of spinning or movement (vertigo), or some other sensation.

In neurology, as in other areas of medicine, a complete history and physical examination also includes past medical history (PMH), family history, social history, and review of systems. The past medical history contains clues based on prior medical problems or *risk factors*. For example, in a patient with abrupt onset of right-sided weakness, a history of rheumatic heart disease, atrial fibrillation, or a prosthetic heart valve would be clues to an embolic stroke. A history of severe hypertension would raise the concern of a cerebral hemorrhage or thrombotic stroke. A history of head trauma would make the interviewer suspect a subdural hematoma. A history of systemic cancer would bring up a metastatic tumor as a possibility, and a history of human immunodeficiency virus (HIV) or immunosuppression might raise suspicion of an abscess or meningeal infection. Past history of surgical procedures, medications, and allergies complete the PMH.

Family history, too, can provide clues, especially in the case of genetic diseases. Neurology has many inherited diseases, of which just a few are hereditary peripheral neuropathies or myopathies, or neurodegenerative diseases such as Alzheimer's disease, Parkinson's disease, or Huntington's disease. Even seemingly sporadic diseases such as stroke have genetically inherited risk factors such as diabetes mellitus, heart disease, and clotting disorders.

The social history contains clues about risk factors such as smoking or use of alcohol or illicit drugs. Toxic exposures might also be relevant. The patient's level of education and highest vocational attainments are important to understanding the significance of lost functions in acquired neurological diseases.

The review of systems can reveal clues to the effects of the disease process on other organ systems. A frequent notation in H&P notes is, "a 12-system review was negative, except as in the HPI." This statement is never literally true. Even healthy patients have occasional headaches, nasal congestion, cough, wear glasses, have hearing loss, have joint pain here and there, and have less energy than in their youth. Almost all of us have mood swings, frustrations, and disappointments. The review of systems should provide a general picture of the health and emotional status of the individual.

HOW TO PERFORM A COMPREHENSIVE NEUROLOGICAL EXAMINATION

The general physical examination

The physical examination of the neurological patient should begin with a general physical examination. Vital signs must always be documented. Physical examination, like the neurological examination, must be tailored to the individual problem to some extent. A few examples will underline the importance of aspects of the physical examination. Fever and stiff neck are invaluable clues to central nervous system infections, especially meningitis. In cases related to stroke or any vascular problem, the cardiovascular examination becomes especially important, including examination of the neck for carotid bruits, the heart and lungs, the abdomen for bruits or abnormally prominent or wide pulsations, and the peripheral pulses. Taking blood pressure in both arms can be important in patients with subclavian steal syndrome. A patient presenting with paraparesis (weakness of both legs) could have an abdominal aortic aneurysm (AAA), and careful palpation of the abdominal aortic pulsation and the pulses in the lower limbs would then be very important. Palpation or percussion over the vertebral bodies of the spine might reveal tender areas in a patient with spinal metastases. The skin examination can reveal congenital malformations such as dimples over the spine related to spinal malformations, hemangiomas, or melanomas which may be metastatic to the nervous system, bruises reflecting coagulopathies or trauma, rashes providing clues to systemic infections or collagen vascular diseases, cyanosis, jaundice, and many other abnormalities. Joint deformities may indicate systemic diseases such as rheumatoid arthritis that can affect the nervous system.

In peripheral nerve syndromes such as carpal tunnel syndrome, it is helpful to elicit signs such as Tinel's sign (tapping over a nerve elicits electric-like paresthesias in the distribution of the nerve) or Phalen's sign (prolonged flexion of the wrist for 30–60 seconds producing numbness in the median nerve territory and pain). Tinel's sign can also be found over the ulnar nerve at the elbow in cases of ulnar palsy. Range of motion testing of the cervical spine can be helpful in evaluating cervical spondylosis. In cases of suspected thoracic outlet syndrome, the Adson's maneuver should be performed; this involves abduction of the arm, while feeling the radial pulse, then having the patient turn the head to the opposite and then to the same side. A positive Adson's test is the disappearance of the radial pulse either with extreme abduction or turning of the head to the opposite side.

The neurological examination

The neurological examination consists of examination of the mental status, cranial nerves, motor system, reflexes, and sensation. We shall consider these parts of the neurological examination in turn.

Table 1-1   **Mental Status Examination**

Level of alertness
Language function (fluency, comprehension, repetition, and naming)
Memory (immediate, short-term, and long-term)
Calculations
Visuospatial processing
Abstract reasoning

MENTAL STATUS

The mental status examination recommended by American Academy of Neurology for the core clerkship curriculum is shown in Table 1-1.

Level of alertness is a description of the patient's level of consciousness. It varies from coma, which designates the lack of any meaningful response to stimulation, through stages of stupor or obtundation, reflecting meaningful responses only with greater than normal stimuli, to milder states of drowsiness, to normal alertness.

Language function can be tested in great detail, especially when a lesion of the left hemisphere is suspected. We generally divide such testing into six parts: (1) a description of spontaneous speech, with emphasis on fluency, word or sound errors, or word-finding difficulty; (2) naming; (3) repetition; (4) auditory comprehension; (5) reading both aloud and for comprehension; and (6) writing. If a patient does not speak in response to invitation, the examiner can try to induce speech by requesting an automatic sequence such as the days of the week or counting from 1 to 10, and then beginning the sequence aloud. In Chap. 2, we shall discuss how abnormalities on the bedside examination of language are useful in localizing lesions and in aiding in the diagnosis of neurological disorders.

Memory encompasses a large number of separate cognitive operations. Immediate or "working" memory is really a measure of attention. It is tested at the bedside by repeating digits forward (the normal digit span is 7), or often by spelling "WORLD" forward and backward. Digits backward or even "WORLD" backward, however, may require some short-term memory. Short-term memory is usually tested antegrade by asking the patient to repeat back three words, and then recall them after a delay of 5 minutes. Short-term memory can be tested nonverbally for locations of hidden objects in the room or reproduction of visual designs (drawings). Short-term memory can also be tested informally in the interview by asking about tests the patient has just had, or details of meals, doctor or relative visits. Long-term memory can be tested for biographical details, provided that a family member can verify the answers, or by asking items of general knowledge such as past presidents.

Calculations are tested because arithmetical reasoning is localized in the left parietal lobe, though written calculations also involve visuospatial functions that may involve the right hemisphere. Serial seven subtractions from 100 can be used as a test of both attention (immediate memory) and calculation ability. Making change from a $5 bill may also be used to test calculation ability.

Visuospatial functions can be tested in a number of ways. The patient can be asked to bisect a line or draw a figure such as a clock (with placement of the numbers and hands to reflect a specific time). Alternative drawings can include a house or a daisy. Visuospatial function can also be tested by asking the patient to draw a map of the United States and locate specific cities or states.

Abstract reasoning tests the patient's ability to plan ahead, to understand the significance of facts or events. Comprehension of irony and humor are also sometimes tested. Finally, the patient's insight into the nature of his or her illness, and his or her reaction to it is important.

Several other functions are not specifically included in the standard mental status examination of Table 1-1. The patient's emotional state is important to gauge, including both the patient's mood (subjective emotional state) and affect (the patient's emotional state as judged by the examiner). If the examiner is in doubt, an estimate of the patient's emotional state can be made by the effect the patient has on the examiner; depressed patients make the examiner feel "down," whereas manic patients may make the examiner laugh or feel elated. Praxis is the ability of the patient to perform learned motor acts, or to pantomime them in response to command. Gnosis is the patient's ability to recognize objects in specific sensory modalities; thus visual agnosia refers to the inability of a patient to recognize a visual object (in the presence of ability to recognize it by touch or sound).

There are a number of standard mental status examinations in use. The most widely used is the Mini Mental State Examination (MMSE) of Folstein and colleagues. This examination is reproduced in Table 1-2. The MMSE has the advantage of a standard format and a quantitative score, but it has several limitations. First, it should not be a straightjacket that keeps the examiner from performing more detailed examinations of language and other functions, when appropriate. Second, it is heavily weighted toward orientation and verbal processes, with only one point on visuospatial functions. Third, it is heavily dependent on education.

The most important aspect of the mental status examination is the importance of performing it. Some patients maintain a "cocktail party" demeanor of social conversation that can mask major deficits in orientation and memory. Focal lesions may affect only visuospatial function, or only language, or even only reading or writing; the correct diagnosis cannot be made without documentation of these specific cognitive deficits.

Table 1-2   **The Mini Mental State Examination**

Item	Points
Orientation—time	
Year	1
Season	1
Month	1
Date	1
Day	1
Orientation—place	
State	1
County	1
Town	1
Hospital	1
Floor	1
Attention	5
Serial 7 subtractions, or	
Spell WORLD backward	
Memory	
Register three items	3
Recall three items at 5 minutes	3
Naming (pencil, watch)	2
Repetition (no ifs, ands, or buts)	1
Following three-step command	3
Following printed command (close eyes)	1
Write a sentence	1
Copy intersecting pentagons	1

Source: Folstein MF, Folstein SE, McHugh PR. Mini-mental state: A practical method for grading the cognitive status of patients for the clinician. *J Psychiatr Res* 1975;12:189–198.

CRANIAL NERVES

Olfactory nerve

The first cranial nerve is the one most frequently omitted in neurological examinations ("cranial nerves II-XII intact"), but testing this nerve can be important for diagnosis. Subfrontal lesions such as olfactory groove meningiomas can affect smell unilaterally, as can traumatic brain injuries; the small olfactory fibers entering the skull through the cribriform plate are highly susceptible to injury. In Alzheimer's disease, olfaction is the only primary sensory modality to be affected early in the disease. In addition, most of what patients call "taste" is actually smell; only the four basic sensations of sour, bitter, sweet, and salty are detected by the "taste" fibers of the 12th cranial nerve.

Pupillary light reflex

The pupillary light reflex involves input via cranial nerve II and output via the pupillomotor fibers of cranial nerve III. The light should be shined in each eye, with examination of both the ipsilateral and contralateral pupil. If the patient has reduced vision because of retinal or optic nerve disease, the afferent arm of the reflex will be reduced. Swinging the flashlight from one eye to the other will serve to compare the direct pupillary reaction in the first eye to the consensual pupillary reaction in the other eye. If the pupil constricts more from the consensual reaction from the other eye than it does to direct light, the patient has an *afferent pupillary defect*. This sign objectively indicates a retinal or optic nerve lesion. If, on the other hand, the efferent arm of the reflex is impaired, as in a III cranial nerve palsy, the pupil will not react to either direct light or light shined into the other eye.

If the examiner has the patient focus on a very near object, the pupil will "accommodate," or constrict. The commonly used acronym "PERRLA" should not be used unless all elements have truly been tested: "pupils equal, round, reactive to light and accommodation."

Extraocular movements

Movement of the eyes is carried out by six muscles in each eye, controlled by three cranial nerves and central systems regulating them. The III cranial nerve innervates the pupil, as we have seen, the upper eyelid (complete involvement of the nerve will produce ptosis, or drooping of the eyelid), and four of the six extraocular muscles: the superior rectus, inferior rectus, medial rectus, and inferior oblique. A complete III nerve palsy will thus result in a droopy eyelid (or the eye completely shut), a dilated, nonreactive pupil, and an eye that is deviated laterally at rest and will not move medially, upward, or downward. The IV cranial nerve innervates only one extraocular muscle, the superior oblique. The nerve exits the midbrain dorsally and goes through a pulley, such that it moves the eye down and in. Patients with IV nerve palsies tilt their heads to reduce double vision. The VI cranial nerve also supplies only one muscle, the lateral rectus.

The examiner should take a small object such as a flashlight or the tip of a pen and ask the patient to follow its movement to both sides, up, and down. The examiner also asks the patient to gaze voluntarily to the right, left, up, and down. If the eye does not move fully in one direction, a single cranial nerve lesion can be diagnosed, most commonly a lateral rectus or *VI nerve palsy*. If the patient describes double vision (diplopia), and the examiner does not see a limitation of eye movement, this does not mean that the diplopia is psychogenic; even a very small degree of disconjugate gaze, too small to see, can produce diplopia. The first task of the examiner is to have the patient close one eye at a time. If the diplopia is still present with only one eye open, then the patient has *monocular diplopia*, usually due to an intraocular problem or possibly a psychogenic origin, and not a cranial nerve deficit. The examiner can then do a *red glass test* to identify the specific nerve involved (see Fig. 1-1).

Many other patterns of extraocular movement abnormalities have been described. Extraocular movement disorders have been divided into infranuclear, nuclear, and supranuclear palsies. Infranuclear palsies refer to disorders of the individual cranial nerves or of the extraocular muscles themselves. Nuclear palsies are less common and have unexpected features. For example, a midbrain lesion that directly affects the III nerve will also affect the other eye; for example, gaze up and to the right will be affected by a left III nerve nucleus lesion because the innervation of the ipsilateral inferior oblique and contralateral superior rectus comes from the ipsilateral III nerve nucleus. Nuclear VI nerve palsies are hard to separate from a conjugate ipsilateral gaze palsies affecting both eyes, since the parapontine reticular formation adjacent to the VI nerve nucleus is thought to be a center for lateral gaze. Internuclear ophthalmoplegias are eye movement problems caused by lesions between the nuclei of the cranial nerves involved with gaze. An internuclear ophthalmoplegia (INO) is a paresis of the ipsilateral medial rectus, with nystagmus of the abducting contralateral eye. The anatomic structure connecting the VI and III nerve nuclei is the medial longitudinal fasciculus, or MLF. A lesion of the ipsilateral MLF will prevent a command for lateral gaze from reaching the adducting eye. The abducting eye jerks laterally, as if trying harder to get the eyes over. INO is a sign of an intrinsic brainstem lesion between the pons and midbrain and is seen frequently in multiple sclerosis (MS), occasionally in other brainstem lesions such as strokes.

Supranuclear palsies usually involve a conjugate loss of either horizontal or vertical eye movements. Lateral gaze palsies can be caused by lesions in the pons adjacent to the VI nerve nucleus. These lesions will prevent movement of the eyes to the side of the lesion. Lesions in the hemisphere, on the other hand, can cause the eyes to stay preferentially to the side of the hemisphere lesion. This type of gaze deviation may not be a true palsy, in that the eyes will sometimes move with stronger stimuli such as oculocephalic (doll's eye) maneuver or ice water calorics (oculovestibular stimulation); these will be discussed under the examination of the comatose patient later in this chapter. Diplopia is also considered in Chap. 10.

The examiner describes not only the full excursion of extraocular movements, but also any adventitious movements such as nystagmus, ocular dysmetria, opsoclonus, or ocular bobbing. Nystagmus is a jerky movement of the eyes, usually on the end point of gaze in the horizontal direction, sometimes with a rotary component, and usually present in both eyes. Nystagmus can be categorized as primary (in only one direction, usually in the direction of gaze), secondary (beating in the same direction both in

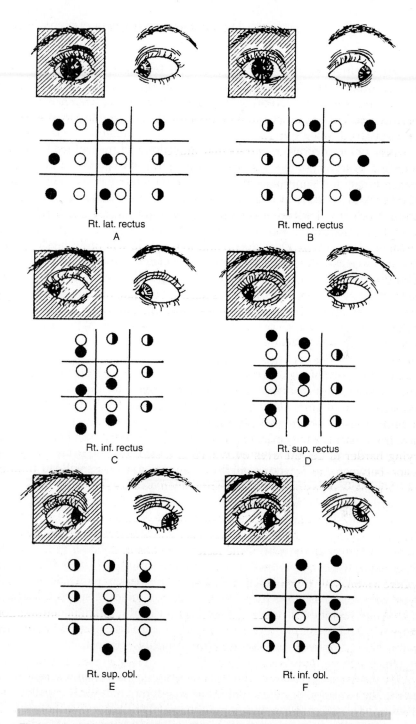

Figure 1-1. **Red glass testing.** (*Source*: Adapted from Victor M, Ropper AM. *Adams and Victor's Principles of Neurology,* 7th ed. 2001, p. 284–285, Fig 14-6.)

primary position and on lateral gaze), and tertiary (beating in the same direction with the eyes turning in the direction of gaze, in the primary position, and even in contralateral gaze). Dissociated nystagmus, or nystagmus present in only one eye, is usually seen in the syndrome of intranuclear ophthalmoplegia. Nystagmus usually has a fast component in the direction of gaze and a slower return phase, but other patterns of nystagmus have been described, such as *pendular* nystagmus, in which movement in both directions occurs at the same speed. Ocular dysmetria refers to the occurrence of several small, corrective movements at the end of gaze, akin to the cerebellar dysmetria seen in the finger during finger-nose-finger testing. It is the ocular equivalent of the incoordination seen in the limbs in association with cerebellar dysfunction. Opsoclonus refers to rapid, seemingly random, usually conjugate movements of both eyes. It is related to myoclonus seen in the limbs. Ocular bobbing is a sudden downward deflection of the eyes, with a slow return to the original position, reminiscent of the movement of a fishing bob when a fish bites the bait on a fishing line. This movement occurs in patients with bilateral lesions of the pons, most commonly pontine infarcts or hemorrhages, and usually it is seen in comatose patients.

Facial sensation, the trigeminal nerve

The sensory examination is always more subjective than any other part of the neurological examination, since the examiner must rely on the report of the patient as to what he or she is feeling. Sometimes patients report minor differences in sensation to pinprick, and the examiner must decide how consistent this finding is, and whether or not it is clinically important. Objective clues can be gained by the occurrence of wincing after a small jab with the sharp object, as opposed to not showing any reaction at all. In the era of HIV and hepatitis, most neurologists use a broken Q-tip with a sharp end, rather than a metal pin. If pins are used, they must be discarded after each use. Older devices such as pinwheels are not safe. The trigeminal nerve has three branches: the ophthalmic, maxillary, and mandibular. Facial sensation can also be affected by supranuclear lesions. Temperature sensation can also be tested. A cool tuning fork will feel less cool to the patient with a deficit in pinprick sensation, and report of a cooler feeling should be suspect. Vibration can also be tested on the skull. Patients who report a difference in vibration sense when a tuning fork is placed a short distance on either side of the midline of the forehead are likely either highly suggestible or outright malingering.

The final objective test related to facial sensation is the corneal reflex. This reflex, like the pupillary light reflex, has an afferent arm via the ipsilateral V cranial nerve and an efferent arm via the ipsilateral VII nerve. If the afferent side of the reflex is impaired, neither eye will blink when one cornea is stimulated. If the efferent arm is affected, only the eye on the side of the VII palsy will not blink.

Facial nerve function

The facial nerve is primarily a motor nerve innervating the muscles of the face. A common finding is that *central* or *upper motor neuron* or supranuclear lesions of the VIIth nerve generally affect mainly the lower face on the contralateral side. Eye closure may be mildly weak, but the elevation or wrinkling of the eyebrow should be normal. A peripheral facial palsy is usually more severe than a central paresis, and it involves both the upper and lower face; many patients with peripheral facial palsy are unable to close the eye or raise the eyebrow at all. In addition, the sensory function of the VII nerve, taste sensation in the anterior two-thirds of the tongue, may be affected. Since taste reflects only the primary detection of saltiness, bitterness, sweetness, and sourness, most of what we perceive as "taste" is actually smell. We can test taste at the bedside by immersing a Q-tip in a concentrated solution of salt or sugar and placing a small amount on the protruded tongue.

Acoustic nerve function

The VIII nerve, or acoustic nerve, carries hearing and vestibular function. An objective screening test for hearing is important to the general neurological examination. This can be the ability to hear the sound of a whispered word or a watch ticking (though contemporary digital watches tend to be silent).

Vestibular function is tested only when the patient complains of dizziness or vertigo. Patients who are actively experiencing vertigo, a sensation of movement, usually rotational or spinning, may have nystagmus. Vestibular nystagmus is almost always horizontal and conjugate in the two eyes, though there may be a rotatory component to the principal direction of the nystagmus. If one suspects vestibular nerve dysfunction, confirmatory physical tests can be carried out, in addition to hearing testing.

The Barany positional maneuver, also referred to by otolaryngologists as the Dix Halpike maneuver, involves having the patient lie straight back with the head below the horizontal plane. The examiner looks for a subjective complaint of vertigo and an objective onset of nystagmus, often a few seconds after the position change. In the case of peripheral vestibular dysfunction, the nystagmus usually lasts well under a minute and then stops. If the patient's head is repeatedly placed back in the same position, the vertigo and nystagmus will fatigue. If there is no vertigo in the straight head back position, then the examiner has the patient sit up, then lie down again with the right side of the head down. Again, the patient sits up after the maneuver and then lies down again, this time in the left head down position. Between the three head down and three head up positions, there are six total positions in which the patient can develop vertigo and nystagmus.

A final vestibular test that can be carried out at the bedside is the ice water caloric test. In this test, ice water is introduced into the external ear canal, stimulating the eardrum with a cold caloric stimulus. The examiner should always examine the ear with an otoscope to make sure that the eardrum is intact and the canal not obstructed before introducing ice water. In testing vestibular responses in an awake patient, very small amounts of ice water, perhaps 2 mL, should be tried. The examiner should proceed cautiously, as the patient may develop nausea and vomiting. The expected ocular response to the cold caloric stimulation is nystagmus, with the fast component in the direction contralateral to the ear that is being infused. For generations, medical students have used the mnemonic "COWS" to indicate "cold-opposite, warm-same" with respect to the direction of the nystagmus after cold water caloric testing. It is important to remember that the ice water caloric test is quite different when used to assess a comatose patient (see below). In that situation, a much larger amount of ice water must be infused, and the response will not involve nystagmus; the normal response in a patient whose cortex is asleep or nonfunctional will be a slow, tonic deviation toward the side of the ice water. The nystagmus, seen in awake patients during cold caloric testing, is a cortical mechanism, a corrective measure to restore the eyes back toward the primary position.

Glossopharyngeal and vagus nerve function

The IX and X cranial nerves function more or less together. Technically, the only function exclusive to the IX nerve is taste sensation over the posterior third of the tongue. In practice, we test these nerves at the bedside by watching the palate elevate when the patient opens his or her mouth and says "ah," testing the gag reflex on each side, listening to the patient's voice quality, and, if necessary, watching the patient swallow a cup of water. When the palate elevates, the weak side (ipsilateral to the X nerve palsy) will elevate less than the other side, and consequently the uvula will "pull up" toward the strong side. The gag reflex should be tested gently, with a Q-tip rather than a tongue blade, so that the patient's sensation can be tested, in addition to a unilateral gag reflex. When the patient speaks, the examiner should listen for hoarseness or nasal quality, which will be much more severe if the X weakness is bilateral.

Spinal accessory nerve function

The spinal accessory nerve is a mixed cranial nerve and spinal nerve, with root contributions emerging from the second through sixth cervical spinal cord segments. The nerve innervates the sternocleidomastoid and trapezius muscles on the ipsilateral side. We test the sternocleidomastoid muscle by having the patient turn the head to the contralateral side, feeling the contraction of the muscle itself (since weakness may be difficult to detect). The trapezius is tested by having the patient shrug the shoulder.

There is some debate about which sternocleidomastoid muscle is weak following a cerebral lesion like a stroke. In practice, it is the ipsilateral muscle that is weak; e.g., patients with a right hemiparesis will be weak in turning the neck to the right. The reason for the ipsilateral involvement is not completely understood; in general, however, the brain is organized more by the side of the direction of movement rather than the side where the muscle is located.

Isolated involvement of the spinal accessory nerve in a peripheral nerve lesion is rare. Cervical lymph node biopsies have inadvertently led to section of the nerve. Rarely, infiltrating tumors may affect the nerve.

Hypoglossal nerve function

The hypoglossal nerve innervates the muscles of the tongue, whose function is mainly to protrude the tongue toward the contralateral side. A hypoglossal palsy will result in atrophy of the tongue on the ipsilateral side, fasciculations in the tongue muscles, and protrusion of the tongue toward the ipsilateral side. The examiner can also ask the patient to push the tongue forcibly into the contralateral cheek, and the force of this movement can be felt with a finger palpating the cheek from the outside. Weakness of the tongue will also be evident in testing the patient's speech, especially rapid, repetitive lingual consonants such as "la la la la."

THE MOTOR EXAMINATION

The motor examination consists of the following items: muscle bulk, adventitious movements at rest, muscle tone, muscle power, coordination, reflexes, stance, and gait. Muscle bulk can be examined by looking at the muscles for signs of atrophy, and noting whether atrophic muscles fall into a specific nerve root, peripheral nerve, or nerve root territory. Any movement of muscles at rest should be noted. These can range from fasciculations, or twitches of individual motor units, to larger movements such as myoclonus, tremor, or involuntary movements such as choreoathetosis (see Chap. 5).

Muscle tone is noted next. The limb should be passively moved through a range of movement at the major joints (shoulder, elbow, wrist, hip, knee, ankle). In general, it is difficult to separate normal tone from decreased tone (hypotonia), though hypotonia may occur in syndromes of diffuse muscle weakness or in cerebellar dysfunction. Increased tone generally follows one of three patterns: cogwheel rigidity, lead pipe or spastic rigidity, and paratonic rigidity. Cogwheel rigidity involves a combination of increased tone and a ratchet-like or cogwheel sensation of a gear going through a series of steps instead of a smooth movement. Although some have considered cogwheel rigidity to be a simple interaction between tremor and rigidity, many patients with Parkinson's disease have cogwheel rigidity in the absence of visible tremor. Movement in a circular direction at the wrist is a very sensitive maneuver for detecting cogwheel rigidity. If the patient makes a large, circular movement with the other arm, this will facilitate the detection of cogwheel rigidity, but the maneuver is so sensitive that it may bring out apparent cogwheeling even in a normal elderly patient. The second type of increased tone, spasticity, is marked by a difference depending on the direction of movement. In the familiar example of a stroke patient with right hemiparesis, extension of the elbow will be met with marked resistance, but once the arm is extended, flexion will be easy. In addition, during extension, there may be a few degrees of unimpeded movement, then a rapid build-up of tone. If the examiner keeps pushing, the arm may suddenly loosen and extend rapidly. This variety of spastic tone is called *clasp-knife rigidity*. The final type of increased tone, paratonic rigidity, feels as if the patient is voluntarily resisting the movement; very slow, easy movement may provoke only normal tone, but the harder the examiner pushes, the more the patient seems to resist. Paratonic rigidity is also referred to by an old German term, *gegenhalten*. It is usually seen in patients with frontal lobe disorders.

Muscle power is a key element of the neurological examination. Neurologists often use the British Medical Research Council scheme for recording muscle strength. This is a 0–5-point scale, where 5 is normal, 4 is weakness with ability to overcome some resistance at a joint, 3 is ability to overcome gravity but not resistance, 2 is some movement but not enough to overcome gravity, 1 is only a flicker or trace of movement, and 0 is no movement. This scheme provides uniformity between different observers, but it is somewhat arbitrary. Some muscle actions do not clearly fit the pattern of overcoming gravity or resistance, such as the hand grip, and the rating scale then becomes a much more subjective grade. The examiner should generally test at least some proximal and distal muscles in each limb. In cases of localized weakness, such as in one limb, much more detailed muscle testing is appropriate. For example, a patient with neck pain and L arm pain and paresthesias would be tested in detail for a radicular weakness. I recently saw an alcoholic, homeless patient brought into our hospital for a possible stroke. He had an obvious left wrist drop and subjective "weakness" involving his L leg as well. When I examined him carefully, all muscles of the upper limb were normal except for the wrist extensors and finger extensors; median and ulnar nerve innervated muscles had normal strength, as did his leg muscles. The diagnosis was a radial nerve palsy, a syndrome caused by leaning his upper arm over the back of a chair and compressing the radial nerve against the humerus, an annoying problem for the patient but clearly less serious than a stroke. Detailed testing of specific muscles in one limb had definite clinical importance in this patient.

COORDINATION

Coordination refers to movements planned and executed in a precise, sequential manner. The cerebellum is the coordinating center in the brain. Cerebellar lesions affect muscle power only minimally, but they disrupt the rhythm and timing of movements, which become irregular and clumsy. In the upper limbs, coordination is commonly tested by finger-nose-finger testing and rapid alternating movements. In the lower limbs, coordination is tested by heel-knee-shin testing, and stance and gait testing. Patients with cerebellar dysfunction typically miss the target slightly in a horizontal direction on aiming for the finger or the nose, and they then make corrective movements. The rapid alternating movement test is done by having the patient slap the front and then the back of the hand in succession on the patient's knee. The rhythm of such rapid alternating movements can be slowed by pyramidal tract lesions with weakness, but cerebellar lesions typically affect the regularity of the rhythm itself. The same pattern of abnormality is seen in heel-knee-shin testing; the heel starts to fall off of the shin, at right angles to the movement. Rapid movements can also be tested by having the patient tap the foot rapidly.

STANCE AND GAIT

The first test of stance is to have the patient stand still, with the feet together and the eyes open. If the patient can stand steadily in this position, the examiner then asks the patient to close his or her eyes. This is called the Romberg test. If the patient can stand, with feet together and eyes closed, the Romberg test is negative. If the patient can stand in this position with the eyes open but becomes unsteady with the eyes closed, this is called a positive Romberg test. The cause of a positive Romberg is classically a loss of position sense, such that the patient can compensate by vision. If the patient cannot stand with the feet together even with the eyes open, this is also an abnormal Romberg test, but it should be described in terms of what the examiner observes rather than being recorded as a *positive Romberg test*. The usual cause is cerebellar ataxia affecting the trunk. It should be noted, however, that patients with mild ataxia can still stand with the eyes open, perhaps with some swaying, but the problem becomes worse with the eyes closed. In borderline Romberg test results such as this, the examiner should describe clearly what was observed, rather than just recording the test as positive or negative.

A second part of the stance examination, not tested in all routine neurological examinations, is testing of postural reflexes. For this examination, the patient stands with the feet a few inches apart. The examiner stands behind the patient and instructs the patient, "I am going to try to throw you off balance, please try to keep from losing your balance." The examiner then pulls back on the patient's shoulders, pulling the patient back (we never push the patient forward or to the side, because we might then have trouble catching the patient, and falls in neurological patients are devoutly to be avoided). A normal patient will make a quick, corrective movement and not lose balance. Patients with Parkinson's disease and related movement disorders (see Chap. 26) will either make several, small corrective movements before regaining balance or will actually fall backward, because they lean so far back before making a corrective movement that they have already lost their balance. The examiner will then have to catch the patient, which is relatively easy to do in this position.

The gait examination is one of the most important aspects of the neurological examination, as gait is affected by so many different neurological lesions in specific patterns. The patient is asked to walk "normally," then on tiptoes, on heels, and finally tandem, or heel-to-toe (the *drunk test* commonly performed by police when a driver is suspected of being intoxicated; in the past, before the decline of circuses, this was referred to as *tight-rope walking*). The task of the neurologist is to describe the gait abnormalities of his or her patients, in a way that helps to localize the disease process causing the gait abnormality.

Examples of gait abnormalities are legion; what follows are a few, common illustrations. If a patient has proximal muscle weakness, the gait will appear "waddling," with an exaggerated rise and fall of the hips with each step. Patients will also have difficulty rising to a standing position from a chair, without "pushing off" with their hands. Patients with bilateral foot drop, from bilateral peroneal nerve palsies, L5 root lesions, or general peripheral neuropathy, walk with a high steppage gait, lifting each foot high to make sure that the toes clear the floor and do not cause tripping. Patients with hemiparesis tend to place weight preferentially on the good leg and then "circumduct" the weak leg, while also holding the weak arm in a flexed posture. Patients with bilateral corticospinal involvement tend to take small steps, scuff their toes, and walk "stiffly"; this is sometimes referred to as a *spastic gait*. Patients with cerebellar lesions and truncal ataxia tend to walk on a very broad base, often lurching to one side or the other (*ataxic gait*). They cannot walk tandem and sometimes cannot stand with their feet together, even with the eyes open. Patients with Parkinson's disease and related basal ganglia disorders tend to stoop forward when standing and take very small steps when walking. There is a poverty of "associated movements," such as swinging of the arms. There may be resting tremor in the hand on one or both sides during walking. Some patients have a tendency to lean forward and to take steps more and more rapidly until they stop themselves with their hands or fall forward, a pattern called *festination*. Finally, when the examiner tests postural reflexes, these patients tend to fall backward into the examiner's arms. A final gait pattern, associated with hydrocephalus, is mainly associated with hesitancy in initiating gait; when the patient gets up to walk, he or she just stands there, as if the feet are glued to the floor, or as if he or she has forgotten how to walk. The patient may gradually get going and walk more normally, until a pause or obstacle stops the patient and initiates the same, hesitant pattern. Further discussion of gait abnormalities is presented in Chap. 6.

Reflexes

The usual reflexes tested on the neurological examination are movements induced by stretching a tendon, as in the familiar examples of tapping over the patellar tendon (*knee jerk*) or over the Achilles tendon (*ankle jerk*). Technically, these reflexes are *muscle stretch reflexes* rather than the older, discredited term, *deep tendon reflexes*, since they do not rely on deep tendons, but rather on stretching of a muscle and firing of muscle spindle afferents.

Similar reflexes can be obtained by tapping the jaw (*jaw jerk*), the biceps tendon (*biceps jerk*), triceps tendon (*triceps jerk*), and brachioradialis tendon on the radial surface of the forearm (*brachioradialis jerk*). Occasionally, reflexes are obtained by striking over the pectoral muscles, deltoid muscle, adductor of the thigh, and finger flexor reflexes. When reflexes are brisk, tapping on the palmar surface of the fingers will elicit a flexion response. A variation of the finger jerk is the Hoffman reflex, elicited by flicking the fingernail of the middle finger, producing flexion of the thumb. All reflexes are graded on a scale of 0–4+. A 0 reflex would mean that no reflex was elicited, either by looking for a visible reflex or feeling for a muscle contraction; 1+ would designate a reflex that is present but less than average size; 2+ would indicate an average, normal reflex; 3+ would mean that the reflex is more active than usual; and 4+ would describe a reflex that triggered further reflexes (*clonus*). Tapping the Achilles tendon or dorsiflexing the ankle, for example, might elicit a series of jerks of the ankle. In normal people, reflexes can vary from 0 to 3+, rarely 4+, and occasionally even a few beats of clonus are seen. Prolonged clonus is abnormal. Spread of a reflex beyond the adjacent reflex (e.g., a brachioradialis reflex causing a biceps contraction may be normal, but spreading down to the leg would be abnormal). The adductor reflex, elicited by tapping on the inside of the knee or just proximal to the knee, should not spread to the other leg unless the reflexes are unusually brisk, usually pathologically so. Normal reflexes are virtually always symmetric, so an asymmetry between the two sides of the body is virtually always abnormal. A common mistake, however, is to assume that the more active reflex is abnormal; since normal reflexes can vary from 0 to 3+, asymmetric reflexes can be abnormal either on the hypoactive or hyperactive side, and other aspects of the examination are needed to determine which side is the abnormal one.

Another class of reflexes is the superficial reflexes. The most commonly tested superficial reflex is the Babinski sign, elicited by stroking the sole of the foot on the outer surface from heel to toe. Normally, the great toe and the other toes curl in flexion. The normal or negative Babinski reflex is referred to as a downgoing or flexor plantar response. Persons who are ticklish may "withdraw" the foot, and as part of this movement, the great toe may go up. Usually a gentler stimulus will then elicit a plantar flexion response. The abnormal response, indicating a corticospinal tract lesion, is an extension of the great toe, accompanied by fanning of the other toes. The Babinski can also be "absent," indicating that no response was observed. This often means that the patient has sensory loss or is unresponsive. Finally, if there is doubt about how to score a Babinski response, it can be called "equivocal," though it is usually more useful to describe what the examiner observed rather than using this confusing term. There are also several variations on the Babinski that carry eponymic names of the neurologists who popularized them. For example, the Oppenheim is a form of Babinski in which the examiner runs a hard object down the anterior shin and watches for flexion or extension of the great toe. The Chaddock's reflex is a similar reflex involving stroking of the lateral surface of the foot instead of the sole. The Bing reflex is elicited by pricking the dorsum of the great toe with a sharp object such as a safety pin or broken Q-tip. If the patient is "withdrawing" from the Babinski stimulus, he or she will not "withdraw" up into a sharp object, but if the extension of the toe is a true Babinski, the toe may extend up into a sharp object.

Another set of superficial reflexes is the abdominal reflexes, elicited by stroking the abdomen in any of the four abdominal quadrants. A positive reflex is a flexion of the rectus abdominus muscle. Acute corticospinal tract lesions cause the reflex to disappear, but occasionally the reflex may become hyperactive, as is true of the muscle stretch reflexes. The absence of lower abdominal reflexes with preserved upper abdominal reflexes would indicate a lesion in the midthoracic spinal cord.

Other important superficial reflexes are the cremasteric and bulbocavernosus reflexes. These reflexes, though not performed on every routine neurological examination, are crucial for the diagnosis of spinal cord lesions. The cremasteric reflex is elicited by stroking upward on the medial thigh in a male patient; the response is a pulling up of the testicle within the scrotum on the stimulated side. This indicates an intact reflex of the lower lumbar spinal cord segments. The bulbocavernosus reflex is elicited by squeezing the glans of the penis and feeling with a gloved hand for a contraction of the anal sphincter.

A last class of reflexes is the *frontal lobe release signs*. These include the grasp reflex (a pathological tendency of the patient to grasp the hand of the examiner when the examiner's hand is placed in that of the patient, and then not to let go), the snout response (the lips pout when a touch stimulus is applied anywhere around the mouth and lips), the suck response (the patient sucks on a tongue blade or other object placed near the mouth), and the rooting response (the patient turns the head toward a touch stimulus just lateral to the mouth).

THE SENSORY EXAMINATION

The sensory examination is the most difficult to write or teach about, because the degree of sensory testing appropriate to a given patient must be based on experience. Some patients describe very minor differences in sensation between different areas of the same or different limbs, and interpretation of such differences is almost an art form. The sensory examination is also "subjective," in the sense that the examiner provides a stimulus and the patient then tells the examiner how it felt. Of course, there are objective elements to the sensory examination if the patient winces or withdraws the stimulated limb. In general, however, we rely more on objective signs such as reflexes than on subjective ones such as the reporting of the sensory examination.

The sensory examination contains a series of types of sensory stimulation. The first is pinprick or sharp-dull sensation. In these days of HIV and hepatitis infections, reusable pins or pinwheels are unsafe. Some neurologists use safety pins, being sure to use a fresh pin for each patient. Others use a wooden Q-tip, broken to create a sharp edge. The first issue is whether or not the patient feels the sharpness, or can tell the sharp end of the Q-tip from the cotton end. Beyond this, the patient reports whether or not the sharpness has full acuity, or whether it differs between one area and another. The details of sensory testing, as mentioned above, will differ between patients. For example, if a patient complains of weakness and numbness of one upper limb, the examiner should deliberately test the major peripheral nerve territories in that limb, as well as nerve root distributions. If the other symptoms and signs suggest a spinal cord localization, then testing of the trunk for a spinal level is critical. If the patient is complaining of headache or dizziness, without sensory symptoms, then the examiner can quickly test both sides of the face and parts of the four limbs. If an entire side is numb compared to the other, it is also useful to test the trunk, especially to see if the sensory loss splits the midline.

Pinprick sensation travels from peripheral nerve to plexus, nerve root, the spinothalamic pathway to the contralateral thalamus, and then on to the sensory cortex. Temperature sensation, along with pinprick sensation, shares the spinothalamic pathway. Testing for temperature sensation changes can be useful in confirming the results of the pinprick examination. The easiest way to test temperature sensation is with a cool object such as a metal tuning fork, which is also used to test vibration sense (see below). In general, the coolness of the tuning fork will be less appreciated in areas of skin where pinprick sensation is also reduced. When a patient says the tuning fork is colder on the numb side, this should raise suspicion about the validity of the sensory examination (unless the pinprick sensory examination suggests a hypersensitivity).

Vibration and position sense share a different sensory pathway from the pinprick and temperature sensory modalities, traveling uncrossed up the posterior columns, then crossing in the medial lemniscus in the medulla. In practice, vibration sense is tested with a tuning fork, ideally 128 Hz. It is tested in the toes and fingers; if absent in the toes, it is then tested in the ankles, knees, or hips, depending on the level. In the trunk, vibration can be tested along the posterior spinous processes of the vertebrae if a spinal level is being sought. Position sense, or proprioception, is tested by moving the great toe (or a thumb or finger) up and down. The toe is squeezed from either side prior to the vertical motion, so that no extra cues of the direction of movement are given. If the patient cannot correctly report a movement of approximately 2 cm, then the examiner moves to the next joint, the ankle. If movement of that joint cannot be reported, then the examiner moves to the knee, then the hip, and in the upper limbs from the fingers to the wrist, elbow, and shoulder. Movement of the shoulder or hip involves movement of the entire trunk, and a patient who cannot report this movement correctly should be suspected of a nonorganic or psychogenic disorder.

HOW TO PERFORM A SCREENING NEUROLOGICAL EXAMINATION

The examination presented in Chap. 1 is a comprehensive examination, one which can take in excess of 30 minutes to complete. Much of the art of neurology is in tailoring this examination to suit the needs of the individual patient. This is the hardest aspect of the neurological examination for the medical student to learn. Students usually start out performing thorough examinations on every patient they see, in order to learn the examination. As they gain experience, they learn to take shortcuts. While I do not want to encourage too many shortcuts too early in the experience, a few suggestions are appropriate. Neurology clinics, where medical student teaching is increasingly taking place, are time-pressured; if a medical student ties up an examining room for 2 hours conducting a history and physical examination on a follow-up patient, neither the patient nor the attending physician will be happy. It is in this spirit that the following guidelines are presented.

Let us first take the example of a patient who presents with symptoms restricted to one limb. A graduate student comes in with a complaint of numbness and pain in the right hand. The history includes no other major positives in the HPI, and a completely benign PMH and ROS. The examination in this patient should include only a very brief mental status examination consisting of observation during the history that the patient recalls historical details well and expresses them in appropriate language, and formal testing only of orientation; if there is any question at all of a mental status abnormality, short-term memory should also be tested. A screening cranial nerve examination should include pupils, extraocular movements, visual field testing, facial sensation to pinprick, facial symmetry and motion, palate elevation, tongue protrusion. The motor examination should be detailed in the right upper limb, and the left upper limb can be tested in key muscle groups for comparison. Strength testing in the lower limbs can be accomplished by watching the patient stand from a sitting position, walk on tiptoes and heels; if all of this is normal, the lower limb strength can be considered to be normal. Reflexes should be tested, at least biceps, triceps, brachioradialis, patellar, and Achilles reflexes, as well as plantar responses. Sensory function should involve detailed pinprick and vibration testing in the R upper limb, cursory testing of the other three limbs, and vibration sense in the toes. This examination should take only a few minutes. Of the "extra" items in addition to the neurological examination, a few musculoskeletal items should be done. The examiner should inspect the wrists for deformities, perform the Tinel's and Phalen's tests (see above) for carpal tunnel syndrome, check the pulse at the wrist and perhaps the Adson's test. Assuming that the motor and sensory deficits are solely within the median nerve territory and the Tinel's and Phalen's tests are at least partly positive, the diagnosis of carpal tunnel syndrome can then be made with confidence.

A second scenario involves the patient who gives no localizing complaints in the history, but has either headaches or seizures. This patient, though not complaining of focal dysfunction in the nervous system, must be evaluated for a possible underlying lesion. In this case, a more detailed mental status examination should be performed on the first visit, including at least orientation, attention, memory, calculations, and at least one visual-spatial or constructional test. The MMSE would suffice for most patients. Cranial nerves should be tested in detail; in addition to the brief survey in the previous paragraph, the optic fundi should be examined and hearing should be tested. Motor examination would include a brief survey of all four limbs, including strength testing in one or two proximal and one or two distal muscles in each limb, gait (including toe, heel, and tandem), reflexes, and sensory testing for pinprick and vibration in the distal portions of each limb. This examination, too, takes only about 10–15 minutes in addition to the history.

A third scenario is a patient presenting with solely cognitive deficits, usually memory loss in an elderly patient. In this patient, complete mental status testing is essential. The MMSE is the standard examination, but I prefer to supplement this with further testing of language, fund of information (presidents or other items more relevant to the specific patient), and sometimes of frontal lobe (*executive*) functions. In the case of language testing, I like to use the six pictures on the NIH Stroke Scale, a test readily available to medical students and residents. This patient should also have the cranial nerve, motor, reflex, and sensory examination referred to in the previous paragraph. Occasionally a patient will present with cognitive deficits but have motor signs of Parkinson's disease or signs of a focal intracranial lesion such as a stroke, brain tumor, or subdural hematoma.

Many other examples of tailored neurological examinations could be envisioned here. Perhaps the best approach is to perform the screening examination for a patient with a headache or seizure, then think about supplementing the examination as directed by other features of the history or examination. For example, the presence of any features suggesting Parkinson's disease should provoke a detailed evaluation for tremor, cogwheel rigidity, handwriting changes, and gait difficulty, including the postural reflex testing described under the gait portion of the comprehensive neurological examination. Any patient whose complaint includes dizziness should be evaluated with orthostatic vital signs and a positional test such as the Barany maneuver (see above) and testing of hearing. Some neurologists would also test for hyperventilation (have the patient breathe deeply in and out at least 20 times, then ask about dizziness or any tingling sensations).

EXAMINATION OF THE COMATOSE PATIENT

Entire books have been devoted to the examination of the comatose patient, and students can spend days reading about the techniques, yet in practice the coma examination takes just a few minutes. The reason for the brevity of the examination can be readily appreciated by going through the major categories of the neurological examination for the awake patient: many parts of the examination simply cannot be performed on an unresponsive patient. Coma is defined as an unresponsiveness from which the patient cannot be aroused. We can start with the mental status examination, which in the comatose patient is generally limited to a statement of the level of responsiveness. If the patient follows any verbal commands, he or she is not comatose. If the patient even responds in a meaningful nonverbal manner, such as fending off a pinch with a brushing movement of the hand, again the patient is not comatose.

Many of the cranial nerves can be examined. Cranial nerve I, the olfactory nerve, cannot be tested effectively unless a strong odor stimulant causes the patient to turn away. The pupillary light reflex tests the afferent arc through the optic nerve and the efferent arc through the III cranial nerve, just as it does in the awake patient. Eye movements cannot be tested by asking the patient to look left or right, or even by having the patient follow a moving flashlight with the eyes, but they can be tested by oculocephalic and oculovestibular reflexes. The oculocephalic, or *doll's head* maneuver involves turning the head forcibly to one side. An awake patient may resist this stimulus, keeping the eyes looking straight ahead. A drowsy or obtunded patient loses this resistance, and the eyes move opposite to the direction of the movement of the head. The term doll's eyes or doll's head is somewhat misleading, since these terms imply that the movement is a passive motion, as in the ball bearing eyes of a plastic doll. In actuality, the doll's eye maneuver involves active firing in the cranial nerve nuclei that control eye movements. If a student is not convinced of this point, try performing doll's eyes on a cadaver; the eyes will not move. If, in an obtunded patient, the eyes move fully and conjugately to the right when the head is moved to the left, and the eyes move conjugately to the left when the head is moved to the right, the doll's head test can be considered "positive," meaning that the pathway from the inner ear, via cranial nerve VIII, to the III and VI nerve nuclei on each side, as well as their interconnections through the MLF and their efferent paths through the cranial nerves III, IV, and VI, are all intact. This finding implies that most of the brainstem real estate is preserved, and in practical terms that the brainstem is not involved in the disease process. If there is a brainstem lesion, it may take the form of an isolated VI nerve palsy (the ipsilateral eye will not abduct), an isolated III nerve palsy (the ipsilateral eye will not adduct, but usually also will not go up or down readily, and the pupil may be dilated), a horizontal gaze

palsy (the eyes will not move to one side), or an internuclear ophthalmoplegia (the ipsilateral eye will not abduct, see above). If no movement of the eyes
is elicited with the doll's head maneuver, this implies a severe brainstem
abnormality, or a very deep coma (*absent doll's head eye movements*). If the
doll's head maneuver elicits movement, the findings should be reliable for
indicating a brainstem or cranial nerve abnormality, or an intact brainstem. If
no movement is elicited with this maneuver, then the examiner should proceed to the oculovestibular or *ice water caloric* test. In this maneuver, the examiner first inspects the ear canal to ensure that the tympanic membrane is
intact, then instills ice water. As mentioned earlier, in an awake patient, the
instillation of just 2–3 mL of ice water will elicit vertigo and nystagmus. The
mnemonic COWS (cold opposite, warm same) refers to the direction of the
fast component of nystagmus elicited by the oculovestibular test. In an
obtunded patient, the nystagmus is not expected. Instead, the normal
response is a slow, tonic deviation toward the side of the ice water. As in the
intact oculocephalic or doll's head maneuver, preserved oculovestibular
responses with ice water in each ear implies an intact brainstem. Abnormal
oculovestibular responses can provide similar localizing information to the
doll's head maneuver (III, IV, and VI nerve palsies, INOs, and gaze palsies).
Ice water in both ears should elicit downward gaze.

Cranial nerves V and VII can be tested by the corneal response, just as in
the awake patient. Similarly, a sharpened Q-tip can be pricked inside the
nostril, often resulting in a grimace response that tests both cranial nerves V
and VII. Cranial nerve VIII can be tested by seeing if the patient responds to
loud noises, such as a hand clap, and also the input through this nerve is
involved in both the oculocephalic and oculovestibular responses. Cranial
nerves IX and X can be tested mainly by the gag reflex. Cranial nerves XI and
XII cannot typically be evaluated in a comatose patient.

The motor examination in the comatose patient includes inspection of
muscle bulk and tone, as in the awake patient. Testing of power can be carried out only by observing responses to noxious stimuli such as pinching the
limb. It is important to record exactly what noxious stimulus was applied
(hard sternal rub, pinch on the inner surface of the upper arm or leg), so that
another examiner can compare his or her examination to yours. Often, in a
comatose patient, the resident or medical student on call at night will be
comparing with examinations recorded during the day, and only if the examination is well specified can the on-call person know whether the patient has
deteriorated or is stable. Reflexes, including the Babinski, can be tested just
as in the awake patient.

The sensory examination is very limited in the comatose patient. The
application of noxious stimuli such as pinprick or pinch on the limbs, or sternal rub, with a description of the movement response elicited, is the only
sensory examination possible.

The examination of the comatose patient should also include a general physical examination. This examination differs much less from that of an awake patient than does the neurological examination. The vital signs, examination of neck stiffness, vascular bruits, heart and lung examinations, abdominal, skin, and extremity examinations are all easily tested.

The coma examination can be interpreted to define a level at which the nervous system is functioning. The monograph by Plum and Posner provides useful guidelines for the localization of disease processes in patients with stupor or coma. The principal findings that lead to this analysis are the status of breathing, the pupillary light reflexes, the extraocular movements, and the motor examination. There are, in general, three anatomic substrates that produce coma. We know that consciousness is maintained by activity of the reticular activating system traveling up the brainstem and into the thalamus on each side, with projections widely into the cerebral cortex. Consciousness can be disrupted by (1) a primary brainstem lesion interrupting the reticular activating system on both sides; (2) a cerebral mass lesion with pressure downward on the brainstem causing brain herniation; and (3) bilateral involvement of the cerebral cortex itself, such that there is no content to be activated by the reticular activating system. In the first lesion, in the brainstem, the localizing neurological signs are usually clear: cranial nerve lesions of the III and VI nerves, VII, IX, and XII nerves, and bilateral involvement of the motor system. In the third substrate, bihemispheral involvement, the neurological examination will be somewhat depressed, but nonfocal. Diffuse, bihemispheral syndromes can be metabolic or structural; for metabolic, think of drug overdoses, uremia, or liver failure. For structural causes, think of bilateral strokes, trauma, or hypoxic-ischemic damage.

In the second of the three scenarios, the herniation syndrome, the key is a temporal progression of symptoms and signs, referred to by Plum and Posner as *rostrocaudal deterioration*. This deterioration can be traced through each of the major neurological signs of the coma examination.

Breathing may be normal in the early stupor phase, then transforms into Cheyne-Stokes respirations during the phase of increased intracranial pressure from a hemispheric lesion. Cheyne-Stokes is a pattern of crescendo-decrescendo breathing, followed by an apneic period, before the crescendo of breathing starts up again. The entire nervous system may seem to wax and wane with the crescendo and decrescendo of Cheyne-Stokes respirations; the patient may respond during the breathing phase, then become unresponsive during the apneic period. As the brainstem becomes compressed at midbrain level, the breathing pattern changes from Cheyne-Stokes to a rapid, regular pattern referred to as *central neurogenic hyperventilation*. This change may appear more comfortable, but it is actually a very ominous change, indicating that irreversible brainstem damage is imminent. Finally, as dysfunction spreads down the brainstem, the pattern of breathing again becomes irregular, with patterns such as ataxic respirations. These patterns are agonal, leading to complete cessation of breathing.

The pupils are the next key part of the examination. Normal pupils can vary in size but are usually equal and reactive to light. As a hemispheric mass expands, there is often pressure downward on the III cranial nerve as it crosses the tentorium. The telltale dilatation of the pupil is a harbinger of impending danger. The pupil first dilates, then loses its reaction to light, and examination of the eye movements at that juncture will show a failure of the ipsilateral eye to adduct. Later, both eyes become non-reactive. The herniation syndrome with an ipsilateral III nerve palsy is termed the *uncal herniation syndrome*, since the uncus of the temporal lobe herniates under the tentorium and then compresses the III nerve. Sometimes, when the pressure downward is more medial, or more balanced on the two sides, the patient will progress to coma without the development of a III nerve palsy. This herniation syndrome is called the *central herniation syndrome*. The pupils are symmetrically midposition and nonreactive.

The eye movements reveal the status of the brainstem cranial nerves III, IV, and VI, and their interconnections, as mentioned. The presence of a third nerve palsy, for example, will be detected by the failure of the eye to adduct, on either the doll's head maneuver or ice water calorics.

The motor examination, too, will change with the rostrocaudal deterioration. Patients on the way to herniation may have a contralateral hemiparesis to begin with. This may worsen as the pressure in the ipsilateral hemisphere increases. As the herniation syndrome progresses, pressure downward may push the contralateral cerebral peduncle of the midbrain against the tentorium. This *Kernohan's notch* may result in an ipsilateral hemiparesis. The motor signs may also include posturing of flexor (*decorticate*) or extensor (*decerebrate*) types. As mentioned earlier, these terms are less important than an accurate description of what noxious stimulus was applied, and what motor response was observed, in order to permit detection of change as the patient is treated.

In general, despite the fact that the description of the neurological examination of the comatose patient occupied several paragraphs, it takes only a few minutes to carry out. It is very important for medical students, no matter what medical specialty or career they plan, to be familiar with the examination of the comatose patient, where timely diagnosis can be critical for successful treatment.

INTERPRETATION OF THE NEUROLOGICAL EXAMINATION

As mentioned at the beginning of this chapter, the neurologist uses the examination findings to localize the lesion in the nervous system, then applies the history to fine-tune the localization and also examine the temporal profile of the illness and the individual's risk factor profile (PMH) to make educated guesses about the etiology of the problem. This process is the key to the interpretation of the neurological examination. A few examples should help the student understand how a neurologist reasons out the diagnosis in evaluating patients at the bedside. It cannot be emphasized enough that this process must be systematically carried out in each patient; the neurologist rarely if ever jumps to a diagnosis just from the examination or from the history. Attempts to do so often lead to error. In a similar fashion, undue reliance on imaging studies or laboratory tests leads to misdiagnoses. We shall return to the issue of laboratory tests later.

There is one exception to the rule of methodically working out the localization of the lesion, then the likely etiologies. This approach can take time, and some medical emergencies need to be dealt with quickly. Emergency medicine physicians take a different approach from that of neurologists. They go through a very rapid-fire differential diagnosis, take out the treatable diagnoses, and initiate treatment coverage for those very rapidly. Neurologists, too, sometimes need to begin treatment before a problem is completely diagnosed. Patients seen in the emergency department need to be stabilized, in terms of airway, breathing, circulation, before an elaborate neurological examination is carried out. Chapter 23 addresses emergency problems in Neurology. Seizures need to be treated quickly, especially if there are repetitive or persistent seizures, as in status epilepticus. Patients with acute stroke symptoms may be taken for a computed tomography (CT) brain scan even before a complete examination is completed to exclude brain hemorrhage, but the examination should be completed as soon as the patient returns. In a patient with fever and stiff neck, the consideration of meningitis must proceed quickly, with a CT scan and lumbar puncture, again even before a detailed examination is completed. In all of these instances, a quick, screening examination is done first, and the rest is completed when time permits.

We shall consider a series of cases in which the history and examination point to lesions in specific areas. We approach each case by taking the examination findings and localizing them one by one, providing the uppermost and lowermost lesion that could account for each sign. We then try to combine the signs together and derive a single lesion localization to account for all of the signs, if this is possible, or a combination of localizations if necessary. We then take into account the patient's history, for any localizing information it provides, as well as the time course of the development of the syndrome and the patient's risk factors. We shall include a few cases in which the examination findings are similar, but the finer analysis of the examination findings or history points to the correct diagnosis.

CASE 1

A 45-year-old man presents with a complaint of difficulty getting up from a chair and walking up steps. These complaints have been slowly progressive over a few months. The patient feels well except for mild fatigue, denies any pain, numbness, or paresthesias. On examination, he is alert and fully oriented. Cranial nerve functions are normal, except for mild weakness in the neck flexors and extensors. There is mild weakness in the shoulder and hip girdles, with minimally reduced strength at the biceps, triceps, and also quadriceps and hamstring muscles, with normal strength in the wrists, hands and fingers, ankles, and feet and toes. The reflexes are 1–2+ and symmetric throughout, with downgoing plantars. Gait has a waddling pattern, with hiking up of the hip on each side during walking, and the patient cannot rise from a squat. He can walk on his toes and heels, and he can do tandem with some difficulty. The sensory examination is completely normal, including pinprick and vibration sense in the toes. The general physical examination is unremarkable.

Discussion: The localization in this case appears to be in the proximal muscles. Peripheral neuropathy usually affects distal muscles and usually involves both sensory and motor nerves. Spinal cord or brain disorders would usually be associated with spastic tone, increased reflexes, upgoing plantars, and other signs, depending on the localization of the lesion. Rarely, a parasagittal mass such as a meningioma between the cerebral hemispheres could cause paraparesis, but there should again be associated hyperreflexia and upgoing plantars. By contrast, muscle disorders often selectively affect proximal muscles. Depending on the history, this could be a muscular dystrophy, an endocrine-associated disorder, or an inflammatory myopathy. Polymyositis would fit the history and findings well. The diagnosis could be confirmed by muscle enzyme assays in the blood (especially creatine kinase [CK] and aldolase), electromyogram (EMG) with nerve conduction studies (NCV), or a muscle biopsy.

CASE 2

A 70-year-old man presents with weakness in the legs and difficulty getting up from a chair, similar to Case 1, slowly progressive over several weeks. In addition, he mentions that his vision seems dim at times, and he has begun having occasional double vision. He states that he does well when he first gets up in the morning, but by the end of the afternoon he is having much more difficulty walking, and this is when he notes the visual disturbances. On examination, he is alert and oriented. On cranial nerve testing, his pupils are equal and reactive, and his extraocular movements appear full, but he has a bilateral ptosis, or droopy eyelids.

If he is asked to look upward for a full minute his lids droop more, and he cannot sustain upward gaze, complaining of double vision. He has intact facial sensation, but his smile seems a bit weak on both sides. His speech sounds nasal and breathy, especially after he has been speaking for a few minutes, and he chokes on liquid when asked to drink a glass of water. He has reasonably good strength in all four limbs, but repetitive extension of his arms shows fatigue of his strength after the first two or three attempts. He can rise from a squat, but he can repeat this performance only one time. His reflexes and sensation are normal, and his gait appears normal for a few steps.

Discussion: This patient, like Case 1, might be thought to have a myopathy, but one with an unusual distribution involving the eyelids, extraocular movements, facial muscles, and swallowing muscles, as well as, by history but not by initial examination, mild proximal muscle weakness. The testing of repetitive extension of the arms or repetitive standing from a squat shows a fatiguing pattern of muscle strength suggestive of a neuromuscular junction disorder. In a man this age, myasthenia gravis would be the most likely diagnosis. Other neuromuscular junction disorders such Lambert-Eaton syndrome might lack the characteristic bulbar muscle weakness, and botulism would usually be more acute in onset and have autonomic signs such as pupillary abnormalities. A typical myopathy would not have the fatiguing pattern, and only a few myopathies would involve both bulbar and extremity muscles as in this patient. The diagnosis could be confirmed by EMG/NCV testing with repetitive stimulation, by assays for antibodies against the acetylcholine receptor, or by an edrophonium test at the bedside (see Chap. 35).

CASE 3

A 44-year-old man complains of awakening one morning with a *foot drop,* with slapping of his left foot and tripping on his toes. The examination shows normal strength everywhere except for ankle dorsiflexion and eversion; plantar flexion and inversion are normal. There is an area of decreased pinprick in the lateral thigh and the lateral and dorsal surface of the foot. All reflexes are intact, including the knee and ankle jerks. Gait shows "high steppage" with the left foot.

Discussion: This case localizes to the peroneal nerve. The most common cause would be a compression of the nerve as it curls around the upper, lateral calf, perhaps because the patient was inebriated and slept heavily on the limb. Other causes would be possible, including diabetic or vasculitic mononeuropathy. The most helpful diagnostic test here would be an EMG with NCVs, which should document a left peroneal nerve palsy.

CASE 4

A 46-year-old man complains of lower back pain, radiating down the buttock, posterolateral thigh, lateral calf, and into the lateral foot. He then notes numbness of the lateral calf, and difficulty walking on his left heel, with occasional tripping on his left toes. The examination shows weakness restricted to ankle dorsiflexion and eversion, but careful testing also shows weakness of the ankle on inversion. The sensory examination shows numbness to pinprick over the lateral thigh, lateral calf, and lateral and dorsal surfaces of the foot. The reflexes are intact, including knee and ankle jerks. The gait pattern shows an "antalgic" avoidance of placing full weight on the L leg, and also a high steppage with that foot.

Discussion: This case seems superficially very similar to Case 1. The difference is that this deficit matches not a peripheral nerve, but rather a nerve root, the left L5 nerve root. This *L5 radiculopathy* is usually the result of a disc rupture or bone spur at the level of the L4–5 disc space. Here the most useful diagnostic test would be a lumbar magnetic resonance imaging (MRI) scan or myelogram. EMG/NCV studies might confirm a left L5 radiculopathy, with denervation in muscles supplied by this root, particularly the peroneal, anterior tibial, and posterior tibial muscles.

CASE 5

A 61-year-old man presents to the emergency department after the abrupt onset of severe midabdominal pain, followed by light-headedness and weakness in both legs, with urinary incontinence. On examination, he is hypotensive, 84/58 systolic, tachycardic, 110/minute, but he is alert, fully oriented, and he has normal cranial nerve findings. On motor examination, he has normal upper extremity strength and reflexes, but the lower extremities are completely paralyzed, flaccid in tone, and with no reflexes at the knees or ankles, with nonresponsive plantar responses. On sensory examination, pinprick sensation is normal in the upper limbs and the chest and upper back, but there is a complete loss of pinprick sensation from about 2–3 cm below the umbilicus, including both lower extremities. Vibration and position sense are preserved, even in the feet and toes. General examination also shows diffuse abdominal tenderness and absent bowel sounds.

Discussion: The complete, flaccid paraplegia and the sensory level below T11–12 indicates a lesion of the thoracic spinal cord. The sparing of vibration and position sense indicates that the posterior columns of the spinal cord are preserved. This fits the pattern of a vascular myelopathy (spinal cord disorder), because the anterior two-thirds of the spinal cord is supplied by one large, anterior spinal artery, whereas the posterior portion of the cord is supplied by several posterior spinal arteries. Vascular myelopathies often occur at lower thoracic level, since there are few radicular arteries to the spinal cord at those levels; in fact, in many persons, there is just one, large radicular artery called the artery of Adamkiewicz. In this patient, the acute onset of abdominal pain and hypotension were caused by the rupture of an abdominal aortic aneurysm (AAA), with dissection or compression of this artery. The patient presented with symptoms of abdominal pain from the local AAA rupture, with hypotension from acute blood loss, and with paraplegia from ischemia of the spinal cord.

CASE 6

A 79-year-old lady complains of painful paresthesias in her feet, as well as poor balance, with occasional falls. Her daughter also mentions that the patient has seemed more forgetful recently. She has been healthy otherwise, so much so that she has rarely visited a doctor, but on previous evaluations she has never had high blood pressure, diabetes, heart disease, or other major illnesses. On examination, she is oriented to person and place but gives the incorrect month and date, and her short-term memory is two out of three memory items in 5 minutes. Her MMSE score is 25/30. She has normal cranial nerve functions except for mildly reduced visual acuity bilaterally. Strength in her arms is normal, but in the legs she has mild weakness of the ankle dorsiflexors. Her reflexes are on the brisk side in her arms, 2+ at the knees, and diminished at the ankles, and her plantars are suggestively upgoing. The sensory examination is grossly normal to pinprick, but she has absent vibration sense in her toes and ankles bilaterally. She is also inaccurate in reporting position changes in the toes. Her Romberg test is positive (she loses her balance with her eyes closed), and she walks somewhat hesitantly, on a mildly broad base. She cannot do tandem gait. She can walk a few steps on her toes but none on her heels. She performs finger-nose-finger and heel-knee-shin testing adequately. The general physical examination is unremarkable.

Discussion: This case is not as simple to localize as the previous cases. First, there is a loss of sensation in the modalities of vibration and position sense, which could reflect either a peripheral neuropathy or involvement of the posterior columns in the spinal cord. Second, there is weakness in ankle dorsiflexion which could also represent peripheral nerve or spinal cord involvement. The upgoing plantars point to an upper motor neuron, or central nervous system etiology for the weakness, excluding a peripheral neuropathy as the sole cause of the syndrome. Within the spinal cord, the signs point to involvement of the posterior and lateral columns. This is our preliminary localization of the lesion, though the abnormal mental status also needs to be considered. We could postulate an incidental dementia, but it would be more parsimonious to consider a disease process that would account for both sets of symptoms.

In interpreting the neurological examination, we first take each sign and make as precise localization as we can, then combine all of the signs and historical features and try to postulate a single localization of the patient's problem. We then consider the history and come up with a differential diagnosis. In this case, the two disease processes that could account for a spinal cord lesion with posterior and lateral column involvement, of subacute or chronic course, would be cervical spondylosis with myelopathy, or subacute combined systems disease (vitamin B_{12} deficiency). Either disorder would fit with a subacute history, but the lack of neck pain or any radicular symptoms or signs in the arms would be somewhat against cervical spondylosis. B_{12} deficiency accounts for all of the symptoms and signs. In this case, we can confirm the diagnosis with a simple blood count, showing anemia and an elevated mean corpuscular volume, or macrocytic anemia. A vitamin B_{12} level will confirm the diagnosis. We could also perform a cervical spine MRI scan to exclude a cervical spondylosis with myelopathy. An EMG and NCV could also be done to exclude a primary peripheral neuropathy.

CASE 7

A 29-year-old woman presents with double vision as her sole complaint, except for some general fatigue over the past few weeks. In answer to the question of whether or not any factors exacerbate the condition, she says that she feels much worse when she is outside on a hot day. Her past medical history is quite benign, but she does recall that she had an episode of pain in the right eye and reduced vision in that eye about 2 years earlier. She had not sought medical attention, since the vision recovered and the pain ceased over a 2–3-week period. On examination, she has normal mentation, but the cranial nerve examination reveals several abnormalities. Visual acuity is 20/20 in the left eye but only 20/25 in the right eye by distant chart. The visual fields are full, but the pupil examination shows that the left pupil has a brisk response, but when the light is shifted to the right pupil, the pupil dilates slightly. Funduscopic examination discloses a pale optic disk on the right, a normal disk on the left. On examination of the extraocular movements, the eyes move fully to the left, but on right gaze the left eye does not fully adduct, and the right eye has nystagmus to the right. She has full up and down gaze. Cranial nerves V and VII–XII are normal, and she has normal motor and sensory examinations except for the fact that her reflexes are diffusely quite active, with flexor plantar responses.

Discussion: This patient has two abnormalities on neurological examination: the double vision, and the mildly reduced visual acuity in the right eye, with an afferent pupillary defect and a pale optic disk. The first finding is diagnostic of a left internuclear ophthalmoplegia, a finding strongly indicative of an intrinsic brain lesion. The second finding is consistent with an optic neuropathy, and the history tells us that this is an old finding. We thus have evidence for two central nervous system lesions: an acute brainstem lesion and an older optic nerve lesion. The combination of lesions, in a young female, is highly suspicious for multiple sclerosis (MS). INO in general is about 90% associated with MS, with most of the rest accounted for by strokes. The diagnosis of MS could be confirmed by MRI scanning of the brain and spinal cord, indicating white matter lesions, by a lumbar puncture, showing immunoglobulin changes (oligoclonal bands and increased [immunoglobulin G] IgG index), and by evoked responses, which would likely indicate changes in the visual evoked response from the right eye in this patient. Further information on MS will be discussed in Chap. 29.

CASE 8

A 62-year-old lady is brought to the hospital because of headaches, confusion, and frequent falling. She had difficulty dressing herself over the past few days, often putting her arm into the wrong sleeve of her blouse. She has bumped into objects, and she had a recent motor vehicle accident in which she struck a car that was parked on the left side of her vehicle. She has been feeling fatigued, and she has lost about 15 lb, which she attributes to poor appetite. On examination, she is a somewhat unkempt appearing woman, who is not sure why she has been brought to the hospital. She is oriented to date and place, has normal attention and only mildly reduced short-term memory, but she cannot draw a clock, omitting some of the numbers on the left side of the clock and placing both hands on the right side of the clock (she was asked to place the hands at "20 minutes till 3"). She also fails the intersecting pentagon test, in that one figure has only four sides, and there is only a small intersection between the two figures. On cranial nerve testing, she has normal pupils, with direct and consensual light reflexes. Her visual fields are full to single stimuli, but when the examiner moves fingers on both sides, however, the patient reports only the movement on the right side ("extinction on the left to double simultaneous stimulation"). The fundi show blurred disk margins, with small hemorrhages and absent spontaneous venous pulsations. The extraocular movements are full. There is grossly normal facial sensation, but the left side of the mouth droops at rest and on voluntary smile. On motor examination, there is a slight pronator drift of the left arm, and strength in the left arm and leg is mildly reduced. The reflexes are increased on the left as compared to the right, and the left plantar response is upgoing. The sensory examination shows grossly intact sensation to pinprick and vibration throughout, but when the examiner taps both sides simultaneously, the patient reports only the right-sided stimuli. This is sensory extinction on the left side, analogous to the visual extinction in the left visual field.

Discussion: All of the signs in this patient point to a lesion in the right hemisphere, especially in the right parietal lobe, with prominent deficits in visual-spatial cognitive function, neglect and extinction in the left visual field and left side of the body on sensory testing. The optic disk swelling indicates the likelihood of increased intracranial pressure, with papilledema. The history provides additional localizing information, in the form of dressing apraxia, also a right parietal lobe syndrome, and the hints of visual neglect on the left. The onset is subacute, most in keeping with a brain tumor, likely a malignant tumor such as a glioblastoma multiforme or a metastasis from a systemic cancer. The differential diagnosis would also include a brain abscess. A stroke would be much less likely, given the subacute onset of the syndrome. Note also the importance of the mental status examination in coming to the correct lesion localization and diagnosis. Diagnostic confirmation would be best accomplished with a brain imaging procedure such as a CT or MRI scan.

CASE 9

A 58-year-old lady is hospitalized for the new onset of a rapid, irregular heart rhythm. She has been given an antiarrhythmic agent. Her husband was with her in the room, went downstairs to get a newspaper and a cup of coffee, and returned to find her in a somewhat agitated state, "talking gibberish." She has been well in the past, except for a history of heart disease. The cardiologist consults Neurology to see if this is a confusional state related to the medication. On examination, the patient is speaking in a rapid, fluent pattern, but the few recognizable words sound like empty phrases, and there are many nonwords. The patient does not seem to understand spoken questions or commands, and the rest of the mental status examination is therefore impossible. Her pupils are equal and reactive. Visual fields are difficult to test, but she seems to blink to visual threat more on the left than the right. She seems to look to both sides in following the examiner. There is no facial weakness or asymmetry, and she seems to withdraw from a sharp object on the right side of the face as well as from the left. She has no arm drift, seems strong in all four limbs, and her reflexes are intact and symmetric, with downgoing plantars. She can walk without apparent difficulty. She has normal sensation, at least as indicated by her withdrawal to pinprick in the four limbs. The general examination is mainly remarkable for the irregular heart rhythm and a diastolic murmur over the mitral valve area.

Discussion: This is a slightly altered version of an actual case, from the days when quinidine was used in atrial fibrillation, and this drug had some potential to cause confusion or delirium. The physical examination, however, points to an aphasia, of fluent type with poor repetition, also called Wernicke's aphasia, rather than to a general confusional state or delirium. There may also be a hint of visual field defect. These findings point to a localization in the left temporal and possibly occipital lobes, and hence a focal brain lesion. The abrupt onset is consistent with a stroke, or acute embolic infarction, the embolus arising from the heart in association with atrial fibrillation. Note the contrast from Case 7, where the onset was subacute versus acute, and the hemisphere lesion was more consistent with a tumor than a stroke. Diagnostic confirmation could come from an immediate MRI scan with diffusion-weighted imaging, which would show the area of acute infarction. Magnetic resonance angiography (MRA) might also show that the left middle cerebral branches do not fill normally, especially the inferior ones. CT scan would not show the acute infarction immediately, but a CT done 1–2 days later would show a low density area corresponding to the bright signal area on the diffusion-weighted MRI scan. CT angiography might also confirm the left middle cerebral branch occlusion. An echocardiogram might show a dilated left atrium with thrombus.

CASE 10

A 69-year-old man is brought to the neurologist for memory loss. He denies any symptoms or problems, insisting that he is doing fine. He is a recently retired officer of a corporation, with a college education. His wife states that he asks her his schedule repeatedly each day, forgetting where he is supposed to be. He has recently become lost in the car, on a route that he has traveled many times. His hygiene has recently begun to suffer; he may wear the same shirt on three consecutive days and he forgets to shave. He has difficulty finding a station he wants to watch on the television. On examination, he is healthy appearing. He knows his age and the year, but is off on the month, the exact date, but he does know the day of the week. He is oriented to the physician's office, city, county, and state, but he does not know the floor. He names the current President but not his predecessors. He names simple objects but misses the hammock and the cactus on the NIH Stroke Scale pictures. He can follow a multistep command, but he needs a reminder of the last step. He spells "WORLD" forward and backward, but on serial 7s he gets only the first two accurately. He recalls only one of three memory words at 5 minutes. He gets one more with hints. He copies the intersecting pentagons figure accurately, but when he attempts to draw a clock he places the numbers appropriately but places both hands on the same side of the clock in showing "twenty minutes till three." His MMSE is 24 if only simple naming tests and the intersecting pentagons figure and spelling WORLD backward are utilized, 20 or below if the examiner uses the serial 7's test and the clock drawing test are chosen, even lower if more sophisticated naming items are used. The remainder of his neurological examination, including cranial nerves, optic fundi, motor, reflex, cerebellar, and sensory testing, is within normal limits. The general physical examination is also unremarkable.

Discussion: In this patient, the mental status examination is the key to the diagnosis. The mental status examination is indicative of a bilateral cortical dysfunction. Note that the extensiveness of the examination is critical; if only the pentagon figure is tested, the MMSE provides no evidence for a right hemisphere abnormality. In addition, the MMSE of 24, when it is given in a very simple form, is borderline for dementia, whereas testing with more sophisticated items indicates a more severe deficit. The patient is highly educated, making more detailed mental status testing imperative. This case exemplifies the arbitrariness of the MMSE, as discussed earlier in this chapter, and it indicates that more detailed mental status testing, including more sophisticated language and visual-spatial testing, is needed in some patients. Taken together, the evidence points to a slowly progressive, bilateral cortical degeneration, typical of Alzheimer's disease. The diagnosis is a clinical one. CT or MRI scanning can be used to exclude alternative diagnoses such as a subdural hematoma, brain tumor, or hydrocephalus, though there are no specific signs pointing to any of these disorders. Blood testing is usually done to exclude hypothyroidism, vitamin B_{12} deficiency, syphilis, or drug intoxication, though the yield of such tests would be low in a case like this, with no symptoms or signs pointing to one of these disorders. Neuropsychological testing indicates a dementing illness consistent with Alzheimer's disease. Positron emission tomographic (PET) brain imaging confirms a biparietal and bifrontal pattern of hypometabolism consistent with Alzheimer's disease.

These cases illustrate the usefulness of the *neurological method* of careful examination and localization of a lesion, followed by consideration of the history, before coming to a diagnostic conclusion. This is the key to the successful practice of neurology. Two cases may present with bilateral leg weakness, but the diagnosis can be a myopathy (Case 1), a neuromuscular junction disorder (Case 2), a spinal cord disorder (Case 5), or even a parasagittal brain tumor, and the distinction must be made by fine points of the examination and history. Similarly, a foot drop can be related to a mononeuropathy (Case 3) or a radiculopathy from a lumbar disk (Case 4). A hemisphere syndrome can be a tumor (Case 8), a stroke (Case 9), or even a dementing illness (Case 10), again depending on the fine points of the examination and history. Neurology may seem "old fashioned" in its emphasis on these principles, but neurologists can do more at the bedside to diagnose their patients than perhaps practitioners of any other medical specialty. In addition, reliance on laboratory testing can be misleading; in the emergency department, a normal CT scan will often yield a puzzled call to the neurologist, when the correct diagnosis, easily made on neurological examination, is a stroke (Case 9) or a dementing illness (Case 10). In fact, the brain imaging studies may be actively misleading. An enhancing mass within the sylvian fissure, seen on CT or MRI scan, may be a slow-growing meningioma, completely incidental to the patient's presenting symptoms. For all of these reasons, medical students should learn to perform a detailed neurological examination, take a careful history, and then make a clinical localization and diagnosis, before proceeding to brain imaging studies and other laboratory tests.

KEY REFERENCE

Folstein MF, Folstein SE, McHugh PR. Mini-mental state: a practical method for grading the cognitive status of patients for the clinician. *J Psychiatr Res* 1975;12:189–198. Gilman S. *Clinical Examination of the Nervous System.* New York: McGraw Hill; 2000.

LOCALIZATION

OF NEUROLOGICAL

LESIONS: SYNDROMES

CEREBRAL HEMISPHERE LESIONS

Localization within the cerebral hemispheres takes place along three spatial axes: left-right, superficial-deep, and lobar (frontal, temporal, parietal, occipital). We shall briefly summarize the syndromes associated with lesions in specific locations within the cerebral hemispheres, without reviewing detailed neuroanatomy.

Frontal lobes

The frontal lobes are large structures, yet much of these massive lobes are remarkably "silent," in terms of obvious effects on the neurological functioning. We can deal with the exceptions first. The precentral gyrus controls motor function in the contralateral limbs, so that a lesion here will cause contralateral hemiparesis, with spastic tone and hyperreflexia. The immediately adjacent Brodmann's area 8, in the superior frontal convexity, controls lateral movement of the head and eyes to the opposite side. An irritative lesion of area 8, as in a seizure discharge, will cause sudden deviation of the head and eyes to the contralateral side, whereas a destructive lesion like a stroke will cause deviation of the eyes to the side of the lesion. Finally, the left hemisphere Broca's area, Brodmann's areas 44 and 45, subserves expressive speech. A lesion here will cause the patient to become mute, or to struggle to speak, with hesitant, single-word or short-phrase utterances. Repetition is not much better than spontaneous speech. Comprehension is intact for single words and for simple sentences, but sentences with complex syntactic relationships and subordinate clauses cause difficulty in language comprehension, just as they do in language expression. The anatomy of the cerebral hemisphere is shown in Fig. 2-1.

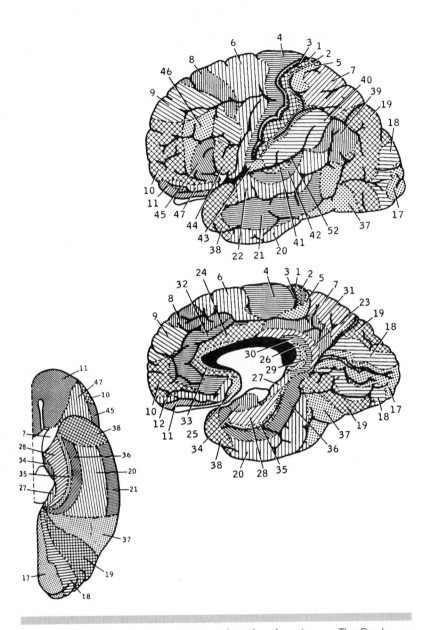

Figure 2-1 **The cerebral hemisphere, functional anatomy.** The Brodmann numbers reflect distinct cytoarchitectonic features of each region of the cerebral cortex. Some of the more common Brodmann numbers are: 3,1,2: somatosensory cortex in the post-central gyrus; 4: primary motor cortex, pre-central gyrus; 8, lateral gaze center, superior frontal lobe; 17: primary visual cortex, occipital lobe;18,19 visual association cortex, occipital lobe; 41,42: primary auditory cortex, Heschl's gyrus, superior temporal gyrus; 44,45: Broca's area, inferior frontal gyrus; 22: Wernicke's area, superior temporal gyrus; 40: supramarginal gyrus, inferior parietal lobule; 39: angular gyrus, inferior parietal lobule (*Source*: Adapted from Victor M, Ropper A, *Adams and Victor's Principles of Neurology*. 2005, Fig. 22-2, p. 387.)

Anterior to these areas of the frontal lobes, localization of function becomes more complex, involving aspects of brain functioning sometimes considered more the province of psychiatry than neurology. Disease of the orbitofrontal and frontal convexity cortex will affect the patient's personality, mood, and behavior more than it will cause any obvious deficit that would be detected on a formal neurological examination. This is the most striking aspect of frontal lobe disease: that the neurological examination can be normal, yet the patient's family may state that the patient is a "completely different person".

Disorders of both orbitofrontal lobes may leave the patient in an *akinetic mute* or abulic state, awake but with staring gaze, not speaking, not interacting with the examiner at all, or only after a delay. Some patients may whisper. This *abulic* state resembles catatonia, as seen in functional psychosis, or it may resemble stupor or coma. Less severe versions of abulia may result in a *pseudodepressed* state, in which the patient seems emotionally flat, interacting little, or responding only after a delay.

Another aspect of frontal lobe disorders is decreased *executive function*. Just as a corporate executive must plan the responses of the company to external developments and lead the future actions of the company, so the frontal lobes are active in determining which of the many incoming stimuli should be attended to, what reactions should be carried out, and how these should be planned sequentially.

Lesions in the left frontal cortex may produce a more selective loss of speech, with intact behavior in other areas, and intact comprehension, a syndrome called *transcortical motor aphasia*. The patient speaks little, as in Broca's aphasia, but unlike Broca's aphasia, the patient with transcortical motor aphasia can repeat long phrases and sentences without difficulty.

Bilateral lesions of the orbitofrontal cortex may lead to a *pseudopsychopathic* rather than *pseudodepressed* pattern of behavior. These patients are uninhibited in their actions and conversation, often breaking social or moral customs. Such behavior is seen often in patients with bifrontal traumatic brain injuries.

Since frontal lobe lesions can be subtle and can produce changes in personality and behavior without producing a formal neurological deficit, the examiner must be sensitive to such changes in taking the history. If there is doubt, neuropsychological testing can evaluate frontal lobe deficits. A simple bedside test is the Luria test (see Fig. 2-2).

Temporal lobes

The temporal lobes are more lateralized in their functions than the frontal lobes. The primary auditory cortex lies in the superior temporal gyrus

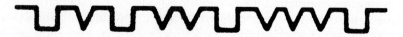

Figure 2-2 **Luria test.** The subject is asked to copy and continue the diagram, adding one more triangle after each square.

(Heschl's gyrus), within the sylvian fissure. Damage to one Heschl's gyrus may be clinically inapparent, but damage to both sides produces either cortical deafness or "pure word deafness," a syndrome in which spoken words cannot be understood, but nonverbal noises can be properly recognized. Bilateral, medial temporal lobe lesions affect short-term memory, as is seen in patients with bilateral posterior cerebral artery strokes or herpes simplex encephalitis. Patients with unilateral, left medial temporal lesions may have impairments in verbal memory, whereas those with unilateral, right medial temporal lesions may have measurable deficits in nonverbal memory, such as memory for pictures or sound sequences. Bilateral temporal lesions can also cause the *Kluver-Bucy syndrome*, in which animals fail to react appropriately with objects in the environment, often failing to show normal fear responses toward predators, and either eating or trying to mate with any object in the vicinity. The Kluver-Bucy syndrome has been described in human patients.

Localized lesions of the left superior temporal cortex produce the syndrome of Wernicke's aphasia. In this aphasia syndrome, patients fail to understand spoken language. Expressive speech is fluent but paraphasic, containing speech errors and often nonwords. Naming and repetition are also deficient.

Lesions of the right temporal lobe are much more subtle to diagnose. Musical appreciation may be affected, and neuropsychological tests of memory for sound sequences, such as the Seashore Rhythm Test, may show deficits.

Parietal lobes

The parietal lobes have a number of localized functions. The postcentral gyrus subserves somatosensory function, and lesions here affect sensation on the contralateral side of the body. Lesions isolated to the postcentral cortex can leave primary sensation for sharp/dull, touch, vibration, and position relatively intact, but *cortical* sensory modalities such as extinction to double simultaneous stimulation, stereognosis (sensory recognition of objects), and graphesthesia (ability to understand letters and numbers "written" on the limb) may be selectively affected by cortical lesions.

The left inferior parietal lobule, comprising the supramarginal and angular gyri, has functions related to language, especially reading and writing, and also calculations. A lesion of the angular gyrus may produce the syndrome of *alexia with agraphia*, in which the patient loses the ability to read or write. This is, in effect, an acquired illiteracy. Patients may have some associated fluent aphasia with paraphasic errors, and sometimes anomia as well. In general, lesions of the left parietal lobe produce various combinations of the symptoms comprising the *Gerstmann's syndrome*. Gerstmann associated lesions in this area with four deficits: agraphia; acalculia, or difficulty with calculations; left-right confusion, or difficulty telling left from right; and finger agnosia, a deficit in the correct identification of one's own or the examiner's fingers (for example, the examiner might ask the patient to "show me your left ring finger"). This deficit may reflect a subtle body image disorder. The four deficits of the Gerstmann's syndrome occur in various combinations and may also be associated with alexia, anomia, and paraphasic speech. The multiplicity of these deficits may mimic a dementing illness.

The right parietal lobe has important functions in the areas of visuospatial, constructional, and body image functioning. Patients with acute lesions of the right parietal lobe often neglect the left side of the body, and often the left side of space. If they have a left hemiparesis they may neglect it entirely, asking to be allowed to go home or to walk to the bathroom. They may say that they could walk if only they were given a cane, or crutches, when they have no use of the left side. This "neglect" of deficit, or *anosognosia*, is a major problem in patients with acute strokes, but also in those with other right parietal lesions such as brain tumors or abscesses. A related deficit is *dressing apraxia*, a disorder in which the patient has difficulty relating a garment, or a sleeve, with the correct part of the body; for example, the patient may try to put on a coat by putting the right arm in the left sleeve and then being unable to get the coat on properly. Patients may even eat half of the food on their plate, missing the left side, or fail to see the dessert on the left side of the dinner tray. In grooming, the patient may comb the right side of the scalp and shave the right side of the face, leaving the left side unkempt. Topographical functions such as drawing a map or recalling the locations of rooms in the house or in the hospital may be deficient. One right parietal stroke patient would call friends across the country and not understand why they could not "come over" and see him in a few minutes. Patients with lesions in the medial parietal and occipital lobes may have isolated topographical difficulty.

Emotions may be affected by localized lesions of the brain, and the right temporal and parietal lobes seem especially involved in the recognition of emotion in others. This *affective agnosia* complements the effect of right frontal lesions in reducing the patient's own emotional expression. A persistently altered emotional deficit amounts to a change in the patient's personality. Many patients suffer such an apparent personality change after strokes or brain injuries affecting the right hemisphere, a major challenge to rehabilitation. Others, particularly those with bilateral strokes, have *emotional incontinence* or *pseudobulbar affect*, in which any fleeting emotion springs out fully in tears or laughter.

Occipital lobes

The occipital lobes are known as specialized areas of the cortex for vision. The primary visual cortex is in the medial occipital pole of each hemisphere, and a lesion here will cause a homonymous hemianopsia on the opposite side. In general, the more congruent the visual field deficit in both eyes, the more likely the lesion is to be in the contralateral occipital lobe. There may be some sparing of macular vision. Bilateral lesions of the medial occipital cortex may produce total *cortical* blindness. Some such patients have *Anton's syndrome*, a disorder in which the patient is not aware of blindness and may confabulate seeing objects or people, yet the same patient may walk directly into a wall. On the contrary, other patients may complain of being "blind" yet behave as if they see objects or avoid obstacles, a phenomenon known as *blind sight* or unconscious vision.

Patients with left medial occipital lesions, especially those with strokes in the distribution of the posterior cerebral artery, may have an inability to read, or alexia, along with a right visual field defect. These patients may have completely normal expressive speech, naming, auditory comprehension, and even writing (inability to read with preserved ability to write is called *pure alexia without agraphia*). The patient may write a sentence and then fail to be able to read it a few minutes later, the hallmark of this syndrome. Many patients also have short-term memory loss, since the left hippocampus is also within the left posterior cerebral artery territory, and some also have *color agnosia*, or inability to associate a perceived color with its name. Such patients can state what color a familiar object is (school bus, apple, and so forth) but fail to name the color of an object or picture placed in front of them.

Cortical syndromes

In this section, we shall discuss some of the common cortical syndromes, aphasia, apraxia, and agnosia. Some examples of these syndromes have come up as we reviewed each lobe of the brain, but some require combinations of lesions.

APHASIA

Aphasia is an acquired disorder of language. It is a separate disorder from dysarthria, an acquired motor speech disorder (see Chap. 11). Most aphasias involve abnormal language in both language expression and comprehension. Because aphasia is such an important problem in clinical neurology, the entire Chap. 16 is devoted to this disorder.

APRAXIA

Apraxias are disorders of learned or skilled movement. In testing for apraxia, the examiner looks at the patient's ability to follow commands to perform a skilled act with the orofacial muscles ("pucker your lips," " lick your lower lip"), or the upper limbs on either side ("show me how you would use a saw, or a hammer"). If the patient fails this test, the examiner can then test the patient's ability to mimic the examiner's own pantomime of the requested action, or finally, the patient's ability to use an actual object such as a saw or a hammer. Apraxias have traditionally been divided into three types, as outlined below.

Ideomotor apraxia involves the inability to pantomime the use of an imaginary object. The patient may perform somewhat better in mimicking the examiner's pantomime, but usually the patient's performance will return virtually to normal in demonstrating the use of a real object. Ideomotor apraxia is usually associated with left hemisphere lesions, and often it is associated with aphasia. Ideomotor apraxia has also been associated with neurodegenerative conditions such as Alzheimer's disease.

Ideational apraxia, also called *conceptual apraxia*, involves the loss of ability to perform actual manipulations of real objects, especially series actions such as filling and lighting a pipe or preparing coffee in an electric percolator. This type of apraxia is more disabling than ideomotor apraxia. The lesions are also usually localized in the left hemisphere and are often associated with aphasia secondary to local lesions or more diffuse, degenerative conditions such as Alzheimer's disease.

Limb-kinetic apraxia refers to a loss of dexterity or deftness in one limb, usually involving fine finger movements. The most common cause of limb-kinetic apraxia is a stroke, in which the patient has recovered gross strength, but the fine dexterity of the finger movements is still impaired.

AGNOSIA

Agnosias are disorders of recognition of perceived objects. The sensory perception itself is preserved, but the meaning of the perception is lost. Agnosias are usually defined in terms of specific sensory modalities such as vision, hearing, and somatosensory function.

Visual agnosia refers to an inability to recognize or understand the meaning of a visual stimulus, which is nonetheless perceived. In most cases, the lesions in patients with visual agnosia are bilateral but spare the primary visual cortex. By one theory, visual agnosia is explained by a disconnection of the occipital cortex from the left hemisphere language cortex. Occasionally, patients have visual agnosia for specific classes of items. The most common such class-specific visual agnosia is *prosopagnosia*, an acquired loss of the ability to recognize people's faces. This very disabling condition also often occurs in patients with bilateral hemisphere lesions, though occasional cases have been reported with right temporoparietal lesions.

Auditory agnosias involve the inability to recognize sound stimuli. They are divided into *pure word deafness*, which will be discussed under the aphasias in chap. 16, and *auditory nonverbal agnosia*. A patient with auditory nonverbal aphasia may understand spoken words but fail to identify animal noises or associate an object such as a bell or a tuning fork with its sound. Both pure word deafness and auditory nonverbal aphasia often result from bilateral temporal lobe lesions and may evolve from an initial syndrome of cortical deafness.

Tactile agnosias involve the failure to identify an object by its feel. A unilateral deficit of failure to recognize objects by palpation is often referred to as *astereognosis*; this deficit could be considered either a primary cortical sensory deficit or a tactile agnosia.

Anosognosia refers to neglect of a deficit such as hemiparesis. The neurobehavioral syndromes of neglect, dressing apraxia, constructional impairment, and topographical deficits were discussed under right parietal syndromes.

Posterior fossa lesions

The structures of the posterior fossa are the brainstem and cerebellum.

CEREBELLAR SYNDROMES

The cerebellum has two main components: the cerebellar cortex and the deep nuclei. The deep nuclei are the sources of cerebellar efferent fibers. Within the cerebellar cortex, three more or less functionally separate regions must be distinguished: (1) the central portion, the vermis, devoted to the control of the trunk; (2) the lateral hemispheres, more devoted to coordination of the individual limbs on one side of the body; and (3) the midline flocculonodular lobe, which projects to the vestibular nuclei in the medulla. The vermis and lateral hemisphere project to their respective deep nuclei, the fastigial nucleus for the vermis, and the dentate nucleus for the lateral cortex. The cerebellar cortex between these two areas projects to the middle two of the deep cerebellar nuclei, the globose and emboliform nuclei. The deep nuclei, in turn, project out via the superior cerebellar peduncle, whereas the middle and inferior cerebellar peduncles are the source of afferent fibers to the cerebellum. The middle peduncle contains principally afferents from the cortex, via the pontine nuclei. The inferior peduncle contains afferents from sensory nerves via the spinocerebellar and trigeminocerebellar pathways. The anatomic layout of the cerebellum is shown in Fig. 2-3.

The clinical effects of cerebellar lesions parallel these anatomic divisions. Lesions affecting the vermis cause predominantly difficulty with balance and walking; at times, the patient cannot stand at all and may lean to one side when sitting. Heel-knee-shin coordination is more affected than finger-nose-finger testing. There may also be abnormalities of the eye movements such as nystagmus. The examination of stance and gait is the key to diagnosis of acute, midline cerebellar lesions such as cerebellar hemorrhage, which most often occurs in the vermis. Patients may present with dizziness, headache, and nausea, and the neurological nature of the illness may not be suspected until the examiner asks the patient to stand and walk. If the patient is examined in a bed or emergency department (ED) gurney, the cranial nerves, strength, and even limb coordination may appear normal. Other midline cerebellar abnormalities include some cerebellar degenerations, particularly alcoholic cerebellar degeneration, and also tumors, such as the medulloblastomas that develop in children and adolescents.

With lesions of the lateral cerebellar cortex, coordination of the ipsilateral arm and leg are typically more affected than the trunk. The patient will show intention tremor on fine movement, as in finger-nose-finger testing. There may be associated eye movement abnormalities such as nystagmus, and

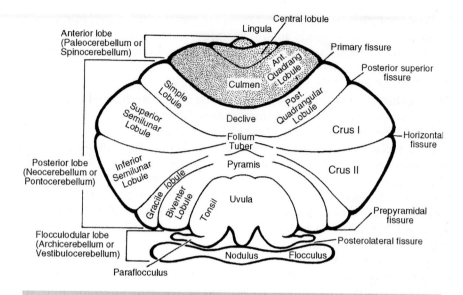

Figure 2-3 **Anatomical layout of the cerebellum.** (*Source*: Adapted from Victor and Ropper, *Adams and Victor's Principles of Neurology.* 2005, Fig. 5-1, p.71.)

there may be ataxic dysarthria, a speech pattern in which the cadence of speech is either slower than normal or irregular. Lateral cerebellar lesions can include strokes, tumors, and infections such as abscesses. Diagnosis of lateral cerebellar lesions can be difficult, in that sometimes the neurological examination is completely normal, despite complaints of dizziness and difficulty with balance and coordination. Younger patients, particularly, are able to compensate well for the effects of cerebellar lesions.

The deep cerebellar nuclei, when involved, produce profound tremor and incoordination on the ipsilateral side of the body. The tremor is usually proximal, and often severe and large in amplitude.

The flocculonodular lobe of the cerebellum is interconnected with the inner ear structures, such that damage there causes vertigo as a prominent symptom. Syndromes of this part of the cerebellum may resemble inner ear disorders, with vertigo and minimal or no focal neurological signs.

BRAINSTEM SYNDROMES

Brainstem localization is the most precise of any area of the central nervous system, because the cranial nerve nuclei and tracts are "eloquent" in terms of producing obvious symptoms and signs, and they are located very close to each other. During the nineteenth century, when small strokes related to neurosyphilis were common, neurologists described syndromes of small brainstem infarctions which still bear their eponyms. I have recommended to generations of medical students that an hour or two spent learning the anatomy of the brainstem is far more worthwhile than memorizing eponymic brainstem syndromes, since most syndromes can be predicted by knowledge of the nuclei and long tracts that are affected by a lesion in a specific location of the brainstem. With this principle in mind, we shall deal here with a few simple patterns of brainstem syndromes.

In general, involvement of cranial nerve nuclei produces ipsilateral cranial nerve symptoms, whereas involvement of the long tracts produces contralateral motor and sensory deficits. This "harlequin" pattern of crossed cranial nerve and long tract signs is the hallmark of brainstem syndromes. As in all stroke syndromes, the precise structures affected depend on the anatomy of the arterial supply to the region of the brain involved. The brainstem is supplied by the vertebrobasilar system. In general, this system respects the midline in branches supplying only one side, but there are two principal exceptions. The first involves disease in the basilar artery itself, which gives rise to branches to both sides of the brainstem. The second involves arterial branches off the top of the basilar or the proximal posterior cerebral artery (*artery of Percheron*), which may have a bilateral distribution.

In the midbrain, the principal cranial nerve nuclei are the III and IV nuclei. The most common midbrain syndrome is an ipsilateral III nerve palsy, with ipsilateral ptosis, pupillary dilatation, and loss of medial, upward, and downward gaze, and a contralateral hemiparesis (Weber's syndrome). There are several variations of this syndrome. Involvement of the red nucleus on the ipsilateral side of the midbrain produces ataxia, often with a marked *rubral tremor*, a violent form of intention tremor involving proximal muscles of the arm. Rubral tremor may occur with ipsilateral III palsy and contralateral hemiparesis (Benedikt's syndrome). Rarely, the ipsilateral rubral tremor is combined with a III nerve palsy but no contralateral hemiparesis (Claude's syndrome). Occlusion of the superior cerebellar artery may produce combined cerebellar and midbrain infarction. Involvement of the cerebellum and/or superior and middle cerebellar peduncles produces ipsilateral ataxia, with contralateral sensory and motor signs (syndromes of basilar branch occlusion). Occasionally, an embolus to the top of the basilar artery (*top of the basilar syndrome*) produces bilateral involvement of the III nerves, often with ptosis, upward gaze palsy, alteration of consciousness or coma, hemianopia or blindness from involvement of the posterior cerebral artery, or hemiballismus. If the small branch called the artery of Percheron is involved, patients may have an infarction confined to the paramedian midbrain and thalamus, with profound alteration of consciousness and memory, sometimes accompanied by unilateral or bilateral III nerve palsies, but without other long tract signs such as hemiparesis or sensory loss. Midbrain anatomy is shown in Fig. 2-4.

The pons is rich with nuclei and pathways. Again, the most common unilateral syndromes involve ipsilateral cranial nerve and contralateral long tract signs. For example, ipsilateral VI, VII, and VIII nerve palsies may accompany a contralateral hemiparesis and sensory loss. Occlusion of the

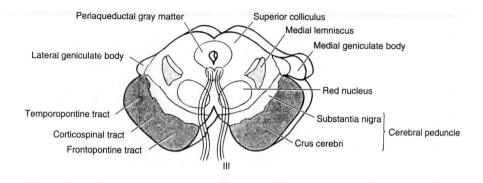

Figure 2-4 **Anatomy of the midbrain.** (*Source*: Adapted from Waxman, *Clinical Neuroanatomy*, Fig. 7-7, part E, p.88.)

anterior inferior cerebellar artery (AICA) may produce ipsilateral ataxia from involvement of the cerebellum or middle cerebellar peduncle, deafness from VIII nerve or cochlear nucleus involvement, ipsilateral Horner's syndrome, ipsilateral gaze paresis, and contralateral motor and sensory signs. Sensory loss from involvement of the spinothalamic tract will usually be associated with loss of pinprick and temperature sensation, without vibration and position sense deficits, and it will also either spare the face or be associated with ipsilateral (crossed) facial numbness. Small infarctions in the pons can produce many variations on this theme. When the basilar artery itself is involved, bilateral infarctions of the pons can result. Symptoms can include coma, quadriparesis, or the "locked-in" syndrome, in which the patient cannot move the limbs, the face, the mouth, or even the eyes in horizontal motion. Patients with *locked-in syndrome* may be mistakenly thought to be comatose, but they are fully conscious and can communicate by blinking the eyes or by looking up and down. Pontine anatomy is depicted in Fig. 2-5.

The medulla is also the site of named stroke syndromes. The most classic syndrome is the *lateral medullary syndrome* of Wallenburg. This is the most common of the brainstem stroke syndromes, because the lateral medulla and inferior, posterior cerebellum are supplied by the only major branch of the vertebral artery, the posterior inferior cerebellar artery (PICA). The occlusion in lateral medullary syndrome can involve either the vertebral artery itself or the PICA. The key signs of the lateral medullary syndrome are ipsilateral ataxia, ipsilateral Horner's syndrome (ptosis, miosis, reduced sweating on the ipsilateral face), ipsilateral facial numbness, ipsilateral dysphagia or palatal paresis (from involvement of the nucleus ambiguus or IX and X fibers), and contralateral pinprick and temperature sensory loss. There is often nystagmus, with the fast component opposite the lesion. Hemiparesis is usually absent. Some patients have hiccups. Much less common is the medial medullary syndrome, which can involve an ipsilateral XII palsy with weakness of the tongue,

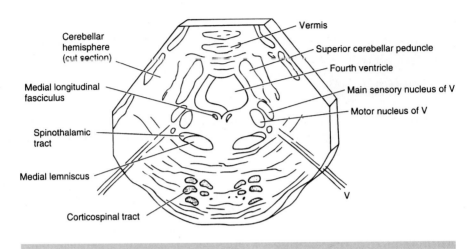

Figure 2-5   **Anatomy of the pons.** (*Source:* Adapted from Waxman, *Clinical Neuroanatomy*, Fig 7-7, part E, p.88.)

ipsilateral vibration and position sense loss from involvement of the medial lemniscus, and contralateral hemiparesis, from involvement of the cerebral pyramid. Medullary anatomy is summarized in Fig. 2-6.

Throughout this brief discussion of brainstem localization, we have used strokes as examples. The principles of anatomic localization apply equally, however, to small brainstem lesions of any etiology. For example, multiple sclerosis has a propensity to produce small brainstem plaques. If plaques occur bilaterally near the dorsal paramedian midbrain or pons, a bilateral

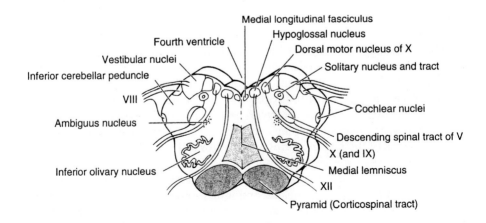

Figure 2-6   **Anatomy of medulla.** (*Source:* Adapted from Waxman, *Clinical Neuroanatomy*, Fig 7-7, part E, p.87.)

internuclear ophthalmoplegia can result. Bilateral internuclear ophthalmoplegia (INO) is caused by multiple sclerosis in over 90% of cases. A unilateral INO, however, could reflect either an MS plaque or a small infarct, or
potentially even a small tumor, abscess, or cavernous angioma.

Spinal cord lesions

To understand the spinal cord, the student need only review a few key pathways. The spinal cord is made up of central gray matter and surrounding
white matter. The anterior gray substance contains the anterior horn cells that
give rise to the axons of the major spinal nerves. Damage to anterior horn
cells produces localized weakness, atrophy of muscles, and loss of the
reflexes in that distribution. Involvement of the spinal cord at C6-7 level, for
example, will produce lower motor neuron signs in muscles innervated by
the C7 nerve root in the ipsilateral arm. The white matter of the spinal cord
can be divided into the posterior, lateral, and ventral columns. Involvement
of the lateral column affects the corticospinal tract, producing weakness and
upper motor neuron signs, including spasticity and hyperreflexia. In acute
lesions of the lateral columns, there may be a period of "spinal shock" with
flaccid tone and absent reflexes. The posterior columns have to do with vibration and position sense on the ipsilateral side. The ventral columns contain
the spinothalamic tracts, carrying information on pinprick and temperature
sensation. The sensory nerve fibers enter through the dorsal nerve root at
each level, synapse, then travel just anterior to the central canal, crossing the
midline in the *central commissure*. They then ascend in the spinothalamic tract
in the contralateral anterior column. Involvement of the spinothalamic tract
produces loss of pinprick and temperature sensation on the contralateral side
of the body, below the level of injury (or one to two segments below the level
of injury). There may also be local sensory deficits at the level of the incoming dorsal root sensory fibers. Spinal cord anatomy is shown in Fig. 2-7.

From this basic anatomy, we can understand the syndromes of injury to
specific regions of the spinal cord.

TRANSVERSE MYELOPATHY

Transverse myelopathy implies involvement of the entire spinal cord at one
vertical level. We would expect to see total paralysis below the level of the
lesion, with upper motor neuron signs possibly coming after the acute *spinal
shock period*; there will also be a sensory level below the injury, involving all
modalities, including vibration, position, pinprick, and temperature sensation. Bilateral spinal cord lesions also cause autonomic involvement, manifest
as bladder and bowel paralysis. Identification of the acute transverse
myelopathy syndrome can be a medical emergency in cases of trauma, mass
lesions such as tumors compressing the cord, or vascular cord lesions. In cancer patients, metastases involving the spinal cord often begin with collapse of
a vertebral body, and often there will be local pain and tenderness with

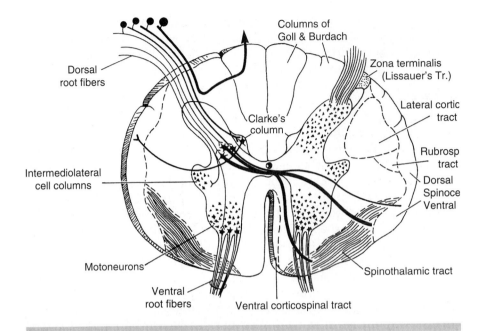

Figure 2-7 **Anatomy of the spinal cord, cervical level.** (*Source*: Adapted from Victor and Ropper, *Adams and Victor's Principles of Neurology*, 2005, Fig. 8-1 p .114)

percussion of the spine, a useful physical sign. Imaging of the spine with magnetic resonance imaging (MRI) or myelography confirms the diagnosis.

ANTERIOR SPINAL ARTERY SYNDROME

The spinal cord receives its blood supply from the anterior spinal artery, which runs just anterior to the cord, except for the posterior columns, which receive blood supply from a plexus of posterior spinal arteries. The hallmark of vascular myelopathies is therefore sparing of posterior column function, vibration and position sense, in the presence of all of the other aspects of the transverse myelopathy syndrome: bilateral upper motor neuron paralysis, bilateral loss of pinprick and temperature sensation below the level of the lesion, and segmental findings of lower motor neuron weakness from involvement of the anterior horn or ventral root at the level of the lesion, localized sensory loss from involvement of the dorsal root, and loss of bowel and bladder function. The syndrome is usually symmetric on both sides of the body, though occasional asymmetries occur. A medical emergency related to anterior spinal artery syndrome is the presentation of a ruptured abdominal aortic aneurysm. As the artery dissects, segmental arterial branches supplying the anterior spinal artery may be compromised, and the patient may present with an acute paraparesis rather than with the abdominal symptoms of the aneurysm. Surgery to repair the aorta may be lifesaving, if the diagnosis can be made rapidly.

BROWN-SÉQUARD SYNDROME

The Brown-Séquard syndrome is the result of a spinal lesion predominantly affecting one side of the spinal cord. Involvement of the lateral column produces ipsilateral upper motor neuron paralysis, again after a period of spinal shock with acute lesions, along with ipsilateral vibration and position sense loss from posterior column involvement, and contralateral involvement of pinprick and temperature sensation, below the level of the lesion. The *crossed findings* of contralateral pinprick and temperature loss, ipsilateral vibration and position sense loss, and ipsilateral motor dysfunction are the hallmark features of the Brown-Séquard syndrome. Again, there can be segmental findings of motor and sensory loss at the level of the lesion, from involvement of the anterior horn and/or ventral root, and the dorsal root. The Brown-Séquard syndrome can result from etiologies as distinct as trauma, tumor, or demyelinating disease. Often the syndromes are not pure, but rather *modified Brown-Séquard syndromes*, with findings predominantly but not exclusively on one side.

COMBINED LATERAL AND POSTERIOR COLUMN INVOLVEMENT

Combined syndromes of lateral and posterior column involvement are the hallmark of two totally different pathological disorders, *subacute, combined systems disease*, seen in vitamin B_{12} deficiency or pernicious anemia, and *Friedreich's ataxia*. In subacute, combined systems disease, the patient usually presents with complaints of tingling in the feet and legs, together with weakness primarily in the legs and in gait. B_{12} deficiency can also produce mental and cognitive symptoms (*megaloblastic madness*) or peripheral neuropathy, so the exact clinical presentation can vary. Early replacement of vitamin B_{12} can prevent permanent neurological damage in this disorder. In Friedreich's ataxia, the onset is usually in childhood or early adolescence, and ataxic gait is the principal presenting sign.

POSTERIOR COLUMN DISORDERS

A rarely seen spinal cord syndrome in the current era is *tabes dorsalis*, a syphilis-related illness in which the dorsal root ganglia cells degenerate and there is secondary degeneration of the posterior columns. The patients present with loss of vibration and position sense, leading to a sensory ataxic gait, often with slapping of the feet because of the profound loss of position sense in the feet and ankles. Patients also complain of lightning or tabetic pains shooting up or down the legs. They may repeatedly traumatize joints such as the knee, leading to *Charcot's joints*, swollen, severely damaged but numb joints.

CENTRAL CORD SYNDROMES

Syringomyelia is a disorder in which a fluid-filled cavity forms within the substance of the spinal cord. A syrinx can form in association with a structural lesion like a tumor or after a traumatic injury such as hematomyelia, or hemorrhage into the spinal cord. Other cases of syringomyelia appear to be congenital, representing an enlargement of the central canal. Such cases are often associated with other genetic, developmental disorders such as the Chiari's malformation at the base of the brain and hydrocephalus. The syndrome produced by a syrinx will depend on exactly which spinal tracts are affected, but the most common presentation is compression of the crossing fibers of the spinothalamic tract in the central commissure by the enlarging central canal. Since most syrinxes occur in the cervical spinal cord, the patient often presents with loss of pinprick and temperature sensation in both upper limbs and in the trunk of the chest and back, a distribution likened to a "cape". Symptoms of numbness, paresthesias, and pain may start on one or both sides within this distribution. As the syrinx expands, the lateral columns or anterior horns may be compromised, leading to upper motor neuron paresis on one or both sides, or segmental lower motor neuron changes at the level of the anterior horn involvement. Surgical procedures to drain or shunt the syrinx cavity may prevent long-term disability.

Another *central cord syndrome* is associated with traumatic injuries, usually in the cervical region. Shear injuries within the cord, from sudden flexion-extension movements, often occur in patients who have preexisting cervical spondylosis. The anterior horn may be affected on both sides, leading to lower neuron weakness in both arms, with milder, upper motor neuron paralysis from corticospinal tract (lateral column) involvement at the same level.

CERVICAL SPONDYLOSIS

Cervical spondylosis is the most common spinal cord syndrome. The term refers to a spinal form of degenerative joint disease, or osteoarthritis. At each level of the spine, bone spurs with associated disc bulges push posteriorly into the spinal canal, compressing the spinal cord, the exiting nerve roots, or both. Patients can present in a variety of ways. First, there may be neck pain, largely caused by compression of exiting nerve roots. The first three cervical nerve roots travel up the back of the head, often producing syndromes of neck pain and posterior headache which are quite common in elderly people. Compression of the C4-C7 nerve roots, all of which exit just below the cervical vertebra of the same number, produces radicular syndromes of pain, sensory loss, and segmental weakness and loss of reflexes, referred to as *cervical radiculopathy*. Compression of the spinal cord develops slowly and insidiously, sometimes presenting with gradually developing weakness of both legs, with hyperreflexia and upgoing toes. Involvement of the posterior columns, with loss of vibration and position sense in the legs, is also common. Most of the time, these slowly progressive myelopathies are accompanied by neck pain and radicular syndromes which make the diagnosis straightforward. Occasionally, however, patients present with a painless myelopathy. Diagnosis is usually accomplished by MRI scanning of the cervical spine, though occasionally myelography is needed. The treatment is largely surgical, involving either posterior laminectomy or anterior cervical diskectomy and fusion. Surgery in this setting can prevent the development of permanent spinal cord damage.

NERVE ROOT/PLEXUS LESIONS

The localization of nerve root and plexus lesions is generally straightforward, a matter of detecting the specific muscles that are weak, specific reflexes that are missing, and specific areas of sensory loss. The examiner must either know the relevant neuroanatomy or have a reference book handy.

Table 2-1 shows the anatomical distributions of the major cervical nerve roots. The principles are straightforward. In the cervical spine, the major roots exit just below the vertebral body of the same number. For example, a C5-6 disk protrusion will affect the C6 nerve root on the same side. The C1, C2, and C3 nerve roots have no major motor innervation and supply a sensory area that runs up the back of the neck, often associated with headache. The C4-T1 roots have motor and sensory distributions in the upper limb. For example, a C5 root lesion, or radiculopathy, produces weakness in the deltoid and biceps muscles, decrease in or absence of the biceps reflex, and a band of pinprick sensory loss over the medial forearm and into the thumb. A C6 radiculopathy is also associated with weakness of the biceps, and also of the wrist extensors, along with a decreased or absent biceps reflex, and a band of sensory loss

Table 2-1   *Cervical Nerve Root Distributions*

Disk Level	Root	Pain	Weakness	Sensory Loss	Reflex
C4-5	C5	Upper back, lat. upper arm	Deltoid, supra- and infraspinatus	Lat. upper arm	–
C5-6	C6	Lat. forearm	Biceps, brachioradialis, wrist extensors	Thumb and index finger	Biceps jerk
C6-7	C7	Upper back, post. upper arm, dorsal forearm, third finger	Triceps, wrist flexors, finger extensors	Post. forearm, third finger	Triceps jerk
C7-T1	C8	Shoulder, ulnar forearm, fifth finger	Thumb flexor, abductors, intrinsic hand muscles	Fifth finger	–

extending into the thumb and first finger. A C7 radiculopathy causes more distal weakness around the wrist extensors and flexors, hand grip, a decreased or absent triceps reflex, and a band of sensory loss extending into the middle finger. A C8 radiculopathy involves the hand intrinsics, a decreased or absent triceps reflex, and numbness along the ulnar side of the hand and forearm. A T1 radiculopathy can also affect the hand intrinsics but will not affect the reflexes and may not be associated with sensory loss in the hand or fingers.

In the thoracic spine, involvement of nerve roots will affect only a band of sensory loss extending around the side from the back. There is no limb muscle innervation from thoracic nerve roots below T1.

In the lumbosacral spine, roots again exit just below the vertebral bodies of the same number. Common lumbar root syndromes are listed in Table 2-2. L1 and L2 radiculopathies are unusual. They do not affect the lower extremity reflexes but may produce weakness in the iliopsoas (hip flexor) muscle. L3 nerve root involvement produces a weak quadriceps muscle (knee extension), a decreased or absent knee reflex, and a band of sensory loss along the medial thigh and into the calf. L4 radiculopathy is very similar to L3, except that the sensory loss involves the lateral thigh and calf. L5 radiculopathy produces weakness in ankle dorsiflexion, ankle eversion, and ankle inversion, but not plantar flexion. There is no reflex affected by an L5 lesion. The sensory loss involves lateral thigh and calf, extending into the dorsum of the foot. S1 radiculopathy produces weakness mainly in plantar flexion of the ankle, though the hip extensors and hamstrings are also affected. The ankle reflex will be reduced or absent. A band of sensory loss may affect the posterior calf and sole of the foot. Below S1, involvement

Table 2-2   **Lumbar Nerve Root Distributions**

Disk Level	Root	Pain	Weakness	Sensory Loss	Reflex
L3-4	L4	Low back-lateral thigh	Quadriceps	Lateral thigh and calf	Knee jerk
L4-5	L5	Low back-lateral thigh and calf, dorsum of foot	Hamstrings, ankle dorsiflexors	Lateral calf, dorsum of foot	–
L5-S1	S1	Low back-posterior thigh, posterolateral calf, sole and lateral side of foot	Ankle plantar flexors	Posterior calf, sole and lateral side of foot	Ankle jerk

of sacral roots is silent in terms of lower extremity muscles, but bilateral involvement can produce abnormalities of bladder, bowel, and sexual function. The dermatomal chart of the spinal nerve roots is shown in Fig. 2-8.

Plexopathies are disorders of the main plexuses of nerves that intermingle with the branches of the spinal nerve roots, predominantly in the cervicothoracic area (brachial plexus, C4-T1 roots) and the lumbosacral area (L1-S1). A lesion of a specific portion of either the brachial or lumbosacral plexus will produce a specific combination of weak muscles. In general, plexus lesions are often noted for pain and weakness, as well as loss of reflexes in the affected limb, usually with only minor sensory symptoms and signs.

The brachial plexus is more commonly the source of neurological syndromes than the lumbosacral plexus. Figure 2-9 shows the anatomy of the brachial plexus, divided into the upper, middle, and lower trunks, giving rise to the lateral, posterior, and medial cords. Careful clinical examination of individual muscles demonstrates a pattern of muscle weakness that can arise

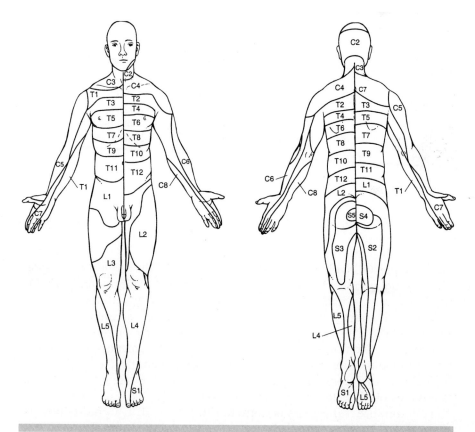

Figure 2-8 **Dermatomal chart of nerv root distributions.** (*Source*: Adapted from Clinical Examination in Neurology. 2nd ed. Philadelphia, PA: W.B. Saunders, 1963, Fig. 49)

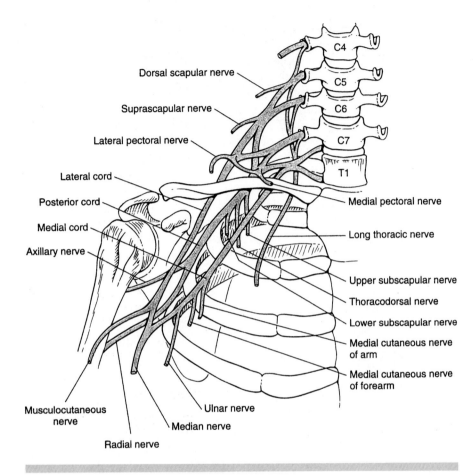

Figure 2-9 **Anatomy of the brachial plexus.** (*Source*: Adapted from Gilman, *Clinical Examination of the Nervous System*, Fig. 7-9, p.202)

only from plexus involvement, rather than a lesion of the cervical nerve roots or individual peripheral nerves or muscles. Traumatic injuries are probably the most common brachial plexus syndromes, especially with forced abduction of the shoulder as is commonly seen in motorcycle accidents, and with fractures of the clavicle or compression syndromes in the presence of a cervical rib or band compressing the axillary artery and elements of the plexus. Autoimmune or idiopathic plexopathies (brachial neuritis, *Parsonage-Turner syndrome*), or tumor involvement are also common. Infiltrating tumors of the plexus are notorious for causing weakness and sensory loss without pain.

The lumbosacral plexus is depicted in Fig. 2-10. Traumatic injuries to the lower back and pelvis can also produce plexopathies in the lumbosacral area, but tumor infiltration by gynecological malignancies is also common.

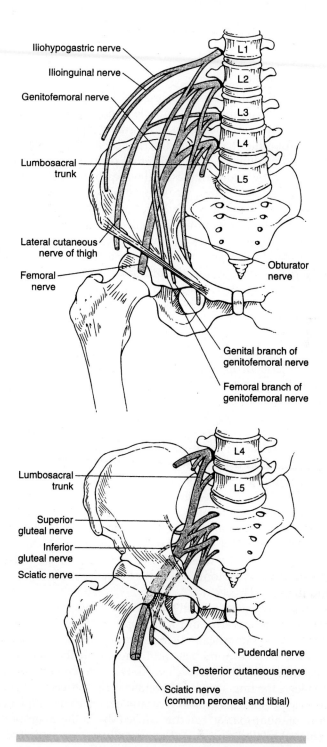

Figure 2-10 **Anatomy of the lumbosacral plexus.**
(*Source*: Adapted from Gilman, Fig. 7-8 parts A&B,
p.200 and 201)

PERIPHERAL NERVE LESIONS

Diagnosis of peripheral nerve injuries, or other *mononeuropathies*, also depends on careful examination of muscle strength, reflexes, and sensory loss, in this case within one nerve territory. Many specific compression and entrapment neuropathies have been described. Case 3 at the end of Chap. 1 was a case of peroneal nerve palsy, with foot drop. Femoral neuropathy is occasionally caused by hemorrhages in the area of the psoas muscle in the retroperitoneal space, with pain, weakness of the iliopsoas and quadriceps muscles, loss of the knee jerk, and sensory loss in the medial thigh. Involvement of the lateral femoral cutaneous nerve causes a syndrome of paresthesias, numbness, and lack of any motor or reflex signs, a syndrome called *meralgia paresthetica*. Involvement of the sciatic nerve, for example from a poorly placed injection in the buttock area, causes severe pain and weakness of both the dorsiflexors and plantar flexors of the ankle, also inversion and eversion, loss of the ankle reflex, and sensory loss on the foot and calf.

In the upper limb, involvement of the radial nerve is often caused by falling asleep with the upper arm over the back of a chair (*Saturday night palsy*). There is a wrist drop, as well as weakness of extension of the fingers. If the wrist is held straight, the flexor and grip muscles remain strong. Ulnar nerve compression at the elbow often causes predominantly numbness and paresthesias in the ulnar distribution of the medial hand and fourth and fifth fingers, and in severe cases, weakness of the ulnar-innervated hand muscles. Tapping over the site of compression at the elbow produces electric-like tingling and pain down the distribution of the nerve (*Tinel's sign*), a sign useful in diagnosis of other compression and entrapment neuropathies. At the wrist, compression of the median nerve (*carpal tunnel syndrome*) is also associated with pain and paresthesias in the medial hand and fingers. In severe cases, weakness of the median-innervated hand intrinsic muscles may also be found (see Chap. 32). In addition to the Tinel's sign produced by tapping on the wrist, prolonged flexion of the wrist (Phalen's sign) also reproduces symptoms. A chart of major peripheral nerve territories is found in Fig. 2-11.

Other peripheral nerve syndromes reflect involvement of multiple nerves (peripheral neuropathy, or *polyneuropathy*, Chap. 33). The most common pattern is a symmetrical, distal, sensory-motor neuropathy. Initial symptoms often involve numbness and tingling in the toes and feet, followed by weakness of distal muscles. As the involvement spreads proximally up the legs, the finger tips and hands become affected. A loss of distal reflexes such as the ankle jerks also typically occurs early in the neuropathy. This pattern of neuropathy can be caused by a number of etiologies. Diabetes, alcohol-related nutritional neuropathies, and toxins are all common causes of this condition, and some are genetic.

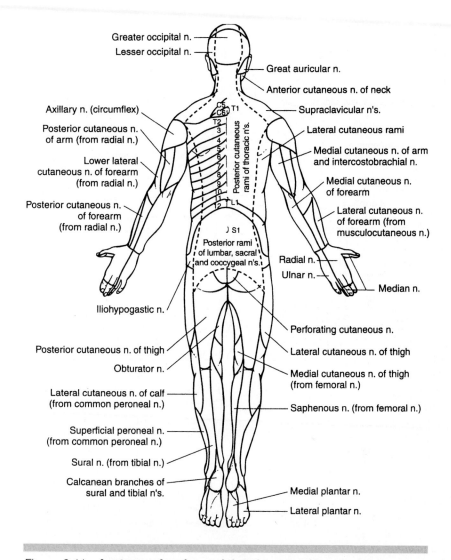

Figure 2-11 **Anatomy of major peripheral nerves.** (*Source*: Adapted from Gilman, *Clinical Examination of the Nervous System*, Fig. 7-3, p. 183.)

Several, more selective patterns of peripheral neuropathy have been described. We shall discuss a few of them here.

Mononeuritis multiplex is a syndrome in which individual mononeuropathies, such as a radial nerve or peroneal nerve palsy, occur sequentially or simultaneously. Such multiple mononeuropathies often reflect a vascular involvement of nerves. The most common causes are diabetes, vasculitis, and sarcoidosis.

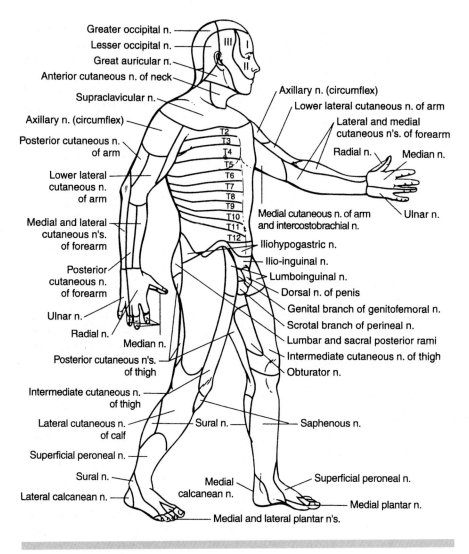

Figure 2-11 **(Continued).**

Acute, ascending polyneuropathy is a syndrome in which a patient goes from a normal state of health, to complaints of numbness and weakness in the feet and toes, to a progressive syndrome of weakness involving the legs, distal arms and hands, then even proximal arms and face. The most common etiology is the Guillain- Barré syndrome (GBS) (see Chap. 33), but similar syndromes can be seen with porphyria, diphtheria, toxic neuropathies, and vasculitides. GBS often begins with predominantly sensory complaints, but progressive weakness soon develops and usually becomes much more severe than the sensory deficits. Many GBS patients are misdiagnosed as having an anxiety disorder when they present in early stages, with only minor sensory complaints in the feet and a grossly normal neurological examination. A high index of suspicion for this disorder is important, and monitoring the patient for the tell-tale loss of muscle stretch reflexes that occurs early in the illness helps in diagnosis. Respiratory monitoring, with measures of vital capacity and negative inspiratory force, is also indicated, as sudden respiratory failure may supervene. Syndromes of pure motor weakness such as tick paralysis, botulism, and myasthenia gravis may be confused with an acute polyneuropathy. The mixture of sensory and motor deficits, loss of reflexes, and distal onset, usually with sparing of autonomic innervation to the pupils and bladder differentiate the neuropathies from these other conditions.

Pure sensory, or small fiber neuropathies produce complaints of numbness and burning paresthesias, often beginning distally in the feet and hands. These disorders may seem largely subjective, since muscle strength and reflexes may be normal, and even *large fiber* sensory modalities such as vibration and position sense may be spared. The differential diagnosis is wide, including paraneoplastic syndromes, heavy metal or organophosphate toxicity, Sjögren's syndrome, and idiopathic neuropathies, to name a few.

Muscle disorders

Muscle disorders generally produce weakness, without sensory loss, cognitive changes, or reflex changes, though reflexes may diminish in profoundly weak muscles. The pattern of weakness is characteristic for most myopathies. The majority of myopathies present with proximal weakness, such as the muscles of the shoulder and hip girdles. This is true in many dystrophies, endocrinopathies such as Cushing's disease and steroid myopathy. Other myopathies are named for their unusual distribution of muscle weakness, such as oculopharyngeal dystrophy, facioscapulo-humeral dystrophy, and others. The subject of myopathy will be discussed in Chap. 34.

KEY REFERENCES

General

Gilman S. Clinical examination of the nervous system. New York: McGraw Hill; 2000.

Victor M, Ropper A. *Adams & Victor's Principles of Neurology.* New York: McGraw Hill; 2005.

Cortical syndromes

Benton AL. Gerstmann's syndrome. *Arch Neurol* 1992;49:445–447.

Caselli RJ. Rediscovering tactile agnosia. *Mayo Clin Proc* 1991;66:129–142.

Cummings JL. Frontal-subcortical circuits and human behavior. *Arch Neurol* 1993;50:873–880.

Damasio AR. Aphasia. *N Engl J Med* 1992;326:531–539.

De Renzi E, Motti F, Nichelli P. Imitating gestures: a quantitative approach to ideo-motor apraxia. *Arch Neurol* 1980;37:6–10.

Fink GR, Halligan PW, Marshall JC, et al. Where in the brain does visual attention select the forest and the trees? *Nature* 1996;382:626–628.

Goldman-Rakic P. The prefrontal landscape: implications of functional architecture for understanding human mentation and the central executive. *Phil Trans R Soc Lond B* 1996;351:1445–1453.

Heilman KM, Maher LM, Greenwald ML, et al. Conceptual apraxia from lateralized lesions. *Neurology* 1997;49:457–464.

Heilman KM, Meador KJ, Loring DW. Hemispheric asymmetries of limb-kinetic apraxia. A loss of deftness. *Neurology* 2000;55:523–526.

Kirshner HS. *Behavioral Neurology: Practical Science of Mind and Brain.* Boston: Butterworth Heinemann; 2002.

Kirshner HS. *Handbook of Neurological Speech and Language Disorders.* New York: Marcel Dekker Inc.; 1995.

Mesulam M-M. *Principles of Behavioral and Cognitive Neurology.* 2nd ed. Oxford: Oxford University Press; 2000.

Na DL, Adair JC, Williamson DJG, et al. Dissociation of sensory-attentional from motor-intentional neglect. *J Neurol Neurosurg Psychiatr* 1998;64:331–338.

Samuelsson H, Jensen C, Ekholm S, et al. Anatomical and neurological correlates of acute and chronic visuospatial neglect following right hemisphere stroke. *Cortex* 1997;33:271–285.

Takahashi N, Kawamura M, Shiota J, et al. Pure topographical disorientation due to right retrosplenial lesion. *Neurology* 1997;49:464–469.

Spinal cord disorders

Carette S, Fehlings MG. Cervical radiculopathy. *New Engl J Med* 2005;353:392–399.

Cheshire WP, Santos CC, Massey EW, et al. Spinal cord infarction: etiology and outcome. *Neurology* 1996;47:321–330.

Geisler FH, Coleman WP, Benzel E, et al. Spinal cord injury. *Lancet* 2002;359(9304); 417–425.

Houser OW, Onofrio BM, Miller GM, et al. Cervical disk prolapse. *Mayo Clin Proc* 1995;70:939–945.

Jahnke RW, Hart BL. Cervical stenosis, spondylosis, and herniated disc disease. *Rad Clin North Am* 1991;29:777–791.

Schiff D. Spinal cord compression. *Neurol Clin* 2003;21:67–86.

Plexopathies, Neuropathies

Cuetter AC, Bartoszek DM. The thoracic outlet syndrome: controversies, overdiagnosis, overtreatment, and recommendations for management. *Muscle Nerve* 1989;12:410–419.

Dawson DM. Entrapment neuropathies of the upper extremities. *N Engl J Med* 1993; 329:2013–2018.

Ferrante MA. Brachial plexopathies. *Muscle Nerve* 2004;30:547–568.

Nakano KK. The entrapment neuropathies. Muscle Nerve 1978;1:264–279.

NEUROLOGICAL SYMPTOM COMPLEXES

WEAKNESS:

GENERALIZED AND FOCAL

One of the most common presentations of neurological illness is with weakness. Analysis of the patterns of weakness and the presence or absence of associated signs is the key to diagnosis.

In any analysis of weakness, the first consideration is the level of the nervous system from which the weakness arises. Lesions can involve, in considering most peripheral to most central causes, the muscle, neuromuscular junction, peripheral nerve, plexus, spinal or cranial nerve root, lower motor neuron (in the brainstem or spinal cord), central nervous system white matter (corticobulbar or corticospinal tract), or cortex. The second consideration is the location on the body of the resulting weakness; does it involve one limb or part of one limb, one side of the body, or both sides of the body? if bilateral, is it symmetric or asymmetric, proximal or distal?

MYOPATHIES

We shall first begin with the patterns of weakness typically seen at each level of the nervous system. First, the muscles are part of a system that includes all four limbs, truncal musculature, and even bulbar muscles in the face, oropharynx, and neck. Myopathies typically produce diffuse weakness, with differing patterns typical for specific myopathies. The most common pattern of weakness in a myopathy is proximal weakness of the arms and legs (often referred to as shoulder girdle and pelvic girdle weakness), and sometimes of the neck flexors and extensors, usually without much involvement of the cranial-nerve-innervated (bulbar) muscles. Patients often present first with difficulty getting out of a low chair, or standing from a squat, because of the pelvic girdle weakness. Not all myopathies follow this pattern; some feature distal weakness (limb girdle dystrophy), or cranial and proximal arm weakness (fascioscapular humeral dystrophy). A few affect bulbar ocular and pharyngeal muscles (oculopharyngeal dystrophy). Patterns of weakness in the myopathies will be discussed in Chap. 34.

The second aspect of myopathy, besides the pattern of weakness, is the absence of involvement of other systems. Myopathy does not affect sensation at all, and the tendon reflexes tend to be normal or diminished only when the muscles participating in the specific reflex are profoundly weak. These "negative signs" help as much as the pattern of weakness in identifying specific myopathies.

NEUROMUSCULAR JUNCTION DISORDERS

Disorders of the neuromuscular junction produce very distinctive patterns of weakness, often with the added feature of fatiguing weakness, or increased weakness with exertion. As in the myopathies, the sensory system is unaffected in neuromuscular junction disorders, and reflexes are diminished only when the degree of weakness is profound. The most common neuromuscular junction disorder is myasthenia gravis, which will be discussed in Chap. 35. This disorder usually produces weakness of the eyelids and extraocular muscles early in the course, so that ptosis and diplopia are common presenting symptoms. The lower cranial-nerve-innervated muscles are also commonly affected, so facial weakness, nasal and breathy voice, dysphagia (difficulty swallowing), and a hanging jaw or hanging head from neck muscle weakness are common. Respiratory muscle weakness, even to the extent of respiratory failure during myasthenic crises, is also common, and limb muscle weakness, usually proximal in distribution, also develops in many cases. Again, the fatiguing nature of the weakness, with better function early in the morning and progressive weakness during exertion during the day, is classic for myasthenia gravis.

Botulism represents a less common neuromuscular junction disorder, but one that medical students and physicians should not miss. Here again, the cranial-nerve-innervated muscles often weaken first, but in botulism, the autonomic parts of the nerves are affected as well, and the patient may have dilated pupils on presentation. Bulbar weakness and limb weakness follow, as in myasthenia.

The Lambert-Eaton syndrome is a rarer neuromuscular disorder. This disorder, often seen as a remote effect of cancers, involves fatiguing weakness of proximal muscles. Like the other neuromuscular disorders, it can be diagnosed on electromyography (EMG) with repetitive nerve stimulation, but the electromyographer must be informed that this diagnosis is a possibility, since the characteristic pattern is a paradoxical increase in amplitude of the compound muscle action potential with rapid rates of stimulation, not tested in a routine EMG.

PERIPHERAL NEUROPATHIES

Peripheral neuropathies are more variable in their symptomatology than the myopathies, since both motor and sensory nerves may be affected. In general, most polyneuropathies produce distal greater than proximal changes in both motor and sensory function, and the reflexes are affected mainly in the areas of weakness. For example, the most common peripheral neuropathy in the United States, diabetic neuropathy, commonly affects sensation first, with loss of both pinprick and vibration sense in the feet, and later hands, with weakness of the ankle and foot muscles and often loss of the ankle reflexes. As the condition worsens, the numbness and weakness gradually ascend, involving hands as well as feet, and in late stages neuropathic sensory loss may even involve the midanterior abdomen. In general, the areas affected are those supplied by the longest nerves in the body, and the nerves going from (sensory) and to (motor) the feet travel as much as 4 ft from the anterior horn cells in the spinal cord, in the case of motor nerves, and to the dorsal root ganglion cells, in the case of sensory nerves.

Other neuropathies have their own patterns of involvement, as will be discussed in more detail in Chap. 33. Some neuropathies involve only sensory nerve fibers, especially the small fiber neuropathies. An example would be the *carcinomatous sensory neuropathy* associated with occult neoplasms, though other diseases such as Sjögren's syndrome may also produce pure sensory neuropathies. Pain is often a disabling aspect of such sensory neuropathies. These conditions may spare the large, myelinated nerve fibers, leaving vibration and position sense, reflexes, and strength completely intact. Other neuropathies preferentially involve motor nerves, as in lead toxicity. In this syndrome, the nerves in the limbs most in use may suffer the most, as in the wrist drop seen in painters who use lead paint. Finally, some neuropathies begin rapidly, and the pattern of involvement can be more variable. The Guillain-Barré syndrome, for example, often presents with sensory symptoms such as numbness in the feet, but then a rapidly ascending paralysis develops, often with respiratory muscle weakness and even acute respiratory failure. In this syndrome, the tendon reflexes tend to disappear all over the body early in the disease. This diagnosis must be made rapidly, since hospitalization and early treatment are mandatory (see Chaps. 33 and 23).

Mononeuropathies often produce weakness in a very focal distribution, as in a wrist drop with radial nerve palsy or a foot drop with peroneal nerve palsy. These syndromes were discussed in the discussion of neurological localization in Chap. 2 and in the case presentations at the end of that chapter.

MYELOPATHIES

Myelopathies often produce both motor and sensory symptoms and signs below the level of the spinal cord involvement. The motor signs include both involvement of anterior horn cells and spinal nerve roots at the level of the lesion (with lower motor neuron signs) and of the corticospinal tracts below the lesion (with upper motor neuron signs). The problem with this analysis, however, is that upper motor neuron signs such as spastic tone and increased reflexes take time to develop, and an acute spinal lesion may cause flaccid weakness below the level of the lesion, a phenomenon called *spinal shock*. This is the presentation to be expected in direct trauma to the spinal cord, or inflammation of the cord, as in acute transverse myelitis.

Other patterns of myelopathy were discussed in Chap. 2. In vascular spinal cord lesions (anterior spinal artery syndrome), the posterior columns are typically spared, so vibration and position sense are preserved. In central cord syndrome, the lower motor neuron involvement of the arms is more severe than the upper motor neuron weakness in the legs (see Chap. 2). In the Brown-Séquard syndrome, the pattern of ipsilateral weakness, ipsilateral posterior column involvement, and contralateral pinprick and temperature sensation loss make the diagnosis straightforward.

BRAINSTEM LESIONS

In brainstem lesions, the key pattern is the ipsilateral involvement of cranial nerves and the contralateral involvement of long tracts (see Chap. 2). When such lesions are bilateral, however, they can cause complete quadriplegia, with initial flaccidity similar to spinal shock, often associated with cranial nerve involvement, and if the lesion involves the brainstem reticular activating system, stupor or coma as well.

CEREBRAL LESIONS

Weakness in cerebral lesions is related to involvement of the central motor pathways beginning in the motor cortex of the precentral gyrus, the descending corticospinal pathways in the cerebral white matter, internal capsule, and then into the cerebral peduncle of the midbrain. The classic hemiparesis of a middle cerebral artery stroke involves the hand and arm more than the leg, often with some involvement of the face on the same side as the limb weakness. Often, cortical symptoms, such as aphasia in left hemisphere lesions and neglect or visual-spatial deficits in right-hemisphere lesions are associated, along with visual field deficits and sensory loss on the same side of the body as the weakness. In anterior cerebral artery territory strokes, the leg is more affected than the arm, and the hand may be spared, sometimes with an involuntary grasp response. Behavior may be affected, as in a frontal lobe syndrome, but sensation and vision are usually preserved. In deeper lesions, as in the internal capsule, the weakness may be profound, but sensation, cortical function, and visual fields are preserved.

A rare pattern of weakness associated with cortical lesions is the bilateral weakness presentation of a parasagittal lesion, such as a meningioma arising from the falx cerebri. The patient may present with bilateral leg weakness, mimicking a spinal cord lesion, but without sensory loss. In this situation, a brain imaging study such as a magnetic resonance imaging (MRI) scan is essential for diagnosis.

FOCAL WEAKNESS

Weakness in a single limb is usually of peripheral origin, though there are exceptions, and the student must employ the same analysis of the level of the nervous system affected as in generalized weakness. Occasionally, a single muscle will be affected, as in a muscle tendon tear or an intramuscular infection or abscess. Neuromuscular junction disorders rarely produce focal weakness in only one limb. Disorders of single nerves often cause focal weakness, as in a foot drop from peroneal nerve palsy or a wrist drop from radial nerve palsy. Bell's palsy, a disorder of the VII cranial nerve, causes focal weakness on one side of the face. A VI cranial nerve lesion produces diplopia, secondary to weakness of one lateral rectus muscle. A single nerve root lesion also produces very localized weakness; for example, a lesion of the L5 nerve root will produce focal weakness of the ankle dorsiflexor, in this case often with associated sensory loss of the lateral calf. An S1 radiculopathy is associated with weakness of the plantar flexor of the ankle, such that the patient cannot walk on the toes, and there will be associated numbness in the lateral calf, lateral dorsum of the foot, and loss of the ankle reflex.

Spinal cord lesions are diagnosed based on the motor, sensory, and reflex changes. Most spinal cord lesions affect both sides of the body below the level of the lesion, with the exception of the Brown-Séquard syndrome, secondary to a unilateral cord lesion. In the cervical spinal cord this would produce weakness of the arm and leg on the same side of the body, numbness on the contralateral side, and perhaps ipsilateral motor and sensory signs in the distribution of the nerve root exiting at the level of the lesion. Posterior column sensory loss would be in the arm and leg ipsilateral to the weakness. In the thoracic cord, a Brown-Séquard lesion could theoretically produce weakness restricted to the lower limb on the same side of the body, but there would be contralateral sensory loss below the level of the lesion, and possibly radicular sensory loss in the nerve root at the level of the lesion.

Brain lesions can occasionally cause very focal weakness. A small lesion of the hand area of the motor cortex in the precentral gyrus can occasionally cause focal weakness of the contralateral hand. The weak muscles will not respect the peripheral nerve anatomy of the median, ulnar, and radial nerves, nor the nerve root dermatomal anatomy. Over time, the development of hyperreflexia may make the central origin of the weakness clear.

KEY REFERENCE

Gilman S. Clinical examination of the nervous system. New York: McGraw Hill; 2000.

CLUMSINESS AND ATAXIA

INTRODUCTION

Ataxia refers to uncoordinated movement. Strength itself is adequate, but the movement is performed without dexterity or smoothness, or the action is jerky, with *intention tremor*, an irregular tremor in which the limb misses the designated target and oscillates back and forth. Most ataxic disorders are associated with disease of the cerebellum or its afferent and efferent connections via the brainstem. A separate type of ataxia, *sensory ataxia*, is associated with a loss of joint position sense, without any other evidence of a motor disorder.

CLINICAL PRESENTATION: SYMPTOMS AND SIGNS

As discussed in the neurological examination in Chap. 1, ataxia can involve the eye movements, with nystagmus; speech, with ataxic dysarthria, or *scanning speech*; swallowing; coordinated limb movements; and truncal movement, including balance and gait. The cerebellum generally functions as a modulator of motor control via the motor cortex. Movements may be decomposed into individual steps, when the movement normally is carried out in one, smooth succession of actions, or there may be frank overshooting or undershooting of a target. This intention tremor, also referred to as dysmetria, involves an oscillation at right angles to the direction of movement, usually taking place at the end of the movement. In the neurological examination, this is best seen on the finger-nose-finger and heel-knee-shin tests. Another revealing part of the neurological examination is *rapid alternating movement* testing, as in slapping first the palm and then the back of the hand on the knee; the movements become slow and dysrhythmic, a pattern referred to as *dysdiadochokinesia*. Ataxic speech, or ataxic dysarthria, refers to speech in which the cadence is altered, with either severe slowing of the speech pattern or with irregular bursts of syllables, interrupted by irregular pauses or "breakdowns" in speech. If the subject is asked to say "papapapa," the cadence may be so irregular that it sounds like popcorn popping.

As mentioned in Chap. 1, the midline of the cerebellum generally controls trunk movements, whereas the hemispheres of the cerebellum control fine movements of the limbs on the ipsilateral side. The vermis of the cerebellum also has connections to the vestibular nuclei, and indirectly to the inner ear, resulting in symptoms of dizziness and vertigo in cerebellar syndromes. Some patients with midline cerebellar lesions complain only of dizziness and difficulty with balance, and their limb coordination is entirely normal.

The gait pattern of cerebellar dysfunction reflects abnormal coordination of the trunk and lower extremities. The patient may have difficulty standing with the feet together, though the unsteadiness is not greatly different with the eyes open or closed. Gait tends to be broad-based, sometimes with sudden lurches from side to side. The patient cannot walk heel-to-toe, or tandem.

DIFFERENTIAL DIAGNOSIS

Patients with severe sensory loss, especially involving position sense, may have a *sensory ataxia* in which they have marked difficulty controlling fine movements. This disorder mimics cerebellar ataxia, in that fine movements of the limbs and truncal balance are both affected, but the nature of the disorder is made clear with the finding of severe sensory loss, especially joint position sense. Sensory ataxia is seen most commonly in peripheral nerve disorders (see Chap. 33), such as diabetic neuropathy.

Another differential diagnosis of cerebellar ataxia is ataxia seen in association with brainstem lesions. The brainstem contains the pontine nuclei that project via the middle cerebellar peduncle to the cerebellum, and lesions in the basis pontis cause ataxia by this mechanism. The vestibular nuclei of the medulla are interconnected with the flocculonodular lobe of the cerebellum, and lesions here produce vertigo and imbalance. In the midbrain, the red nuclei are involved with the cerebellar outflow, and lesions here cause coarse intention tremor and incoordination. Finally, vascular lesions of the brainstem may be associated with infarction also in the cerebellum, as the major arteries: the posterior inferior cerebellar artery (PICA), anterior inferior cerebellar artery (AICA), and superior cerebellar artery (SCA), each supply both portions of the brainstem and portions of the cerebellum. Brainstem lesions producing ataxia can usually be diagnosed readily by the presence of focal signs associated with the involvement of cranial nerves and long tracts within the brainstem.

The third differential diagnosis with ataxia is the clumsiness that accompanies corticospinal tract disorders, sometimes called *pseudoataxia*. In general, corticospinal tract disorders are associated with weakness and spasticity, rather than clumsiness. Mild corticospinal deficits, however, may leave gross strength intact but interfere with fine movements, especially the fine movements of the fingers. The key differential point between ataxia and clumsiness from corticospinal tract lesions is in the rhythm of the movement; corticospinal lesions generally make the movement slower, whereas cerebellar lesions make the rhythm irregular.

A related point is the presence of clumsiness out of proportion to weakness in a patient with a corticospinal tract lesion, usually a stroke. One of the lacunar stroke syndromes, termed by Dr. C. Miller Fisher *ataxic hemiparesis*, involves weakness and clumsiness of movement on the same side of the body, usually secondary to a small infarction in the pons. Such patients often do appear to have weakness in the contralateral limbs, but also clumsiness or ataxia out of proportion to the degree of weakness. Since corticospinal tract lesions above the pyramidal decussation produce contralateral weakness, and cerebellar lesions usually produce ipsilateral ataxia, it is difficult to explain the presence of weakness and ataxia on the same side of the body. Critics have argued that patients with weakness are clumsy, and that the whole concept of clumsiness out of proportion to weakness is invalid. Many clinicians, however, continue to find the concept useful in localizing small infarctions in the pons.

A final differential diagnosis concerning cerebellar disorders is the occurrence of gait disorders with lesions in other areas of the nervous system besides the cerebellum. Frontal lesions sometimes produce difficulty walking, often with difficulty initiating gait, as if the feet are "glued to the floor." This phenomenon is sometimes referred to a Brun's ataxia or frontal ataxia. Similar gait ataxia is seen with hydrocephalus. In these conditions, the rest of the cerebellar function is normal, and there may be evident deficits associated with frontal lobe dysfunction such as poor attention, reduced short-term memory, and urinary incontinence. Gait disorders are also associated with disorders of the extrapyramidal system, as in Parkinson's disease, dystonia, and choreoathetosis (see Chaps. 5 and 6).

In terms of disorders of the cerebellum itself, a wide variety of disease states can be involved. Strokes of the cerebellum often present with seemingly nonfocal symptoms such as vertigo or dizziness, headache, and imbalance with walking. This is especially true of cerebellar hemorrhages, which have a predilection for the vermis of the cerebellum. Patients with cerebellar hemorrhage may have a normal neurological examination while lying on a stretcher, but once they try to stand and walk, their truncal ataxia becomes evident. It is thus essential to get such patients up and test stance and gait. Occasionally, patients with cerebellar infarctions have normal neurological examinations, even including stance and gait testing. A general phenomenon in cerebellar disorders is that the cerebellum seems to have considerable reserve, such that lesions can be compensated for, especially in younger patients. Imaging studies are thus necessary for the diagnosis of cerebellar lesions in patients with suspicious symptoms.

Cerebellar disorders can also be divided by their time course into acute, subacute, and chronic disorders. Acute cerebellar syndromes are seen in cerebellar hemorrhages and infarctions, also in traumatic brain injuries. In children, a syndrome of *acute cerebellitis* often follows varicella (chicken pox) infections, or occasionally other viral illnesses.

Subacute cerebellar ataxia has a wider differential diagnosis. Cerebellar tumors and abscesses can develop over days or weeks. Demyelinating diseases such as multiple sclerosis can present with predominantly cerebellar symptoms. Occasionally, these disorders can be associated with an acute onset, but more typically they develop over days and weeks. The demyelinating disease progressive multifocal leukoencephalopathy can present with ataxia of subacute, progressive form. Creutzfeldt-Jakob disease also begins occasionally with cerebellar symptoms, especially in the hereditary form called *Gerstmann-Straussler-Schenker disease*, as does the prion disease *kuru*, originally discovered in New Guinea. Paraneoplastic cerebellar degeneration is a long-described disorder associated with systemic cancers such as lung and ovarian carcinoma. These paraneoplastic disorders, originally referred to as "remote effects of cancer on the nervous system," are now thought to result largely from the production of antibodies that cross-react with cerebellar neurons. Drug intoxications and side effects can also produce ataxia, and alcoholic intoxication can mimic acute cerebellar disease. The antiepileptic drug phenytoin (Dilantin) is a frequent cause of ataxia when the blood level is above therapeutic levels, and a chronic cerebellar degeneration is suspected with chronic phenytoin toxicity. Excessive doses of lithium also cause both acute cerebellar dysfunction and chronic cerebellar degeneration. Hypothyroidism is also associated with ataxia.

Chronic, progressive cerebellar disorders are numerous. Chronic, progressive ataxias are often associated with neurodegenerative diseases affecting the cerebellum, sometimes in combination with other neural systems. Cerebellar degenerations were originally divided according to the presence or absence of signs in other neurological systems, but these patterns are so variable that they have not formed a useful classification scheme. Age of onset was another traditional way of dividing the cerebellar ataxias. This, too, is variable, but the diseases with childhood onset are somewhat distinguishable from other cerebellar degenerations. The most helpful classification is based on heredity; the hereditary ataxias are increasingly being classified based on specific genetic mutations, whereas the sporadic ataxias are still largely of unknown cause.

Cerebellar diseases beginning in childhood include ataxia telangiectasia, which usually begins at age 1–2 years, with deterioration of previously acquired gait, along with slurred speech and incoordination of hand movements. Milder forms of the disease may present later in childhood. Difficulty with voluntary gaze (*optic apraxia*) may be associated. The cutaneous telangiectasias may not be present until after the ataxia has begun.

Friedreich's ataxia (FA), the most common hereditary ataxia, usually begins later in childhood but can also present in adult life. FA usually begins with gait unsteadiness, often with associated scoliosis, and later limb ataxia. The posterior columns are also affected in most cases, with loss of position sense, and some cases have associated optic neuropathy or deafness. Cardiomyopathy and congestive heart failure are also associated. The pathology of FA is a degeneration of the dorsal columns of the spinal cord, along with pyramidal tracts, Clarke's columns, and dorsal root ganglia. The genetic basis of FA is a GAA trinucleotide repeat, leading to abnormal variants of the gene product *frataxin*. There are many other cerebellar ataxias, some hereditary, others sporadic.

A rare, recessively inherited condition is vitamin E deficiency, in which alpha-tocopherol levels are low in the serum, and the ataxia improves with vitamin E supplementation.

The spinocerebellar ataxias (SCAs) are a group of dominantly inherited ataxias, of which the genes are currently being discovered at a rapid pace. In all of these disorders, there is a great variety of ages of onset, clinical deficits, and courses, sometimes related to the nature of the genetic defect. Most patients with SCA1 have a combination of cerebellar ataxia, nystagmus, and pyramidal tract signs. Late in the disease, magnetic resonance imaging (MRI) scans show cerebellar and pontine atrophy, and pathology involves loss of Purkinje cells and neurons in the dentate nuclei, inferior olives, and cranial nerve nuclei, with demyelination of cerebellar white matter pathways. SCA1 is a CAG trinucleotide repeat disorder; the gene product is called *ataxin-1*. SCA2 is a similarly variable disorder, often presenting with ataxia, supranuclear gaze paresis, leg stiffness, and other changes. SCA2 is also a CAG repeat disease, and the gene product is called *ataxin-2*. SCA3, also called Machado-Joseph disease, has a variable presentation with ataxia, sometimes loss of eye movements, facial twitching, dystonia and Parkinsonism, and peripheral neuropathy. It is seen more commonly in Portuguese populations. As the reader may have already guessed, Machado-Joseph disease is a CAG repeat disease, and the gene product is called ataxin-3. Several other SCA diseases have been classified, not all of them representing CAG repeat changes. These disorders are being discovered on a frequent basis, and no medical student would be expected to remember all of them. The interested student is referred to the Online Mendelian Inheritance in Man (OMIM) or Geneclinics Web sites (see references at the end of this chapter) for the latest information on these disorders.

About a third of progressive ataxias occur as sporadic disorders, and genetic testing for all of the known hereditary ataxias is negative. Some represent relatively pure, progressive ataxias, beginning later in life and resembling the known hereditary ataxias. Another large group has associated signs of Parkinsonism or autonomic nervous system degeneration with orthostatic hypotension. This disorder, formerly referred to as *Shy Drager syndrome*, is now increasingly called *multisystem atrophy*. Ataxia may be seen in association with celiac sprue, along with antigliadin antibodies. This syndrome has been thought to underlie some cases of multisystem atrophy, but the association has not been confirmed. Vitamin E deficiency may also be associated with ataxia. Probably the most common progressive cerebellar ataxia is alcoholic cerebellar ataxia, which may be mixed with other effects of alcohol on the nervous system, such as thiamine deficiency-induced peripheral neuropathy.

LABORATORY AND RADIOLOGICAL INVESTIGATION

Aside from the physical examination, the most useful diagnostic test in cerebellar disease is a brain imaging study, either computed tomography (CT) or MRI scanning. CT scanning has the disadvantage of bony artifacts rendering the posterior fossa difficult to image accurately. MRI serves both to confirm the localization of the lesion in the cerebellum and to provide clues as to the etiology of the lesion, such as stroke, tumor, or abscess. In stroke syndromes, magnetic resonance angiography (MRA) or CT angiography may be helpful in identifying the location of a vascular occlusion causing an infarction in the cerebellum. In the case of demyelinating disease or multiple sclerosis, immunoglobulin studies of the cerebrospinal fluid and evoked response tests (see Chap. 29) are helpful. Autoantibodies are helpful in the diagnosis of the paraneoplastic cerebellar disorders. In the cerebellar and spinocerebellar degenerations, the combination of the clinical course and the pattern of atrophy on MRI scanning may be helpful in classification, but ultimately the diagnosis depends on the documentation of a specific genetic defect. The number of diseases diagnosable by genetic testing of the blood is increasing rapidly.

TREATMENT

The treatment of ataxia is usually that of the underlying cause of the disorder, if such treatment is available. Cerebellar tumors and abscesses are often helped by surgery. In the case of multiple sclerosis, high-dose corticosteroid treatment for acute exacerbations and immunomodulating treatments (see Chap. 29) to prevent new attacks are helpful in reducing disability. Treatment of ataxia itself, in the way of "symptomatic" drug therapies, is very limited. Intention tremor may be dampened by use of benzodiazepine drugs, buspirone, or isoniazid, though these treatments are very limited in efficacy. Patients who have other neurological systems involved can be treated symptomatically for some of the associated deficits, such as baclofen or tizanidine for spasticity, levodopa for Parkinsonism, meclizine for vertigo, and antiepileptic drugs for patients who also have epileptic seizures. Rehabilitation techniques, particularly occupational therapy adaptive equipment such as wide handles for utensils, cups with tops, and also physical therapy devices such as walkers, may help the patient adapt to the disorder.

KEY REFERENCES

Charness ME, Simon RP, Greenberg DA. Ethanol and the nervous system. *N Engl J Med* 1989;321:442–454.

Darnell RB, Posner JB. Paraneoplastic syndromes involving the nervous system. *New Engl J Med* 2003;349:1543–1554.

Delatycki MB, Williamson R, Forrest SM. Friedreich ataxia: an overview. *J Med Genet.* 2000;37:1–8.

Geneclinics: Hereditary Ataxia Overview. http://www.geneclinics.org/profiles/ataxias/details.html

Martin JB. Molecular basis of the neurodegenerative disorders. *N Engl J Med* 1999;340:1970–1980.

Online Mendelian Inheritance in Man http://www.ncbi/nlm.nih.gov/Omim/

Spacey SD, Gatti RA, Bebb G. The molecular basis and clinical management of ataxia telangiectasia. *Can J Neurol Sci* 2000;27:184–191.

Tan E, Ashizawa T. Genetic testing in spinocerebellar ataxias: defining a clinical role. *Arch Neurol* 2001;58:191–195.

C H A P T E R 5

INVOLUNTARY
MOVEMENTS

INTRODUCTION

Involuntary movements refer to a diverse group of *movement disorders* having in common the presence of abnormal movement patterns, usually but not always featuring increased movement compared to normal, in the absence of gross weakness or ataxia. The disorders are classified by the type of abnormal movement and by the etiology. Movement disorders can be hyperkinetic, usually involving involuntary movements, or hypokinetic, involving reduced movement. We shall discuss specific diseases such as Parkinson's disease and essential tremor in later chapters. In this chapter, we will consider a series of involuntary movements, along with a description of the movements, the disorders in which they occur, diagnostic procedures, and treatments. These disorders include dystonias, dyskinesias including choreoathetosis, tics, akathisia and the restless legs syndrome (RLS), myoclonus, and tremors.

TICS AND TOURETTE SYNDROME

Tics are defined as brief, involuntary or semivoluntary movements or vocalizations, usually nonstereotyped. Some patients have an uncomfortable feeling or urge, relieved by performance of the tic. The patient can suppress the tics briefly, but a psychic pressure then builds up, leading to more tics later. Tics may be lessened by concentration on a task such as a video game, increased by stress or boredom. The suppressibility of tics makes them different from other movement disorders, in that they are at least in part under voluntary control. Tics may involve jerking of a limb, more prolonged movements of the eyelids or eyes, or more complex tics such as throwing movements, brushing hair movements, or occasionally obscene gestures. Vocalizations can include simple grunting or barking sounds, or socially inappropriate phrases (coprolalia). In order for a patient with tics to be diagnosed as Tourette syndrome, he or she must have multiple motor tics and one or more phonic tics, with either frequent tics or intermittent tics over a period in excess of 1 year. In addition, the tics must be witnessed by a knowledgeable observer, must have started before age 21, and must not be explainable by other medical conditions. Usually the disorder begins in childhood, before age 11. Most patients have less tics after puberty, though some have persistent difficulty. Tics may occasionally occur in older individuals as part of other neurological diseases such as Alzheimer's disease. The neurological examination in a young patient with tics or Tourette syndrome should be normal except for the tics themselves. Many patients have coexisting symptoms of attention deficit hyperactivity disorder (ADHD), and some studies have found that stimulant treatment for ADHD may worsen tics. There is also an overlap between Tourette syndrome and obsessive-compulsive disorder. Tourette patients often have subjective urges not only to produce the tic movements and vocalizations, but also to perform ritualistic behaviors such as checking and rechecking and compulsive counting.

The pathogenesis of tics and Tourette syndrome is not fully understood. Genetic studies support an inherited, organic basis for the disorder, though the precise gene locus of the condition has not been established. Routine brain imaging studies are typically normal, but detailed comparisons of the basal ganglia and functional imaging with functional magnetic resonance imaging (fMRI) and positron emission tomography (PET) scans have shown abnormal patterns of activation in the basal ganglia, and abnormalities of dopamine release and uptake.

Treatment of tics involves both counseling and reassurance and specific pharmacological therapies. Dopamine-blocking drugs such as haloperidol and pimozide are effective but should be prescribed in as low doses as possible to avoid long-term side effects. Atypical antipsychotic drugs also hold promise in this condition. Clonidine may reduce tics to a modest extent. Associated neurobehavioral symptoms of attention deficit disorder and obsessive-compulsive disorder can be treated with stimulants and with selective serotonin reuptake inhibitors (SSRIs), respectively.

DYSKINESIAS, DYSTONIAS, ATHETOSIS, CHOREA, BALLISMUS, HEMIBALLISMUS

The word *dyskinesia* involves any type of involuntary movement in which there is excessive or hyperkinetic movement, but the term is often reserved for drug-induced movement disorders. Dystonias are abnormal movements involving a fixed posture at least for a brief period, though spasmodic dystonias involve excessive movements associated with dystonic postures. A related condition, *athetosis*, refers to slow, writhing movements; this term has been largely abandoned in favor of dystonia. *Chorea* refers to the rapid, irregular, seemingly random movements, without any sustained postures. It typically involves distal muscles such as the hand intrinsics. Some patients have both the proximal, slower, and distal, more rapid involuntary movements, a combination sometimes referred to as *choreoathetosis*. Sudden, proximal movements of a limb are called *ballismus*, and when these types of movements involve the arm and leg on one side, the movement is called *hemiballismus*.

Dystonia is a varied condition, including both slow movements, writhing in type, with sustained abnormal postures, and also fast, jerky movements. The movements are repetitive and stereotyped, unlike the random, non-stereotyped movements of chorea. They are often worsened by anxiety, sometimes leading to the misdiagnosis of these conditions as psychogenic. Some patients discover peculiar movements, such as touching the affected limb or body part, that allow them to eliminate or reduce the dystonic movements; these maneuvers are called *sensory tricks*, and they also sometimes give the impression of a volitional nature of the abnormal movements, which is not truly present. Dystonias are often task-specific, such as the abnormal posture of the wrist and hand only during writing in "writer's cramp," or the abnormal posture of the mouth and lips in a trumpet player with a musician's dystonia. Sometimes dystonic postures follow traumatic injuries or occur in association with pain disorders. It can be difficult to sort out true dystonias from psychogenic disorders in this setting. Worsening of movements under stress, use of sensory tricks, and inconsistency of abnormal movements in the same muscle groups with different tasks all serve to make the examiner suspect a psychogenic origin to the movements, which may be unjustified. If distraction by another task makes a movement stop, that truly suggests a psychogenic cause.

Dystonias are divided into focal, segmental, and generalized forms. Focal dystonias include blepharospasm, or forced eye closure; oromandibular dystonia, in which the lips, mouth, and tongue have writhing movements, including bruxism, or chewing, or trismus, a spasm of the jaw; spasmodic dysphonia, in which the vocal folds are primarily affected; torticollis (cervical dystonia), or turning of the neck; or focal dystonias of the limbs, such as writer's cramp, musician's dystonias, and so forth. Cervical dystonia can involve lateral, anterior, or posterior movement (torticollis, laterocollis, retrocollis, anterocollis). Dystonias of the trunk can result in scoliosis, exaggerated lordosis, and so forth. These dystonias can be primary but are also frequently seen in Parkinson's disease. Focal dystonias often begin in adult life, and in such cases, the dystonia usually remains focal. Childhood-onset dystonia, on the other hand, is more often generalized. Some dystonias are paroxysmal, coming and going. An example is the oculogyric crisis. Dystonias can also be analyzed according to whether they are primary or secondary to another neurological disease, such as Wilson's disease or Parkinson's disease (see Chap. 27).

Generalized dystonias often begin in childhood. Many are genetic disorders such as dystonia musculorum deformans, or DYT1 dystonia. This begins focally in distal muscles, then spreads to proximal muscles and generalizes throughout the body, leaving the affected children in twisted, uncomfortable postures. This type of dystonia is most commonly encountered in Jews of Ashkenazic origin. The most common genetic defect is a 3-base pair deletion in chromosome 9. Children with DYT1 dystonia have recently been treated successfully with deep brain stimulation of the globus pallidus. Another generalized dystonia is L-dopa-responsive dystonia, which also occurs in families. Generalized dystonias also occur in association with Wilson's and Parkinson's diseases, Huntington's disease, neurodegeneration with brain iron accumulation (formerly called Hallervorden-Spatz disease), some metabolic diseases in childhood such as lipidoses (metachromatic leukodystrophy, ceroid lipofuscinosis, Niemann-Pick disease, and so forth) and in diseases like multiple sclerosis.

Treatment of the focal dystonias is only modestly successful with drugs such as anticholinergic agents (trihexyphenidyl, or Artane), beginning with 1–2 mg at bedtime and gradually increasing to doses as high as 30–60 mg, especially in children. Benzodiazepines such as clonazepam, dopaminergic drugs such as levodopa, and dopamine-blocking drugs have all been tried. Dopamine-blocking drugs have a high tendency to cause tardive dyskinesia and are hence not favored. Levodopa or Sinemet is most effective in the DOPA-responsive dystonic syndrome, seen primarily in children. Finally, the most effective and commonly used therapy for focal dystonias is botulinum toxin (BTX). This toxin is injected directly into muscles that are overacting, thereby leading to weakening of the muscles. This weakness reaches a peak at about 7–10 days after the injection, lasting typically for about 3 months. Surgery for focal dystonia has become less frequently attempted in the BTX era, but occasional local procedures such as rhizotomies, or central procedures such as "deep brain" basal ganglia stimulation, have been used in refractory cases.

Chorea

Chorea involves rapid movements, often beginning in distal muscles of the hands, but later flitting from one limb or one part of the body to another. The movements are nonstereotyped and often seemingly random in occurrence and location. They may interfere with normal movement if severe. Related to the choreiform movements is an impersistence of motor activity, such that a patient with chorea may not be able to maintain a fixed posture, such as keeping the tongue protruded for more than a few seconds.

Chorea occurs in many different disorders. It can be seen in infancy in association with cerebral palsy or kernicterus, and also in late life as *senile chorea*. Chorea gave the original name to Huntington's disease, a condition in which chorea is often severe and disabling (see Chap. 27). Other causes include Wilson's disease, Machado-Joseph disease, neurodegeneration with brain iron accumulation, other neurodegenerative disorders, in chorea gravidarum (chorea of pregnancy), postinfectious causes (e.g., Sydenham's chorea), in systemic lupus erythematosus, multiple sclerosis, and stroke. For the diagnosis of Huntington's disease, a family history is very helpful, and the diagnosis can now be confirmed by a genetic blood test.

Treatment of chorea involves dopamine-blocking drugs such as haloperidol, also dopamine-depleting drugs such as tetrabenazine.

Ballism

Ballism refers to involuntary movements of the proximal limb muscles, such that the limb appears to be flung into the air. The movements are similar to those of chorea, except for the proximal location. Hemiballism, or hemiballismus, denotes the involvement of the arm and leg on one side of the body. The movements of hemiballismus are dramatic, exhausting to the patient, and a major medical treatment problem. The most common cause is a stroke, either infarction or hemorrhage, classically located in the subthalamic nucleus. Rarely, hemiballismus is caused by a brain tumor, encephalitis, multiple sclerosis lesion, or induced by a drug, e.g., phenytoin given after a stroke.

The treatment of ballism, or ballistic movements, involves dopamine-blocking agents such as haloperidol.

RESTLESS LEGS SYNDROME

RLS is a disorder in which unpleasant sensations in the legs result in an urge to move them for relief. The patient may be able to suppress or resist the desire to move only briefly, after which the urge to move becomes irresistible. The symptoms are usually worst at night, when the patient is trying to go to sleep. Some patients describe pain or discomfort, which is relieved only by moving the legs or standing up and walking around. RLS is similar to the drug-induced movement called akathisia, also an irresistible impulse to move, but a reaction to dopamine antagonist medications. RLS is a common disorder. The disorder is frequently familial, but it may be associated with peripheral neuropathy or iron deficiency. RLS responds to dopaminergic treatments such as pramipexole (Mirapex) or ropinirole (Requip), also to benzodiazepines such as clonazepam (Klonopin).

DRUG-INDUCED MOVEMENTS

Many different patterns of abnormal or involuntary movements can be caused by drug effects. The most common variety is tardive dyskinesias. These movements are most commonly seen in association with dopamine-blocking drugs such as neuroleptics, especially the older phenothiazines and butyrophenones such as chlorpromazine (Thorazine) and haloperidol (Haldol). Dopamine-blocking agents used for other purposes, such as prochlorperazine (Compazine) for nausea or metoclopramide (Reglan) for improving gastrointestinal motility are sometimes unsuspected as causes of tardive dyskinesia.

The movements of tardive dyskinesia can be variable, including rapid, stereotyped movements such as movements of the lips and tongue, and also dystonias and tremors. The movements are usually rapid, resembling chorea but more stereotyped and repetitive. Patients do not have the motor impersistence seen in chorea; even if the tongue is flitting in and out like a frog's tongue, patients can usually keep it voluntarily protruded if requested. The movements begin insidiously, more commonly in older than younger patients, and more commonly in women than men. If the offending drug is discontinued early in the course, the movements may cease, but after a period of dyskinesias, the movements may become permanent. The term *tardive* means that the movements do not begin immediately after a dopamine-blocking drug is started, but only after days, weeks, or months of therapy. Newer, "atypical" antipsychotic agents such as clozapine (Clozaril), risperidone (Risperdal), olanzapine (Zyprexa), quetiapine (Seroquel), ziprasidone (Geodon), and aripiprazole (Abilify) are generally less likely to cause tardive dyskinesia, akathisia, acute dystonic reactions, and parkinsonism (*extrapyramidal side effects*), as compared to the older phenothiazines and butyrophenones.

The theory of tardive dyskinesia is that prolonged blockade of the dopamine receptors results in postsynaptic hypersensitivity, such that drugs that ordinarily reduce movement patterns become associated with overactivity of movements. If the causative drug is stopped, the movements may initially flair and then gradually lessen and disappear. Dopamine-depleting agents, such as reserpine and tetrabenazine, have some beneficial effect. BTX can help the dystonic movements associated with tardive dyskinesia.

Dyskinesias can also occur as a result of dopaminergic agents such as levodopa-carbidopa (Sinemet) or direct dopamine agonists. In this case, reducing the dose of the drug may result in disappearance of the dyskinesias.

Other movements developing as a result of drug treatments include acute dystonic reactions, akathisia, and parkinsonism. Acute dystonic reactions are very incapacitating and uncomfortable, involving peculiar, dystonic movements of the tongue, turning of the head, and movement of the jaw. They can be stopped easily by injection of a variety of medications, including anticholinergic medications (trihexyphenidyl, Artane, or benztropine, Cogentin), dimenhydrinate (Benadryl), or benzodiazepines such as diazepam (Valium), lorazepam (Ativan), or clonazepam (Klonopin).

Akathisia is an inward need to move, resembling idiopathic RLS (see above). Akathisia often develops during neuroleptic therapy, and inexperienced examiners may mistakenly conclude that the patient is anxious and needs more neuroleptic medication. The movements can be helped by removing the offending agent and treating with anticholinergic medications.

Drug-induced parkinsonism includes many of the cardinal features discussed in Chap. 27 on Parkinson's disease. Early signs include bradykinesia or slowed movements, cogwheel rigidity of the limbs, small-stepped gait, reduced facial expression, stooped posture, and finally, resting tremor (see below). This movement pattern, too, can be induced by dopamine-blocking neuroleptic drugs or nonneuroleptic dopamine-blocking drugs such as prochlorperazine or metoclopramide. Stopping the offending drug early in the course will reverse the symptoms, but these movements, too, can become permanent with long use of the drugs.

Closely related to drug-induced parkinsonism, but more severe, is the condition termed *neuroleptic malignant syndrome*. In this syndrome, patients on neuroleptic medications develop symptoms of severe rigidity and bradykinesia, as well as tremor, and they often become febrile, sometimes to very high body temperatures. Patients are often encephalopathic or obtunded. The other principal piece of evidence needed to make the diagnosis is the creatine kinase (CK) enzyme in the blood, which is typically severely elevated. Leukocytosis and elevated liver function tests are also commonly encountered. Prompt diagnosis is essential, since the disorder has as high as 20% mortality in some series. Neuroleptic malignant syndrome can develop either early or late in the neuroleptic drug therapy, and it is not clearly related to dose. Treatment includes supportive care, liquids, antipyretics and cooling blankets, and use of dopaminergic drugs such as levodopa-carbidopa, bromocriptine (Parlodel), or other direct-acting dopaminergic agents. Dantrolene, a direct muscle relaxant used in the related condition, malignant hyperthermia, may also be of some benefit, in doses of 2–3 mg/kg.

While the preceding four movement disorders—acute dystonic reactions, akathisia, tardive dyskinesia, and parkinsonism—are the most common drug-induced abnormal movements, many other examples can be found. Lithium carbonate, commonly used for bipolar affective disorder, also causes tremor of both resting and action type, ataxia, and rigidity, and at times these signs can closely mimic Parkinson's disease. Valproic acid (Depakote), used for epilepsy and migraine, also produces an action tremor as a side effect. Any drug with adrenergic effects such as stimulant drugs, beta-agonists used for asthma, and even tricyclic antidepressants can induce tremor.

TREMOR

Tremor refers to an oscillatory movement of a body part, usually with a regular periodicity. Tremor is further described according to the position or activity in which it occurs, as well as the amplitude and frequency of the movements.

There are many different types of tremor, but in general tremors fall into three principal categories: *resting, postural,* and *action* or *intention.* All tremors typically worsen when the patient is angry, anxious, or under stress.

Resting tremor is by definition a tremor occurring when the limb or body part is at repose. It is usually a large amplitude, slow frequency (2–5/second) tremor. Resting tremor is most commonly present at the fingers and hand (*pill-rolling tremor*), but occasionally in the ankle and foot. Resting tremor tends to diminish or go away completely during volitional movement. This type of tremor is most commonly seen in Parkinson's disease, and it may be the first symptom of the disease, occurring only intermittently. Spread from the hand to the foot on the same side is even more specific for Parkinson's disease. Tremor in the head and neck (titubation tremor) appears to be at rest, but the neck muscles are often tensed. This location of tremor is more commonly seen in essential tremor or tremors associated with cervical dystonia (see below). Resting tremor can be seen in secondary parkinsonism (see Chap. 27), Wilson's disease, or in association with cerebellar outflow tremor (see below). The treatment of resting tremor is generally that of Parkinson's disease (dopaminergic agents, see Chap. 27), but consideration should also be given to secondary (drug-induced) parkinsonism and Wilson's disease.

The second type of tremor, postural tremor, usually begins in the hands and fingers, both with the arms outstretched (hence the name, postural tremor) and during skilled actions. In the neurological examination, this tremor is seen best during drift testing and finger-nose-finger coordination testing. Compared to resting tremor, the amplitude is small ("fine"), and the frequency high (5–10/second). When severe, the tremor can also affect the voice and the head and neck. Strictly speaking, we all have a slight tremor of the outstretched hands, termed *physiologic tremor.* Many other factors may worsen physiological tremor, including hypoglycemia, hyperthyroidism, adrenergic conditions such as pheochromocytoma or extreme anxiety or anger, drugs such as amphetamines, beta-agonists, lithium, valproic acid, theophylline and caffeine, heavy metal toxicity, and alcohol withdrawal. Essential tremor is the occurrence of an exaggerated action tremor, without these aggravating factors. Essential tremor is usually a genetic disorder of autosomal dominant inheritance. Occasionally, a head and neck tremor resembling essential tremor may occur in association with cervical dystonia or *torticollis*; this tremor can be diagnosed by the co-occurrence of dystonic posturing of the neck, or of neck pain, that is rarely present with essential tremor. Exaggerated physiologic tremors are generally treated by removal of the offending drug or condition, if possible, and by a variety of other drug therapies. Alcohol often diminishes essential tremor. The pharmacological treatment of essential tremor will be discussed in Chap. 28.

The third principal type of tremor, intention or action tremor, occurs during a skilled act such as finger-nose-finger testing, as in cerebellar dysmetria.

The movement does oscillate, at right angles to the plane of the movement, most typically at the end of the movement, as the finger approaches the target. More coarse, proximal intention tremors, often so marked as to be called *wing-beating* tremor, are called *cerebellar outflow tremor* or *rubral tremor*, because the causative lesions often involve the deep cerebellar nuclei or the vicinity of the red nucleus in the midbrain. Rubral tremor is also referred to under the name *Holmes tremor*; this coarse tremor is present both at rest and with sustained posture. These tremors are often so severe that they are present at rest, but they increase with volitional movement and often make finely coordinated movements impossible. These are very disabling conditions. Such tremors are seen in multiple sclerosis, in Wilson's disease, and occasionally in heavy metal toxicity. The treatment of both intention tremor and cerebellar outflow tremor is problematic, not responding well to pharmacologic therapy. The tremor may respond to deep brain stimulation, usually in the thalamus.

A few other, less common types of tremors deserve mention. There are a few "task-specific" tremors, of which the most common is writing tremor, resembling postural or essential tremor except that it is present only during writing. It may or may not be associated with writer's cramp, a dystonia. The primary writing tremor may respond to drugs used to treat essential tremor, but those writing tremors related to writer's cramp may not respond. Another task-specific tremor is orthostatic tremor, a tremor of the trunk and legs seen only during walking. This tremor may subside if the patient holds onto an object, or if he or she can walk freely; the tremor is most noticeable when the patient first gets up, or when the patient is about to encounter an obstacle or the end of the course of walking.

MYOCLONUS

Myoclonus refers to lightning-like, twitching movements. Myoclonus is classified first by its distribution in the body; it can be generalized, multifocal, or focal (segmental). Myoclonus can be spontaneous or can be provoked by stimuli such as loud noises, or during voluntary movements (*action myoclonus*). Myoclonus can be an epileptic phenomenon, originating in the cerebral cortex, but it can also arise from the brainstem or spinal cord. Research studies involving "back averaging" of the electroencephalogram (EEG) may be necessary to prove whether or not a myoclonic discharge originates from spikes in the cerebral cortex. Myoclonus can occur as a normal phenomenon, as a part of an epileptic seizure disorder, or as an aspect of a neurological disorder of degenerative or vascular type.

Examples of normal (*physiologic*) myoclonus would include hiccups, single jerks of the head and neck on falling asleep (*hypnagogic jactitation*), and occasional, single twitches in the limbs. Focal or segmental myoclonus occurs in the palate (referred to preferentially as *palatal tremor* and also as *palatal myoclonus*), in association with brainstem strokes and neurodegenerative disorders. This is a rhythmic twitching of the soft palate, sometimes accompanied by twitching of the neck visible from the external surface. Action myoclonus is sometimes seen in association with metabolic disturbances such as the hyperosmolar nonketotic state seen in severe hyperglycemia. Another cause of action or intention myoclonus is a hypoxic injury to the brain, as seen in survivors of cardiac arrest. Some such patients have a combination of ataxia and intention myoclonus (the Lance-Adams syndrome). Generalized myoclonus may occur in some epileptic disturbances, degenerative diseases such as dentatorubrothalamic atrophy (Ramsey Hunt syndrome), Lafora's body disease, dementing illnesses, infections such as encephalitis, and metabolic disturbances such as uremia, hypoxia, and drug-induced or toxic encephalopathies. In Creutzfeldt-Jakob disease, patients often have an exaggerated startle response to noises that includes myoclonic jerks. This list is a much simplified account of the many conditions that can be associated with myoclonus.

The treatment of myoclonus is somewhat dependent on the specific cause of the disorder. Epileptic myoclonus will often respond to antiepileptic drugs such as valproic acid (Depakote) or clonazepam (Klonopin). In the postanoxic intention myoclonus (Lance-Adams) syndrome, large doses of the serotonin precursor 5-hydroxytryptophan may also be helpful, though it is difficult to obtain, and many cases are treated with the antiepileptic agents.

Asterixis

Asterixis is considered a "negative myoclonus," meaning that whereas myoclonus is associated with an active twitch of a muscle on an electromyogram, asterixis is associated with a period of silence in the muscle. If the patient holds the hands outstretched with the palms up and the wrists dorsiflexed (the "stop traffic" position), there will be a sudden "flap" downward of the hands, followed by renewed extension, from time to time. The most common cause of asterixis is hepatic failure (*liver flap*), though it can also be seen in renal insufficiency.

KEY REFERENCES

Bain PG, Findley LJ, Britton TC, et al. Primary writing tremor. *Brain* 1995;118:1461–1472.

Barnes TRE, McPhillips MA. Novel antipsychotics, extrapyramidal side effects and tardive dyskinesia. *Int Clin Psychopharm* 1998;13(Suppl 3):S49–S57.

Burke RE, Fahn S, Jankovic J, et al. Tardive dystonia: late-onset and persistent dystonia caused by antipsychotic drugs. *Neurology* 1982;32:1335–1346.

Caviness JN. Myoclonus. *Mayo Clin Proc* 1996;71:679–688.

Earley CJ. Restless legs syndrome. *N Engl J Med* 2003;348:21032109.

Guze BH, Baxter LR. Neuroleptic malignant syndrome. *N Engl J Med* 1985;313: 163–166.

Hallett M. Classification and treatment of tremor. *JAMA* 1991;266:1115–1117.

Hyde TM, Weinberger DR. Tourette's syndrome. A model neuropsychiatric disorder. *JAMA* 1995;273;498–501.

Jancovic J. Tourette's syndrome. *N Engl J Med* 2001;345:1184–1192.

Jancovic J, Brin MF. Therapeutic uses of botulinum toxin. *N Engl J Med* 1991; 324:1186–1194.

Louis ED. Essential tremor. *N Engl J Med* 2001;345:887–891.

Saltz BL, Woerner MG, Kane JM, et al. Prospective study of tardive dyskinesia incidence in the elderly. *JAMA* 1991;266:2402–2406.

Silber MH, Ehrenberg BL, Allen RP, et al. An algorithm for the management of restless legs syndrome. *Mayo Clin Proc* 2004;79:916–922.

Tarsy D, Simon DK. Dystonia. *N Engl J Med* 2006;355:818–829.

Thompson PD, Rothwell JC, Day BL, et al. The physiology of orthostatic tremor. *Arch Neurol* 1986;43:584–587.

CHAPTER 6

GAIT DISORDERS

INTRODUCTION

Examination of gait is an important aspect of the neurological examination. An expert observer can learn a great deal about the patient's deficit from just watching the patient walk, and neurologists are fond of diagnosing people they see walking on the street. The techniques of gait examination were discussed in Chap. 1. This chapter will focus on specific disorders that can be diagnosed on the basis of abnormal walking patterns.

CLINICAL PRESENTATION: SYMPTOMS AND SIGNS

Patients may walk abnormally for a host of reasons. We shall begin with more caudal portions of the nervous system, and then progress centrally.

The most caudal part of the nervous system is the muscle. Myopathies commonly affect gait. Most myopathies involve proximal muscles, and hence the gait disorders to be expected in myopathy usually involve a "waddling gait," associated with the patient having to hike up a hip with each step. Other signs of a myopathic gait would include difficulty rising from a low chair, difficulty squatting down and then standing up, and weakness of the hip flexors and extensors on the muscle strength examination. Pertinent negatives would include the absence of sensory loss and the absence of major changes in reflexes, diminished only in muscle groups that are severely weak.

Next come the disorders of the neuromuscular junction. Patients with myasthenia gravis (see Chap. 35) often walk well when rested, but they develop weakness when fatigued. Repetitive squatting and standing (deep knee bends) can induce weakness through progressive fatigue of the proximal muscles. Similar findings are seen in botulism, though the involvement of the autonomic nervous system (such as dilatation of the pupils) helps in diagnosis. Patients with the Lambert-Eaton syndrome, a paraneoplastic neuromuscular junction disorder, may also develop proximal weakness, and occasionally they improve rather than fatigue with exercise, a phenomenon that can be documented by electromyogram (EMG) with repetitive stimulation. In all of these neuromuscular junction disorders, sparing of sensation and of reflexes are helpful signs.

The next level of the neuraxis is the peripheral nerves. Peripheral neuropathies typically affect the distal parts of the body, supplied by the longest nerves, preferentially. If the neuropathy is purely sensory, the gait disorder might represent a *sensory ataxia*, in which the patient has a strongly positive Romberg test and walks cautiously, looking down and watching the feet. Patients may adopt a broad-based gait suggestive of cerebellar ataxia (see below). In a sensorimotor neuropathy, the patient may also have distal weakness, most commonly taking the form of bilateral foot-drop. The gait then takes on a *high-steppage pattern*, in which the patient must lift each foot higher than normal to prevent tripping on the plantar-flexed foot and toes. A mononeuropathy of the peroneal nerve might cause this pattern just on one side.

With spinal cord lesions, the gait pattern depends on the level of the myelopathy. Lumbosacral lesions cause varying degrees of paraparesis, with both motor and sensory involvement, but with flaccid tone and hyporeflexia. The patient may be unable to walk at all, or may have partial weakness. Patients with poliomyelitis usually have asymmetric involvement, with weakness in specific muscle groups, making for a variable pattern of lower motor neuron gait difficulties. Patients with thoracic and cervical spinal cord lesions will have either paraparesis or quadriparesis, depending on the level of the lesion. After the initial period of flaccidity associated with *spinal shock*, increased tone will develop, and the gait pattern takes on *spastic* or stiff-legged features. In a unilateral or Brown-Séquard cord syndrome, only one leg is affected, but in a bilateral cord lesion a bilateral spastic gait pattern develops. The patient holds the legs stiff, shifting weight from one to the other leg very slowly. The diagnosis of a spastic gait is aided by the presence of increased reflexes, upgoing plantars, spastic tone, and a sensory level corresponding to the level of the spinal cord lesion.

Cerebellar lesions often have profound effects on gait. As mentioned in Chap. 4, cerebellar hemispheral lesions affect limb coordination more than truck coordination, whereas cerebellar vermis lesions affect stance and gait more than limb movements. A bilateral cerebellar vermis lesion may produce a broad-based gait, in which the patient staggers unpredictably from side to side. This may occur acutely, as in a cerebellar hemorrhage, or chronically in cerebellar degenerations such as that associated with alcohol abuse. Some patients have a tendency to retropulsion, or falling backward, which leads to falls, even when the patient is using a walker. Limb ataxia and dysdiadochokinesia aid in the diagnosis of cerebellar disorders, as well as the sparing of strength, sensation, and reflexes.

Unilateral lesions of the brainstem or cerebral hemisphere are often associated with a hemiparesis, and the gait pattern associated with such lesions takes the form of a *hemiparetic gait*. The affected leg is stiff and spastic, and the patient often has to swing it out, away from the body, a phenomenon termed *circumduction*. In addition, the arm is often flexed at the elbow and held against the body in a spastic posture. This gait pattern is very familiar in survivors of stroke. Involvement of sensory function makes the gait pattern less steady, as the patient cannot feel where the affected leg is and must look before placing the foot with each step. Training a hemiparetic patient to walk is a major goal of rehabilitation therapies.

Bilateral gait abnormalities associated with brain diseases take several patterns. Bilateral cerebral lesions may produce a quadriparesis, with a bilateral spastic gait resembling the spastic gait associated with spinal cord lesions.

Parkinson's disease affects gait in characteristic ways, as will be discussed in Chap. 27. Patients lose postural reflexes, losing their balance if they are pulled backward. They walk with a characteristic flexed posture of the trunk, small steps, reduced associated movements such as arm swing, and sometimes a pattern of more and more rapid steps, until the patient begins to fall, a phenomenon called *festination* . Of course, the severity of the gait disorder varies from patient to patient, and in early stages of Parkinson's disease the gait may be virtually normal. Increased tendency to take small steps and lose balance while turning is characteristic. Resting tremor also comes out during gait, since the arm and hand are "at rest" during walking.

In hyperkinetic movement disorders such as dystonia or Huntington's disease, the gait may be affected by sudden, involuntary movements which nearly throw the patient off balance. Diagnosis of these conditions rests on the documentation of involuntary movements.

A final gait disorder is the phenomenon termed *gait apraxia*. This disorder is most closely associated with hydrocephalus, such as the syndrome of normal pressure hydrocephalus. The patient appears to have forgotten how to walk. He or she may stand as if the feet are glued to the floor, unable to initiate the first step. Once the patient starts walking, the gait pattern may improve. Some examiners find it useful to have patients demonstrate the movements of walking while lying down or holding the legs up in the air to demonstrate bicycling movements. Patients with gait apraxia may also have difficulty with these maneuvers. In addition, patients with normal pressure hydrocephalus typically manifest slowed cognitive function, sometimes with dementia, and urinary incontinence. Many have reduced speech and motor output, along with frontal lobe release signs. Apraxic gait, as described above, can also occur in patients with multifocal vascular lesions of the white matter of the brain.

It should be apparent from this brief, somewhat simplified discussion that observation of gait is a rich source of information about the status of a patient's nervous system. Careful observation and description of gait early in the neurological evaluation will often help to focus diagnostic thinking.

There is no substitute, however, for a detailed neurological examination in specifying what neurological deficits are actually contributing to the gait problem.

GAIT DISORDERS IN THE ELDERLY

Gait disorders in the elderly often represent mixtures of the deficits described above, along with non-neurological contributions such as the effects of degenerative arthritis of the spine and peripheral joints, reduced visual acuity, and perhaps fear of falling. Pain in the limbs or back can result in an *antalgic* gait pattern, in which the patient seems to limp or reduce weight bearing on the affected leg. Postural hypotension is a common cause of gait instability, dizziness, or falling in the elderly. Other neurological disorders contributing to gait difficulty in elderly patients include strokes, Parkinson's disease or drug-induced Parkinsonism, cervical spondylosis with myelopathy, reduced joint position sensation related to peripheral neuropathy, reduced vision, and reduced vestibular function. Sedative medications such as benzodiazepines also appear to contribute to falls in the elderly. Even depression may cause a slowing of the gait pattern. Senile gait disorders often comprise more than one element (*multifactorial gait disorder*), in which the diagnostic evaluation must consider a number of separate etiologies.

TREATMENT

Treatment of gait disorders depends on the cause of the disorder. Examples of specific treatments for causes of gait difficulty would include vitamin B_{12} replacement for B_{12} deficiency (subacute combined systems degeneration), ventriculoperitoneal shunting for normal pressure hydrocephalus, and levodopa therapy for Parkinson's disease. For those patients who do not have a specific neurological disorder, especially elderly patients, simple measures such as glasses to improve vision and use of assistive devices such as walkers, canes, and corrective shoes to ensure good posture may be helpful in preventing falls. Physical therapy and balance assessments may also be helpful.

KEY REFERENCES

Sudarsky L. Geriatrics: gait disorders in the elderly. *New Engl J Med* 1990;322: 1441–1445.

Tinetti ME, Speechley M. Prevention of falls among the elderly. *New Engl J Med* 1989;320:1055–1059.

BLADDER, BOWEL, AND SEXUAL DYSFUNCTION

INTRODUCTION

Bowel, bladder, and sexual dysfunction are aspects of the history and physical examination that neither medical students nor patients are eager to discuss, because of the embarrassing or private nature of these functions. In terms of what they mean to the normal health and functioning of a patient, however, these functions are critically important, and they are also crucial to the diagnosis of disorders at varying levels of the nervous system, both central and peripheral. When questions about bladder, bowel, and sexual functions are answered in a way suggesting abnormal function, detailed examinations should follow. As the television commercial for Viagra states, what is needed to diagnose erectile dysfunction, and also most bowel and bladder problems, is not a complicated laboratory test, just a conversation.

BLADDER DYSFUNCTION

The ability to urinate, in normal volumes, at normal intervals, is one of the most important of bodily functions. The bladder, a storage repository for urine, is filled via the two ureters from the kidney on each side. Emptying of the bladder, on the initiative of the patient, requires a complex neurological system to function properly. A brief review of the neuroanatomy of bladder function is necessary before we discuss the way this system goes awry in neurological disorders (see Fig. 7-1).

First, sensory inputs from the bladder, which detect the degree of bladder filling, exit the bladder via the pelvic nerves and sacral roots, especially S2 and S3. These sensory inputs ascend through the spinal cord and then synapse in the *pontine micturation center*. Secondary sensory fibers travel to the thalamus, and ultimately to the cerebral cortex. When the sensory input indicates a full bladder, the pontine micturition center initiates the reflex of

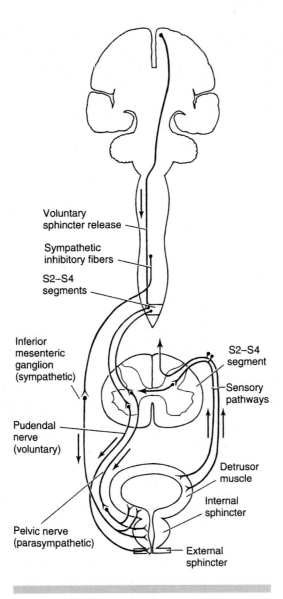

Figure 7-1 **Neurological control of the urinary bladder.** (*Source*: From Waxman SG, Clinical Neuroanatomy, Lange, Figure 20–9, p. 259)

voiding. The motor control of the bladder begins in the paramedian frontal cortex, which projects down to the pontine micturition center. Secondary efferent motor fibers descend through the spinal cord. The urinary bladder is a smooth muscle structure, with a muscle called the detrusor at the bladder neck, to force emptying of the bladder into the urethra. The detrusor is innervated by parasympathetic fibers, originating from the intermediolateral cell columns of the S2-S4 spinal segments in the conus medullaris, projecting to the *pelvic ganglia* in the bladder wall, near the ureteral entry zones. Postganglionic neurons are thought to be both adrenergic and cholinergic. A separate, sympathetic innervation of the bladder, originating from lower thoracic and upper lumbar segments, involves the internal bladder sphincter or *bladder neck* , also comprised of smooth muscle. The bladder neck and detrusor act oppositely, the internal sphincter contracting to preserve continence when the detrusor is relaxed, then relaxing to permit urine flow when the detrusor contracts. The external sphincter, a striated muscle, is innervated by the pudendal nerve and is under voluntary, pyramidal tract control. The relaxation of the internal and external sphincters must be timed with the contraction of the smooth muscle detrusor for proper voiding to take place.

Bladder dysfunction may not always be neurological. The most common cause of incontinence in multiparous, middle-aged and elderly women is stress incontinence, in which the pelvic floor is weakened, and any cause of increased intra-abdominal pressure such as straining, laughing, or sneezing will result in leakage of urine. Other structural disorders of the bladder or urethra can likewise affect urinary continence.

Neurogenic bladder dysfunction, like other neurological functions, can be divided into syndromes, based on the level of the lesion within the neuraxis. A pure sensory neuropathy, first, could prevent sensation of bladder filling until the bladder is full enough to overflow, leading to small, frequent voids and incontinence. A peripheral neuropathy of the more common, mixed sensorimotor neuropathy type, as in diabetic neuropathy, interferes with both the sensation of bladder filling and with the active emptying of the bladder. Again, the bladder will overdilate, resulting in frequent, small voids and incontinence. This type of neurogenic bladder is called a *flaccid bladder*.

Syndromes of bladder dysfunction from nerve root, spinal cord, and brainstem or hemispheric brain lesions can be quite complicated. Involvement at the level of the sacral nerve roots of the cauda equina can paralyze the bladder even more severely than a peripheral neuropathy. With lesions higher in the spinal cord, the bladder reflexes become overactive or spastic, as do the limb reflexes. The bladder is small but empties every time it begins to fill, a *spastic bladder*. Since the bladder empties often, spastic bladder, like flaccid bladder, is associated with frequent, small voids and incontinence. It can thus be difficult to distinguish a flaccid bladder from a spastic bladder, unless the examiner measures a post-void residual urine volume by catheterizing the patient immediately after a void. Ultrasound devices can be used to *scan* the bladder noninvasively after voiding. More elaborate testing of bladder function can be achieved through a test called a cystometrogram, in which the volume, pressure, and contractions of the bladder can be measured during infusion of fluid into the bladder.

A few examples of clinical neurological disorders and their effects on the urinary bladder may be useful in gaining an understanding of neurogenic bladder dysfunction. In a stroke, the bladder may initially seem flaccid, just as the limb muscles do in the paralyzed limb after a stroke. Many stroke patients have to be catheterized because of incontinence. This phenomenon tends to occur in large strokes, and bladder incontinence is a marker of poor recovery after stroke. Over time, however, the bladder may become spastic. In spinal cord injury at cervical or thoracic level, the bladder involvement may likewise evolve from a flaccid to spastic state, as the *spinal shock* resolves. In multiple sclerosis (MS), involvement of lower levels of the spinal cord may result in a flaccid bladder. Others with MS have spastic bladder, and still others have dyssynergia between the detrusor and the voluntary muscle of the external sphincter. The bladder neck may contract, but the sphincter may be closed, leading to uncomfortable bladder spasms and incontinence.

Treatment of bladder incontinence is important to neurologists. The first principle of management of bladder dysfunction in neurological patients is to make sure that the problem is truly neurogenic, and not caused by a drug effect on bladder function (such as an anticholinergic drug), by a urinary tract infection, or by an obstruction such as benign prostatic hypertrophy. In flaccid bladder, intermittent catheterization appears to be the best treatment. Drug therapy for flaccid bladder, with agents such as urecholine, is not effective. Newer surgical techniques such as bladder stimulators have shown promise. The bladder can also be rerouted from the urethra to a surgically created stoma in the abdominal wall, through which a catheter can be introduced. For patients who require catheterization to void, use of intermittent catheterization is generally safer in terms of infection risk than an indwelling catheter, though both carry a risk of infection over time.

For spastic bladder, anticholinergic drugs such as oxybutynin (Ditropan), tolterodine (Detrol), or trospium (Sanctura) can be used to inhibit bladder contractions. Trospium is a large molecule, a quarternary amine, which does not cross the blood-brain barrier and hence does not cause as much central anticholinergic effect as the other agents. Oxybutynin and tolterodine are available as long-acting preparations.

BOWEL DYSFUNCTION

Bowel problems are often not a central focus of neurologists, who generally prefer to treat the other end of the body. Neurological conditions, however, frequently affect bowel function. For the purpose of this discussion, bowel dysfunction will be divided into constipation and bowel incontinence.

Constipation is traditionally defined by the passage of fewer than three bowel movements per week. Associated symptoms include straining to produce a stool, difficulty or pain with defecation, and hard stools. As in urinary dysfunction, constipation is often the result of non-neurological causes such as disorders of the rectum and anus. Medications, especially opiate analgesics, anticholinergic agents, tricyclic antidepressants, and calcium channel blockers can also provoke constipation. Lesions in the brain or spinal cord commonly result in constipation. This is particularly a problem in hospitalized patients after stroke and other neurological illnesses, at least partly because exercise is important to healthy bowel function. Parkinson's disease is also frequently associated with constipation, possibly because of loss of autonomic function in the large intestine. Multiple sclerosis, spinal cord injury, and even peripheral neuropathies, especially those with autonomic dysfunction, are often associated with constipation.

The treatment of constipation does not differ greatly between patients with neurological causes of constipation and those without such etiologies. We recommend exercise and addition of fiber to the diet, as well as the use of stool softeners and laxatives. Patients with impactions in the rectum should have manual disimpaction before the heavy use of laxatives.

Fecal incontinence is a less common problem than constipation. Minor fecal incontinence may result from diarrhea or from anorectal disorders such as hemorrhoids or rectal prolapse. One cause of fecal incontinence that must be excluded is incontinence of liquid stool passing around an impaction. Treatment of the impaction must precede any other management. More severe incontinence may result from autonomic neuropathies, such as diabetes, spinal root disorders such as cauda equina syndromes, or spinal cord disorders such as spinal cord injuries, tumors, or multiple sclerosis. Treatment involves use of bulk-formers such as fiber, antidiarrheal agents such as loperamide, and timed trips to the bathroom.

SEXUAL DYSFUNCTION

Sexual dysfunction is the third aspect of the triad of bladder, bowel, and sexual dysfunction. The neuroanatomy of sexual function closely parallels that of bladder function. In the male, reflex erection begins with sensory stimulation of the penis, via the dorsal penile nerve, which projects via the pudendal nerve to the sacral spinal cord. The erection reflex involves parasympathetic efferent fibers, S2-S4, projecting via the pelvic nerves to the smooth muscle surrounding the corpora cavernosa. Relaxation of the smooth muscle, likely via nitric oxide as the neurotransmitter, allows the vascular channels to engorge with blood. Detumescence and ejaculation involve the sympathetic nervous system. Psychogenic stimuli leading to erection presumably involve limbic cortical areas, the hypothalamus, and descending tracts to the spinal cord.

Sexual dysfunction may be induced by drugs, especially blood pressure medications (especially beta blockers and alpha blockers such as prazosin, sympatholytics such as clonidine, vasodilators, and diuretics), and antidepressants. Peripheral vascular disease or peripheral neuropathy, as in diabetes, can also interfere with the normal functions of erection and ejaculation. Spinal cord lesions may cut off the mental stimuli that lead to erection from the peripheral nerve mechanism of erection. Impotence also occurs commonly after stroke, and in neurological diseases such as Parkinson's disease and multiple sclerosis. In the case of stroke, studies have shown that sexual interest is little affected in both males and females, but in a large series of stroke patients, ability to achieve an erection declined from 75% before the stroke to 46% afterward, and ejaculations declined from 88% before the stroke to 29% afterward. Women are also less likely to achieve orgasm after stroke. Partial recovery of sexual dysfunction after stroke is usual. Counseling is essential for patients who wish to resume sexual activity after a stroke. Drugs such as sildenafil (Viagra), vardenafil (Levitra), or tadalafil (Cialis) enhance vasodilation and improve erectile function in males.

A less common subject is alteration of sexual interests and behavior after brain lesions. Most focal lesions either diminish sexual dysfunction or leave it unchanged. Occasionally, frontal lobe lesions produce disinhibition and inappropriate sexual behavior, occasionally directed at nurses and female medical students and physicians in the hospital setting. Bilateral temporal lesions may also lead to inappropriate sexual interest and behavior, as in the Kluver-Bucy syndrome (see Chap. 2).

KEY REFERENCES

Bladder dysfunction

Blok BFM, Holstege G. The central nervous system control of micturition in cats and humans. *Behav Brain Res* 1998;92:119–125.

Blok BFM, Willemsen ATM, Holstege G. A PET study on brain control of micturition in humans. *Brain* 1997;120:111–121.

Chutka DS, Fleming KC, Evans MP, et al. Urinary incontinence in the elderly population. *Mayo Clin Proc* 1996;71:93–101.

Fowler CJ. Neurological disorders of micturition and their treatment. *Brain* 1999;122:1213–1231.

Iqbal P, Castleden DM. Management of urinary incontinence in the elderly. *Gerontology* 1997;43:151–157.

McGuire EJ. The innervation and function of the lower urinary tract. *J Neurosurg* 1986;65:278–285.

Ouslander JG. Management of overactive bladder. *N Engl J Med* 2004;350:786–798.

Bowel dysfunction

Prather CM, Ortiz-Camacho P. Evaluation and treatment of constipation and fecal incontinence in adults. *Mayo Clin Proc* 1998;73:881–887.

Romero Y, Evans JM, Fleming KC, et al. Constipation and fecal incontinence in the elderly population. *Mayo Clin Proc* 1996;71:81–92.

Rudolph W, Galandiuk S. A practical guide to the diagnosis and management of fecal incontinence. *Mayo Clin Proc* 2002;77:271–275.

Sexual dysfunction

Goldstein I, Lue TF, Padma-Nathan H, et al. Oral sildenafil in the treatment of erectile dysfunction. *N Engl J Med* 1998;338:1397–1404.

Korpelainen JT, Nieminen P, Myllyla VV. Sexual functioning among stroke patients and their spouses. *Stroke* 1999;30:715–719.

Miller BL, Cummings JL, McIntyre H, et al. Hypersexuality or altered sexual preference following brain injury. *J Neurol Neurosurg Psychiat* 1986;49:867–873.

Murray FT, Geisser M, Murphy TC. Evaluation and treatment of erectile dysfunction. *Am J Med Sci* 1995;309:99–109.

Levy A, Crowley T, Gingell C. Non-surgical management of erectile dysfunction. *Clin Endocrinology* 2000;52:253–260.

Lue TF. Erectile dysfunction. *New Engl J Med* 2000;342:1802–1813.

Nehra A, Barrett DM, Moreland RB. Pharmacotherapeutic advances in the treatment of erectile dysfunction. *Mayo Clin Proc* 1999;74:709–721.

Steers WD. Neural pathways and central sites involved in penile erection: neuroanatomy and clinical implications. *Neuroscience and Biobehav Rev* 2000;24:507–516.

DIZZINESS AND VERTIGO

INTRODUCTION

Dizziness and vertigo are among the most common complaints of mankind. One of the difficulties of this symptom is the subjectivity of the complaint, and the fact that people use quite different terms and descriptions when they complain of dizziness. We shall start by dividing the complaint of dizziness into three separate categories: (1) light-headedness or presyncopal feeling, (2) vertigo, and (3) miscellaneous symptoms that do not fit into either of the other two categories. Syncope and light-headedness are described in much greater detail in Chap. 20; these symptoms reflect decreased blood flow or perfusion to the brain and have a much different connotation from vertigo. The third category includes the peculiar sensations that are part of metabolic disturbances such as hypoglycemia, carcinoid syndrome, systemic mastocytosis, transient ischemic attacks (TIAs), epileptic seizures, movement disorders, sleep disorders, and psychiatric manifestations. These symptoms are also discussed briefly in Chap. 20. This chapter will be dedicated primarily to a discussion of vertigo.

CLINICAL PRESENTATION: SYMPTOMS AND SIGNS

Vertigo is defined as a sensation of movement of the self or the environment. The term is derived from a Latin verb "to turn," and most often, vertigo has a turning or spinning component. In current usage, however, any sensation of movement counts as vertigo. Some patients will describe a "swimming" or "swaying" movement, or they feel as if the floor or ground is moving, or objects are moving in their vision. In fact, vertigo is a symptom complex with four separate components: (1) a vertiginous, dizzy sensation; (2) a visual disturbance with objects moving in one's vision (*oscillopsia*, the subjective equivalent of nystagmus, or jumping of the eyes), or just blurring of vision, difficulty focusing, or even transitory double vision; (3) a gastrointestinal sensation of nausea; and (4) a balance disturbance, with staggering when one starts to walk. Patients may emphasize one or more of these four elements.

For example, a football player presented with a complaint of repeated nausea and vomiting, precipitated by movement. In this case, a positional testing maneuver in the office produced a sudden sensation of nausea, during which the patient had easily observed nystagmus. For unclear reasons, this patient complained of only the gastrointestinal aspect of the symptom complex, and not of dizziness. Other patients complain of just the dizziness, just the visual complaints, just the balance loss, or varying combinations of the four symptoms. Vertigo is often precipitated by movement, and a history of exactly when the symptom occurs, what it is like, what stimuli appear to trigger it, how long it lasts, and how the patient tries to avoid the symptom, are all important to the correct diagnosis.

DIFFERENTIAL DIAGNOSIS

The first point in differential diagnosis is to separate vertigo from a light-headed or presyncopal symptom. This will usually be clear from a careful history, but there are occasional patients who seem to endorse both types of dizziness or cannot clearly distinguish between the two. In that case, the patient should be evaluated for orthostatic hypotension, cardiac arrhythmia, pulmonary embolism, and the like, as outlined in Chap. 20, in addition to vertigo.

The third type of dizziness, miscellaneous symptoms that do not fit easily into either the light-headed or vertiginous categories, is the hardest to diagnose. A careful history is essential. Dizziness and vertigo can be a prodrome of migraine, epileptic seizure, or transient ischemic attack, but usually associated symptoms will clarify the diagnosis. In migraine, the characteristic throbbing headache, with nausea, will usually follow a dizzy sensation. In epilepsy, the vertigo may evolve into an altered state of consciousness, with peculiar psychic sensations (unusual smells, feelings of strangeness or familiarity), motor automatisms or even full-blown tonic-clonic activity. In vertebrobasilar TIA, vertigo will usually be associated with other brainstem symptoms such as diplopia, dysarthria, dysphagia, unilateral numbness or weakness, or ataxia. Hypoglycemia will usually include a sense of hunger as well as *cold sweats*, light-headedness, and other symptoms. Carcinoid syndrome and systemic mastocytosis may produce unusual dizzy sensations, along with flushing, hypotension, and other manifestations. Hyperventilation predominantly causes a presyncopal sensation, but there may be associated anxiety symptoms of dyspnea, tachycardia, and sweating.

Once the symptom has been identified as vertigo, the next crucial decision is whether the abnormality arises from the peripheral or central vestibular system. Statistically, about 90% of patients with vertigo have a peripheral vestibular or *inner ear* etiology of their vertigo, and these conditions, while bothersome in terms of symptoms, are usually not life-threatening. The central vestibular disorders, on the other hand, can be warning signs of serious conditions, and prompt diagnosis is therefore paramount.

Peripheral vestibular disorders involve the classic symptom complex of vertigo, visual symptoms, nausea, and gait imbalance, as outlined above. In addition, there may be otic symptoms such as hearing loss, tinnitus, and ear pain. In many cases, the symptoms are "positional," meaning that they are precipitated by movement. Such symptoms can be reproduced on physical examination by a positional test, often referred to by neurologists as the Nylen-Barany maneuver, by otologists as the Dix-Hallpike maneuver. The patient sits upright, then lies down, with the head below the horizontal level by about 15°. The examiner asks the patient about symptoms and observes the eyes for nystagmus. In peripheral vestibulopathy, there is usually a latent period of a few seconds before the vertigo and nystagmus begin. These manifestations also typically last less than a minute, more typically 10–30 seconds. The examiner then sits the patient back up and watches for similar symptoms and signs. The maneuver is then repeated in the left-head-down and right-head-down positions. Reproduction of the patient's symptoms will make both the patient and physician confident that the symptom is clearly understood and represents a peripheral vestibulopathy. In addition, repeated positional testing will cause the vertigo to fatigue. The cause is most often benign, such as a viral illness such as vestibular neuronitis, an acute attack of inner ear symptoms lasting days or weeks. Another benign peripheral vestibular disorder is *benign positional vertigo*, a positional syndrome in which an otolith repeatedly activates the vestibular mechanism in certain head positions. Meniere's disease is a condition in which there is a buildup of endolymphatic fluid in the inner ear (*endolymphatic hydrops*). The symptoms are attacks of vertigo, tinnitus and hearing loss, often lasting days or weeks, and leaving the patient with some permanent hearing loss in the affected ear. Other inner ear disorders include labyrinthitis, an infection affecting both the acoustic and vestibular portions of the inner ear; a vascular syndrome of infarction of the inner ear mechanism; and tumors such as acoustic neuroma. Acoustic neuroma usually produces unilateral hearing loss before vertigo, a key to diagnosis. Another cause of peripheral vestibulopathy is drug intoxications. Alcohol causes vertigo because of differential changes in osmolarity between blood and endolymph. The anticonvulsants, phenytoin (Dilantin), carbamazepine (Tegretol), and Phenobarbital can all cause vertigo when present in levels above the therapeutic range. Aminoglycosides, cis-platinum, and quinidine can all produce a toxic vestibulopathy.

Central vestibular disorders are somewhat more complicated in diagnosis and treatment. These may be episodic, as in vertebrobasilar transient ischemic attacks (TIAs), or chronic, as in patients with structural lesions of the brainstem or cerebellum, such as tumors, infections, or multiple sclerosis. Strokes, including brainstem or cerebellar hemorrhages or infarctions, can produce both vertigo and ataxia. In neurological disorders associated with vertigo, there are often other neurological symptoms such as diplopia, visual field defects, dysarthria or dysphagia, unilateral or bilateral sensory loss, weakness, and ataxia. Gait ataxia or nystagmus without vertigo is always a central nervous system manifestation. The neurological examination may also reveal evidence of a structural lesion. In the Nylen-Barany maneuver, vertigo may begin without a latent period, nystagmus may occur without vertigo, and the nystagmus and vertigo may last more than a full minute after the position change. The vertigo and nystagmus may fail to fatigue on repeated testing. Direction-changing nystagmus in the same position is occasionally seen in central vestibular disorders. Any of these features should make the clinician suspect a central cause of the vertigo and embark on a more detailed diagnostic work-up.

LABORATORY AND RADIOLOGICAL INVESTIGATION

When the diagnosis is thought to be a peripheral vestibulopathy, further laboratory testing may not be necessary. More precise diagnosis can be obtained by electronystagmography, which represents a more sensitive version of the positional testing done as part of the physical examination. The patient is placed in a rotating chair, and responses to specific movement, as well as to cold caloric stimulation, can be measured. Eye movements are monitored by electrodes, with the eyes closed. Eye opening, as done in positional testing, inhibits nystagmus. In addition, an audiogram can be done to test hearing.

Suspicion of a central cause of vertigo should always lead to diagnostic testing. Brain imaging with magnetic imaging resonance (MRI) is usually the first step, since the posterior fossa structures are better visualized on MRI than computed tomography (CT). If TIA or stroke is suspected, magnetic resonance (MR) angiography, CT angiography, or catheter angiography is indicated. If multiple sclerosis or an infectious cause is suspected and a mass lesion has been excluded, lumbar puncture should be performed. Evoked response tests can also be performed in the diagnosis of multiple sclerosis. Brainstem auditory evoked responses are also helpful in detecting VIII cranial nerve and brainstem lesions.

TREATMENT

The treatment of a peripheral vestibular dysfunction is primarily reassurance. Drug therapy is not very effective, but such agents as meclizine (Antivert), glycopyrrolate (Robinul), or a transderm scopolamine patch can be used to reduce the activity of the vestibular end organ. Minor tranquillizers such as diazepam (Valium) may also help, but the addiction potential must be kept in mind. For simple benign positional vertigo, a positioning maneuver called the *Epley maneuver* can be tried. The object is to dislodge

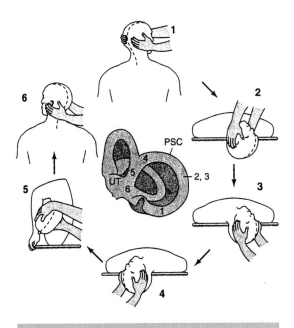

Figure 8-1   **The Epley maneuver, repositioning treatment for benign positional vertigo. An otolith is removed from the posterior semicircular canal of the right ear and into the utricle. The numbers (1–6) refer to the position of the patient and also to the location of the otolith material within the inner ear. The patient is seated, and the head is turned 45° to the right (1). The head is lowered quickly to below horizontal (2). The head is rotated rapidly to 90° in the opposite direction, remaining at 45° to the right for 30 seconds (4). The patient rolls onto the left side, without turning the head, and stays there for another 30 seconds (5). The patient sits up (6). The maneuver can be repeated until the vertigo is absent. The patient should avoid the supine position for the next two days.** (*Source*: Figure 3-7 from Aminoff, Greenberg, and Simon, Clinical Neurology, 2005, p. 109).

the otolith that is repeatedly stimulating the inner ear end organ. This simple maneuver is surprisingly effective. The Epley maneuver is shown in Fig. 8-1. In Meniere's disease, diuretics can be tried, or surgery can be performed by an otolaryngologist.

The treatment of central vestibular disorders depends critically on the precise diagnosis. These issues are considered in the chapters on the specific disorders.

KEY REFERENCES

Baloh RW. Vestibular neuritis. *N Engl J Med* 2003;348:1027–1032.

Brandt T. Management of vestibular disorders. *J Neurol* 2000;247:491–499.

Hotson JR, Baloh RW: Acute vestibular syndrome. *N Engl J Med* 1998;339:680–686.

VISION LOSS

INTRODUCTION

Loss of vision is a common and extremely worrisome symptom, since we depend to such a large extent on our ability to see the environment. Localization of a lesion causing visual loss is dependent on a knowledge of the anatomy of the visual system. Disorders of the eye and retina affect only vision from that eye, though some eye conditions such as glaucoma may be bilateral. The lens of each eye reverses the visual image, such that light from the superior part of the visual field falls on the inferior part of the retina, that from the inferior part falls on the superior retina, that from the left side of the visual field falls on the right side of the retina, and so on. The optic nerve carries visual information from the retina through the optic chiasm, where the fibers from both eyes subserving the opposite field of vision come together on each side to form the optic tract. The optic tract extends back to the lateral geniculate body, from which the optic radiations project to the occipital lobe. This anatomy is shown in Fig. 9-1.

CLINICAL PRESENTATION: SYMPTOMS AND SIGNS

Vision loss is a part of many different neurological disorders. We will divide vision loss syndromes into prechiasmatic (retina or optic nerve) lesions, chiasmatic lesions, optic tract lesions, and retrogeniculate lesions. The symptoms of a lesion of the retina or optic nerve will be a loss of vision in the ipsilateral eye. The clinical presentation is usually with loss of vision in part of the visual field in that eye, sometimes with pain in the eye. Disorders affecting the macula often cause a *positive* symptom of a black spot in the vision of that eye, or even of active visual scintillations, photopsias, or metamorphopsia (distortions in shape), whereas optic nerve lesions are more often the cause of *negative* visual symptoms. Optic nerve lesions are often associated with red desaturation or reduced red-green color vision, as well as with reduced pupillary light reflexes. Lesions directly in the vicinity of the optic chiasm will cause defects in both eyes, but not congruous between

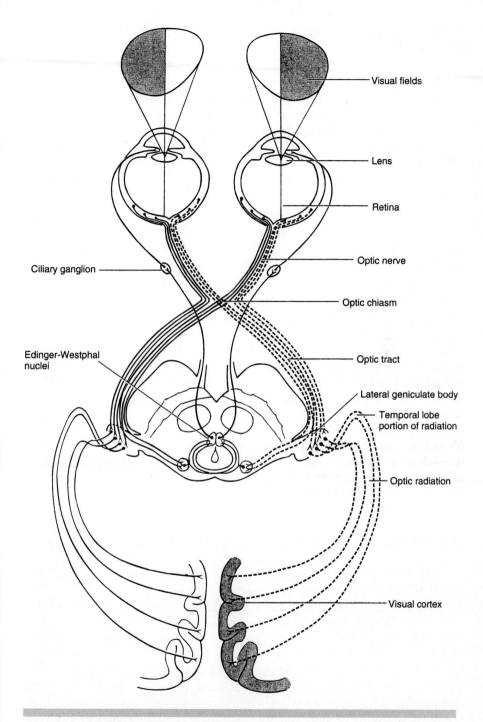

Figure 9-1 **Anatomy of the visual system.** The visual pathways. The solid blue lines are from the right half of the visual field, the broken blue lines from the left half of the visual field. The black lines represent the efferent pathway for the pupillary light reflex. (*Source*: Figure 15-14 in Waxman SG, Clinical Neuroanatomy 25th edition, p. 216)

the two eyes. A lesion of the crossing fibers of the central optic chiasm produces a typical, bitemporal visual field loss, most commonly associated with a pituitary neoplasm. Retrochiasmal lesions usually cause homonymous visual field defects in both eyes.

Transient, monocular visual loss in one eye is usually of vascular origin, a transient ischemic attack in the internal carotid artery or ophthalmic artery distribution. More rarely, monocular visual loss can be a symptom of *retinal migraine*.

DIFFERENTIAL DIAGNOSIS

Optic nerve lesions

The differential diagnosis of optic nerve lesions includes optic neuritis, ischemic optic neuropathy, and compressive optic nerve lesions. In addition, glaucoma is a very common cause of optic nerve disease.

Optic neuritis is a syndrome of optic nerve inflammation, occurring either as a single illness or as an attack of multiple sclerosis. It typically occurs in young patients. The onset can vary from instantaneous to a worsening deficit over a few days, often with a central scotoma and pain on moving the eyes. The examination may show optic nerve swelling if the inflammation involves the optic disk (*papillitis*); if the inflammation is retrobulbar (*retrobulbar neuritis*), the optic nerve head will look normal during the acute attack, then gradually become pale and atrophic. The pupillary light reflex will often be diminished, or the swinging flashlight test will reveal an afferent pupillary defect (formerly, erroneously referred to as a Marcus Gunn pupil) in the affected eye. The prognosis of optic neuritis is for gradual improvement, but studies have shown that high dose, intravenous corticosteroid treatment (methylprednisolone, 1000 mg daily for 5 days) improves outcome over the first several months, and delays the occurrence of a new attack of multiple sclerosis. The percentage of patients with optic neuritis who go on to develop multiple sclerosis has varied in published series, from less than 20% to almost 80% with longer follow-up.

Ischemic optic neuropathy usually occurs in middle aged or older people, often with vascular risk factors such as diabetes mellitus and hypertension. The onset of loss of vision is usually abrupt and painless. It may involve the entire vision of the eye or a partial nerve fiber bundle defect, as would typically be seen in a central retinal artery embolus. Ischemic optic neuritis is usually not caused by an embolus, but rather by disease in the ophthalmic or central retinal arteries themselves. One subtype is the syndrome of temporal or giant cell arteritis, which typically causes both severe headaches and sudden episodes of visual loss, with an elevated erythrocyte sedimentation rate. Other associations with temporal arteritis are jaw claudication and polymyalgia rheumatica, or diffuse muscle and joint aching.

The prognosis for return of vision in ischemic optic neuropathy is limited, though some improvement is possible. In temporal arteritis, there is a high risk of later involvement of the other eye, and corticosteroid treatment may prevent this. In non-arteritic ischemic optic neuropathy, there is a somewhat smaller risk of recurrence in the other eye, but no clear treatment has been shown effective. Decompressive surgery, popular in the past, not only fails to benefit patients, but may reduce visual recovery. Radiation therapy to the brain or pituitary region can cause radiation vasculopathy, a type of ischemic optic neuritis.

Compressive lesions can affect the optic nerve, producing a slowly progressive loss of vision and often an afferent pupil. Meningiomas of the optic nerve sheath or of the subfrontal region can compress the nerve. Pituitary tumors, though they typically affect the optic chiasm, may affect a single optic nerve. Intrinsic optic nerve tumors such as optic nerve gliomas occur mainly in children and adolescents. Occasionally, an intraorbital tumor or infection will impinge on the optic nerve, usually with associated proptosis. Rarely, an aneurysm of the internal carotid or ophthalmic artery may cause a compressive optic neuropathy.

Other causes of optic nerve lesions are much less common than the ones above, but there are multiple etiologies. These include vitamin B_{12} deficiency; drug therapy with agents such as the antituberculous drug ethambutol, the antiepileptic drug vigabatrin, the antiarrhythmic agent amiodarone, and hydroxychloroquin (though the damage may be more prominent in the retina than in the optic nerve); other inflammatory conditions such as sarcoidosis or infectious meningitis or fungal infections such as mucormycosis; and the hereditary condition Leber's hereditary optic atrophy (LHON). Leber's optic atrophy is a mitochondrially inherited disorder, with male predominance and onset usually in the twenties. The vision loss appears abruptly in one or both eyes, usually stabilizing within a few months. Optic disc swelling may be seen acutely. This diagnosis can be made by a mitochondrial DNA test. A rare paraneoplastic syndrome can result in optic neuropathy.

Chiasmatic lesions

Most lesions affecting the optic chiasm are compressive and develop gradually over weeks or months. The classic cause is a pituitary tumor growing up into the central portion of the chiasm, producing a bitemporal hemianopsia. Not all cases, however, have a symmetric lesion. A large lesion of the anterior chiasm may predominantly affect one eye, resembling a compressive or inflammatory optic nerve lesion, but careful visual field testing may reveal a superior temporal defect respecting the midline in the visual field of the contralateral eye (Fig. 9-2). Most lesions of the optic chiasm are pituitary adenomas, occasionally a craniopharyngioma. Rarely, an optic nerve glioma or multiple sclerosis plaque may extend into the optic chiasm and mimic a pituitary tumor. Pituitary apoplexy, or sudden hemorrhage and necrosis in the

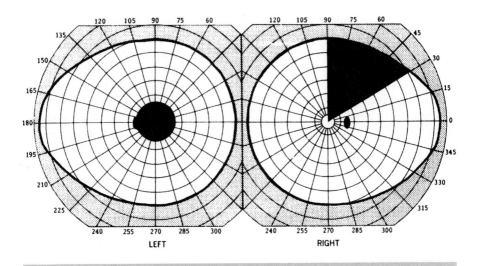

Figure 9-2 **Junctional scotoma** A lesion of the left optic nerve at the junction of the chiasm produces a central scotoma in the affected (left) eye and a small superior scotoma in the other eye. (Courtesy of Dr. Patrick Lavin)

pituitary gland, can cause a sudden optic chiasm lesion, sometimes associated with thyroid or adrenal failure.

Retrochiasmatic lesions

Lesions behind the optic chiasm typically produce a homonymous visual field defect in both eyes. The closer to the occipital lobe, the more congruent the visual field defect will be in the two eyes. The differential diagnosis of a homonymous visual field defect would include the gamut of diseases of the cerebral hemispheres. A brain tumor or abscess will cause a slowly progressive visual field defect. Ischemic strokes in the middle or posterior cerebral artery territory will cause a homonymous hemianopsia or quadrantanopsia (see Chap. 24). In some series, the more anterior the lesion causing a visual field defect, the more likely the cause is to be tumor, whereas the more posterior the lesion, the more likely is a vascular etiology. In the case of occipital lesions, the hemianopsia may be unaccompanied by any motor or sensory abnormalities, whereas these will usually be present in lesions of the temporal and parietal lobes.

LABORATORY AND RADIOLOGICAL INVESTIGATION

A visual field examination can document the visual field defect, in terms of the localization to prechiasmatic, chiasmatic, or postchiasmatic location. A few simple blood tests may be useful, including a sedimentation rate and C reactive protein for giant cell (temporal) arteritis and related vasculitides, a vitamin B_{12} level, an angiotensin converting enzyme (ACE) test for sarcoidosis, and thyroid function tests. If giant cell (temporal) arteritis is strongly suspected, a temporal artery biopsy should be performed. The rare, paraneoplastic optic neuropathy can be tested with paraneoplastic antibodies. A magnetic resonance imaging (MRI) scan is invaluable for diagnosis of mass lesions such as optic nerve glioma or meningioma, chiasmatic lesions, or retrochiasmatic lesions such as strokes, brain tumors, and brain abscesses. A vascular imaging study such as ultrasound, magnetic resonance (MR), computed tomography (CT), or catheter angiography may be necessary for diagnosis of carotid artery lesions, aneurysms compressing the optic nerves, or occlusive vascular disorders affecting the cerebral hemispheres.

KEY REFERENCES

Burger SK, Saul RF, Selhorst JB, et al. Transient monocular blindness caused by vasospasm. *New Engl J Med* 1991;325:870–873.

Hayreh SS. Anterior ischemic optic neuropathy: trouble waiting to happen. *Ophthalmology* 2000;107:407–409.

Howell N, Bindoff LA, McCullough DA, et al. Leber hereditary optic neuropathy: identification of the same mitochondrial NDI mutation in six pedigrees. *Am J Hum Genet* 1991;49:939–950.

Liu GT, Glaser JS, Schatz NJ, et al. Visual morbidity in giant cell arteritis: clinical characteristics and prognosis for vision. *Ophthalmology* 1994;101:1779–1785.

Newman NJ. Optic neuropathy. *Neurology* 1996;46:315–322.

DIPLOPIA

INTRODUCTION

Diplopia is typically binocular, indicating that the two eyes are not moving in tandem, and one is pointing in a slightly different direction from the other. We shall omit any discussion of monocular diplopia, which indicates either intraocular pathology or less commonly a nonphysiologic, psychiatric disorder. Binocular diplopia can occur close to the subject, if the near reflex is incomplete; this would be an example of physiological, or normal diplopia. Occasionally, patients with nystagmus may describe "double vision," by which they may mean oscillopsia or jumping of objects in vision; fixed diplopia should not occur in this setting. Assuming that the patient truly has an extraocular motor abnormality producing diplopia, the cause can be at one of three anatomic locations: (1) in the extraocular muscles themselves or in the cranial nerves supplying the extraocular muscles (infranuclear ophthalmoplegia, (2) in the brainstem between cranial nerve nuclei (internuclear ophthalmoplegia), or (3) in the brainstem above the individual cranial nerve nuclei (supranuclear ophthalmoplegia).

CLINICAL PRESENTATION: SYMPTOMS AND SIGNS

Patients often give little more description of diplopia than that they "see double." The examiner must first ensure that the diplopia is binocular, and that it disappears if the patient covers one eye. Next, the examiner should ask if the separation of the two images is horizontal, vertical, or oblique. Most diplopia increases with the distance of the object from the eyes. The examiner should ask whether the diplopia is worse with gaze in one direction. In some conditions, such as myasthenia gravis, diplopia may come on or worsen with fatigue. Finally, associated symptoms should be fully characterized.

DIFFERENTIAL DIAGNOSIS

Intranuclear ophthalmoplegias

A number of myopathic diseases affect the extraocular muscles. These would include thyroid ophthalmopathy, mitochondrial disorders such as *progressive external ophthalmoplegia* (PEO), a few muscular dystrophy syndromes such as oculopharyngeal dystrophy, and myasthenia gravis. PEO is a hereditary disease, including progressive loss of extraocular muscle function, but with a host of other, associated symptoms such as blindness and deafness. In oculopharyngeal dystrophy, there is usually a family history, and the muscle weakness involves not only the eye muscles, but also the eyelids and lower face and pharyngeal muscles. Myasthenia gravis differs from other causes of diplopia in that the symptoms come and go, worsening with fatigue, and often producing inconsistent patterns of diplopia. Ptosis of the lid is usually present, and other, fatiguable muscle weakness may develop.

Lesions of cranial nerves III, IV, and VI cause diplopia. The pattern should be easily discerned by examination of the extraocular movements, including use of the red glass test (see Chap. 1). A diagram of the eye muscles and their actions is shown in Fig. 10-1, and the three cranial nerves

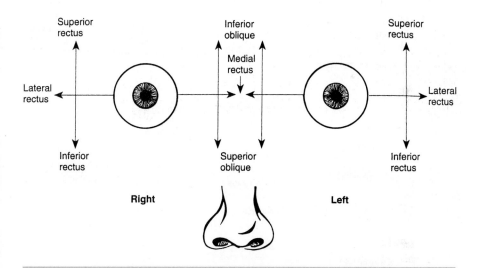

Figure 10-1 **Actions of the extraocular muscles** The six extraocular muscles and the directions of eye movement. Note that the superior, medial, and inferior rectus, as well as the inferior oblique are innervated by the III cranial nerve; the superior oblique is innervated by the IV cranial nerve, and the lateral rectus is innervated by the VI cranial nerve. (*Source*: From Waxman SG, Clinical Neuroanatomy, 2003, p. 109, Fig 8-5)

responsible for extraocular movements are shown in Fig. 10-2. A VI nerve palsy is the easiest to diagnose, since the diplopia is purely horizontal and increases with gaze in the direction of the eye with the weak lateral rectus muscle. Many different lesions can result in a unilateral VI nerve palsy. Involvement of the VI nerve can be seen in diabetes or hypertension, or as an idiopathic cranial nerve palsy, usually with good improvement over time. Mass lesions in the nasopharynx or closer to the eye, in the cavernous sinus, superior orbital fissure, or orbital apex can compress the nerve. Because of its long course from the pons to the eye, the nerve may be affected by any disorder associated with increased intracranial pressure, a phenomenon often referred to as a *false localizing* cranial nerve VI palsy. Finally, lesions within the pons can affect the VI nerve, though a nuclear VI lesion more typically produces a *lateral gaze palsy*, in which neither eye will move to the affected side.

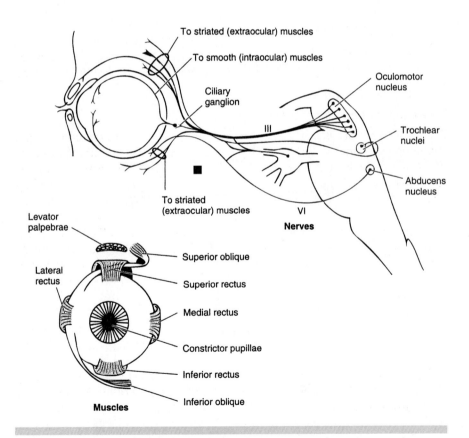

Figure 10-2 **The III, IV, and VI cranial nerves** (*Source*: From Waxman SG, Clinical Neuroanatomy, 2003, p. 107, Fig 8-4)

A IV nerve palsy affects the superior oblique muscle and causes a verti-cal diplopia. The patient often adopts a head tilt to minimize diplopia. Trochlear nerve palsies are often caused by trauma in the vicinity of the orbit, though idiopathic IV nerve palsies, or IV nerve palsies related to dia-betes are also relatively common.

III nerve palsies are potentially more serious. Like IV and VI palsies, iso-lated III nerve palsies are common in diabetic patients, usually with sparing of the pupillary fibers and involvement of the eyelid and III nerve-innervated extraocular muscles (inferior oblique, superior rectus, inferior rectus, medial rectus). The nerve can also be affected by compressive or inflammatory lesions in the orbital apex or superior orbital fissure (Tolosa-Hunt Syndrome), or in the cavernous sinus. Mucormycosis is a fungal infec-tion in diabetics that can affect the III nerve in the orbit or cavernous sinus. The III nerve can be compressed in the subarachnoid space by an aneurysm of the internal carotid artery at the posterior communicating artery take-off. This syndrome is a *painful ophthalmoplegia*, usually with pupillary involve-ment. Prompt diagnosis of the aneurysm is critical, since surgery or endovascular intervention before the aneurysm ruptures will spare the patient all of the complications of subarachnoid hemorrhage. Occasionally, the pupil is spared in a compressive lesion, so this sign cannot be relied on completely.

Internuclear ophthalmoplegias

The most common *internuclear ophthalmoplegi* (INO) is a lesion affecting the medial longitudinal fasciculus between the III nerve in the midbrain and the VI nerve in the pons. As discussed in Chap. 2, an INO involves incomplete adduction of the ipsilateral eye, usually with nystagmus of the abducting eye. If the patient can move the eye medially during convergence (the near reflex) better than on attempted lateral gaze to that side, this confirms that the lesion does not lie in the medial rectus muscle or in the III nerve branch innervating it, but rather as part of a higher lesion. INO is most commonly seen in multiple sclerosis (MS), though occasionally a small stroke or tumor in the brainstem can cause an INO. Bilateral INO is a sign of MS in about 95% of cases, with the other 5% representing brainstem strokes. In bilateral INO, upward beating nystagmus is often an associated sign.

Lesions in the pons can also produce a horizontal (lateral) gaze palsy to the ipsilateral side. Lesions associated with a lateral gaze palsy can involve either the VI nerve nucleus or the parapontine reticular formation (PPRF) adjacent to the VI nerve nucleus. In this syndrome, the eyes deviate away from the side of the lesion and fail to abduct to the side of the lesion.

A rare oculomotor syndrome is the *one-and-a-half syndrome*, a combina-tion of a lateral gaze palsy and an INO. The one-and-a-half syndrome is caused by a lesion in the pons that affects both the VI nerve nucleus or PPRF and also the medial longitudinal fasciculus (MLF). The eyes fail to look toward the side of the lesion; on attempted gaze to the contralateral side, only the lateral rectus of the contralateral eye moves, not the medial rectus of the ipsilateral eye. There may be nystagmus of the abducting eye. This syndrome is most commonly caused by brainstem strokes. Brainstem lesions, especially in the medulla, can result in the eyes being dysconjugate, but with the same relative position to each other throughout the excursions both horizontally and vertically. This pattern is called a *skew deviation*.

Supranuclear ophthalmoplegias

The most common supranuclear syndrome affecting the extraocular movements is a *gaze preference*, often seen in patients with large lesions of the frontal lobe, including ischemic strokes and brain tumors. The patient will gaze mostly to the side of the lesion, occasionally straight ahead, but rarely if ever to the contralateral side. This syndrome is traditionally explained by involvement of the lateral gaze center (Brodmann's area 8 in the superior frontal cortex), with the contralateral gaze center then becoming dominant. The term *gaze preference* is somewhat unfortunate, in that the tendency to look toward the lesion and away from an associated hemiparesis is not truly a voluntary preference, but the term does distinguish this pattern from a horizontal gaze palsy of pontine origin. In a gaze preference, the patient may be able to look to the opposite side if stimulated strongly enough, or with reflex eye movements in the oculocephalic and oculovestibular reflexes (see Chap. 2).

Vertical gaze palsies are more complex than horizontal ones. Upward gaze palsies are often seen with lesions in the rostral midbrain or the junction between the midbrain and thalamus. In Parinaud's syndrome, an upward gaze palsy is combined with mid-sized, poorly reactive pupils, often presenting in a child with premature puberty. This syndrome can be a sign of a tumor in the pineal region, with pressure downward on the upper midbrain.

Downward gaze palsies are relatively rare but can be seen in lesions near the red nuclei and periaqueductal gray matter. Downward gaze paresis is perhaps best described in the disease progressive supranuclear palsy (PSP), in which loss of downward gaze may be the first symptom of the disorder. Upward gaze loss follows, and only late in the course are the horizontal eye movements affected. Patients with PSP also manifest a wide-eyed "look of perpetual astonishment," a cervical dystonia in extension, dysarthria, dysphagia, and Parkinson-like rigidity (see Chap. 27).

LABORATORY AND RADIOLOGICAL INVESTIGATION

It should be clear from the preceding discussion that clinical assessment of the patient with diplopia, especially a careful history and physical examination, is essential for the diagnosis of extraocular movement disorders.

In some centers, extraocular movement studies can be performed to confirm the diagnosis, or referral to a neuroophthalmologist can be considered. Laboratory tests are helpful in some instances, such as a sedimentation rate for the diagnosis of arteritis, a tensilon test or electromyogram (EMG) with repetitive nerve stimulation for myasthenia gravis, or a lumbar puncture for an infectious disease. A brain imaging study, usually a magnetic imaging resonance (MRI) scan, can be helpful for diagnosis of mass lesions, strokes, and infectious disorders. If an aneurysm compressing the III cranial nerve is suspected, a magnetic resonance angiography (MRA), computed tomographic angiography (CTA), or catheter angiography is urgently indicated.

TREATMENT

Treatment of the patient with an extraocular motor disorder depends on an accurate diagnosis of the problem. For those cases of diplopia for which no specific treatment exists, such as the aftermath of a brainstem stroke, referral to a neuroophthalmologist is appropriate. Prism glasses may be of help in eliminating or reducing diplopia, and surgery on the extraocular muscles can also be considered. Generally these measures are deferred for at least 3 months after an acute illness such as a stroke, to allow for spontaneous recovery.

KEY REFERENCES

Brazis PW. Localization of lesions of the oculomotor nerve: recent concepts. *Mayo Clin Proc* 1991;66:1029–1035.

Brazis PW. Palsies of the trochlear nerve: diagnosis and localization—recent concepts. *Mayo Clin* 1993;68:501–509.

Brazis PW, Lee AG. Acquired binocular horizontal diplopia. *Mayo Clin Proc* 1999;74:907–916.

Leigh RJ, Zee DS. *The Neurology of Eye Movements*. 3rd ed. F. A. Davis Co., Philadelphia, PA, 1999.

Spector RH, Troost BT. The ocular motor system. *Ann Neurol* 1981;9:517–525.

DYSARTHRIA

INTRODUCTION

Dysarthria refers to abnormal articulation of speech phonemes, with or without an associated abnormality of language function. Dysarthria can result from non-neurological causes, such as cleft palate, absence or thickening of the tongue, laryngectomy, or abnormalities of the temporomandibular joint such as trismus. Neurogenic dysarthria implies that the cause of the articulatory disturbance reflects an abnormality of the nervous system, usually associated with weakness or incoordination of the muscles of articulation. A patient with pure dysarthria, and no aphasia, should have abnormal spontaneous speech, repetition, naming, and reading aloud on the bedside mental status examination, but auditory comprehension, reading comprehension, and writing should all be normal. If any of these is abnormal, an aphasic disorder should be suspected (see Chap. 15). In general, if the examiner transcribes the speech output of a dysarthric patient and then reads it aloud, it should sound normal. Neurogenic motor speech disorders are generally divided into dysarthria and apraxia of speech.

CLINICAL PRESENTATION: SYMPTOMS AND SIGNS

Neurogenic dysarthrias have been divided by the Mayo Clinic group into six main categories: flaccid, spastic, ataxic, hypokinetic, hyperkinetic, and mixed (Darley, Aronson, and Brown, 1969). These disorders represent the effects on speech of neurological disorders affecting specific levels of the neuraxis. Table 11-1 lists a summary of the classification of dysarthria. The astute medical student can utilize speech characteristics to help in the localization of neurological lesions and in the diagnosis of neurological disorders. Subsequently, the Mayo Clinic group (Duffy, 1995) has added a subtype of spastic dysarthria called *unilateral upper motor neuron dysarthria*.

TABLE 11-1 **Classification of the Dysarthrias**

Type	Level of CNS	Features	Examples
Flaccid	Bilateral lower motor neuron	Breathy, nasal voice, imprecise consonants	Stroke, myasthenia gravis
Spastic	Bilateral upper motor neuron	Strain-strangle, harsh voice; slow rate; imprecise consonants	Bilateral strokes, tumors, primary lateral sclerosis
Unilateral upper motor neuron	Unilateral upper motor neuron	Consonant imprecision, slow rate, harsh voice quality	Stroke, Tumor
Ataxic	Cerebellum	Irregular articulatory breakdowns, excessive and equal stress	Stroke, cerebellar degenerations
Hypokinetic	Extrapyramidal	Rapid rate, reduced loudness, monopitch and monoloudness	Parkinson's disease
Hyperkinetic	Extrapyramidal	Prolonged phonemes, variable rate, sudden silences, voice stoppages	Dystonia, Huntington's disease
Spastic-flaccid	Upper and lower motor neuron	Hypernasality, strain-strangle, harsh voice, slow rate, imprecise consonants	Amyotrophic lateral sclerosis, multiple strokes

Source: Adapted from Darley, Aronson, and Brown, 1969; and Duffy, 1995.

Flaccid dysarthria

Flaccid dysarthria reflects lower motor neuron weakness of the muscles of articulation. The voice is soft, breathy, and hypernasal. Consonants may be articulated imprecisely.

Diseases associated with flaccid dysarthria include bulbar disorders such as bulbar myopathies (oculopharyngeal dystrophy), neuromuscular disorders such as myasthenia gravis or botulism, and peripheral nerve disorders such as the Guillain-Barre syndrome.

Historically, acute poliomyelitis was a common cause of flaccid dysarthria.

Spastic dysarthria

Spastic dysarthria is the speech pattern associated with bilateral, upper motor neuron motor involvement, often seen as part of the pattern called *pseudobulbar palsy*. Pseudobulbar palsy is a syndrome of dysarthria, dysphagia, and emotional lability, or pathological laughter and crying. The dysarthria itself has a "strain-strangle" quality, usually a slower than normal rate, and consonant imprecision. "Papapapa" might be distorted into something sounding more like "Babababa." This type of dysarthria can be seen with any bilateral lesion affecting the corticobulbar tracts. The most common such disorder is bilateral stroke, but spastic dysarthria can be seen after traumatic brain injuries, bilateral tumors, or degenerative disorders such as primary lateral sclerosis.

Unilateral upper motor neuron (UUMN) dysarthria

This pattern of dysarthria results, as the name implies, from a unilateral, upper motor neuron lesion. The auditory signs are similar to the spastic type, but less severe: (1) harsh voice, (2) slow rate, and (3) imprecise consonants. Common causes of UUMN dysarthria are a unilateral hemisphere stroke or brain tumor.

Ataxic dysarthria

This speech pattern results from damage to the cerebellum or its connections. The auditory signs are (1) irregular articulatory breakdowns; and (2) excessive and equal stress, also referred to as *scanning speech*. Irregular breakdowns cause a patient saying "papapapa" to sound like he is popping popcorn. In general, the articulation pattern is slow, but sometimes there are staccato, excessively rapid syllables. Possible causes include cerebellar degenerations, strokes, and tumors. Multiple sclerosis frequently produces ataxic dysarthria, but it may be mixed with elements of flaccid, spastic, or unilateral upper motor neuron dysarthria.

Hypokinetic dysarthria

This dysarthria is associated with basal ganglia diseases. The auditory characteristics are: (1) rapid rate, (2) soft voice (reduced loudness), (3) monopitch (unvarying pitch level), and (4) monoloudness (unvarying loudness level). The most common cause of hypokinetic dysarthria is Parkinson's disease. Occasionally, strokes involving the basal ganglia can mimic this pattern.

Hyperkinetic dysarthria

This type of dysarthria is also associated with extrapyramidal disorders, but those with increased rather than decreased movement. The auditory signs include: (1) prolonged phonemes (individual speech sounds are stretched out); (2) variable rate (sometimes too fast and sometimes too slow); (3) harsh voice quality; (4) sudden, inappropriate silences (abnormal pauses in the flow of speech); and (4) sudden voice stoppages (inappropriate absence of phonation). Common causes of hyperkinetic dysarthria are dystonia (e.g., dystonia musculorum deformans), Machado Joseph disease, and Huntington's disease.

Mixed dysarthria

This last subcategory of dysarthria can take several forms. The speech characteristics vary, depending on which neurological systems are involved. Mixed, spastic-flaccid dysarthria results from involvement of both the upper and lower motor neuron systems. The auditory characteristics are: (1) hypernasality; (2) strain-strangle, liquid sounding voice quality (phonation is accompanied by a gurgle); (3) extremely slow rate; and (4) severe consonant imprecision. Spastic-flaccid dysarthria is typically caused by amyotrophic lateral sclerosis (ALS) but may be seen in multiple strokes. Multiple sclerosis may produce a mixed ataxic-spastic-flaccid dysarthria resulting from involvement of the cerebellum, corticobulbar tracts (upper motor neuron), and cranial nerves (bulbar weakness, lower motor neuron). The ataxic features (excessive and equal stress, slow rate) may be most prominent. Similarly, Wilson's disease may produce auditory characteristics of hypokinetic, ataxic, and spastic dysarthrias.

APRAXIA OF SPEECH

Apraxia of speech is a disorder which can be thought of as intermediate between the dysarthrias and the aphasias. It is more often diagnosed by speech-language pathologists than by neurologists. The concept of this disorder is that of an apraxia for producing rapid sequences of phoneme articulations, especially consonant shifts, in the absence of weakness, slowness or incoordination of the muscles of articulation. Apraxia of speech is a motor speech disorder, not a language disorder or aphasia, although it is frequently mixed with aphasia, and often with dysarthria.

In practical terms, speech apraxia causes articulatory errors that, in contrast to dysarthric mispronunciations, are inconsistent. The subject may pronounce the same word differently, and sometimes normally, in different utterances.

Table 11-2 lists the key features of apraxia of speech. The patient makes effortful, trial and error, groping attempts at articulation. The patient seems hesitant, with particular difficulty in the initiation of speech. Errors are often followed by attempts at self-correction. The speech pattern is dysprosodic, with disruptions in the rhythm, stress (emphasis), and intonation of speech. The most important feature is that the speech is inconsistent. For example, a patient may make different errors in pronouncing the same word several times; this is especially evident with polysyllabic words, such as

---

TABLE 11-2 **Auditory Features of Apraxia of Speech**

Effortful, groping, trial-and-error articulation, with attempts at self-correction
Difficulty with initiation of utterances
Difficulty most evident on initial phonemes of multisyllabic utterances
Dysprosody
Inconsistency on repeated productions of the same word

"impossibility," "artillery," or "catastrophe." A patient trying to say "catastrophe" five times might produce: "capastrophy, catastroophy, catastrophe,
caphastromy, calastrothy."

Localization of apraxia of speech

The motor programming of speech sequences is thought to take place in
Broca's area in the left inferior frontal gyrus, since patients with Broca's
aphasia frequently have an associated apraxia of speech. In a study by
Dronkers (1996), apraxia of speech appeared to be associated with lesions of
the insula; 25 stroke patients who displayed apraxia of speech all had lesions
involving the left insula, whereas none of the 19 patients without apraxia of
speech had lesions in this area. In this study, the insula appeared to be specialized for the motor planning of speech. Research in acute stroke, however,
continues to provide evidence that apraxia of speech is associated with acute
lesions affecting Broca's area in the left frontal cortex (Hillis et al, 2004).

Etiology of apraxia of speech

In Duffy's large series of patients with apraxia of speech, the great majority
of cases had left hemisphere strokes. Less common causes of apraxia of
speech included degenerative diseases of the nervous system such as corticobasal degeneration (see Chap. 27), traumatic brain injury, and brain tumors.
In general, apraxia of speech is less useful in practical neurological diagnosis
than either dysarthria or aphasia, but it continues to be analyzed as a part of
motor speech disorders, and it influences speech therapy treatments provided
by speech-language pathologists. It should be suspected when a patient has
marked and inconsistent difficulty with articulation, in the absence of major
language comprehension deficits.

Muteness

A special problem in the diagnosis of speech and language problems is the
mute patient. The mute patient may have dysarthria of severe degree
(anarthria), apraxia of speech, a nonneurologic disorder such as a laryngeal
obstruction, a frontal lobe syndrome with akinetic mutism, an extrapyramidal

disorder such as severe Parkinson's disease, stupor, a psychogenic state such as catatonia, or simple uncooperativeness. In general, some language output must be present before the examiner can confidently evaluate the speech pattern and make a diagnosis of dysarthria, apraxia of speech, or aphasia.

The examiner uses other cognitive and neurological functions to help in diagnosing the speech or language problem. Normal performance in writing and in language comprehension makes aphasia unlikely. Muteness and inability to follow commands in a patient who is seemingly alert may signify severe aphasia, but care must be taken in this diagnosis. Of course, other "neighborhood signs" of left hemisphere injury such as right hemiparesis, right-sided sensory loss, and right hemianopsia aid in the diagnosis of aphasia. In general, the aphasic patient tries to communicate by gesturing, grunting, or pointing; he or she is mute in speech but not in other behaviors.

The medical student should see from this chapter that motor speech disorders are complex, and it is not sufficient just to say that a patient has *slurred speech* or even *dysarthria*. Characterization of the specific pattern of abnormal articulation can help to localize neurological disorders and diagnose specific disease processes.

KEY REFERENCES

Darley FL, Aronson AE, Brown JR. Differential diagnostic patterns of dysarthria. *J Speech Hear Res* 1060;12:246–249.

Dronkers NF. A new brain region for coordinating speech articulation. *Nature* 1996;384:159–161.

Duffy JR. Motor Speech Disorders. Substrates, Differential Diagnosis, and Management. St. Louis, MO: Mosby; 1995.

Hillis AE, Work M, Barker PB, et al. Re-examining the brain regions crucial for orchestrating speech articulation. *Brain* 2004;127:1479–1487.

DYSPHAGIA

INTRODUCTION

Dysphagia is an inability to swallow. This chapter will consider neurogenic causes of swallowing difficulty, not those due to local anatomic problems such as esophageal stricture, surgery on the oral or pharyngeal structures, or gastroesophageal reflux disease. Like speech, swallowing can be affected by various neurological disorders at different levels of the nervous system, including muscle diseases, neuromuscular junction disorders, neuropathies, abnormalities of the cranial nerves IX and X, or lesions of the brainstem, cerebellum, or cerebral hemispheres.

Dysphagia is a major cause of morbidity in patients with neurological diseases. Patients can choke on food or fluids, regurgitate fluids into the mouth and nose, and suffer recurrent respiratory infections, weight loss, dehydration, and malnutrition. Identification of dysphagia is therefore important to the treatment of neurological patients.

We must begin with a brief review of the neuroanatomy and physiology of swallowing. The voluntary act of swallowing begins in the cerebral cortex, where a *frontal swallowing center* has been localized in front of the face area, at the foot of the precentral gyrus. Electrical stimulation of this area in animals induces swallowing activity in muscles of the mouth and pharynx. The corticobulbar fibers from this swallowing center project to the swallowing center in the medulla. The medullary swallowing center receives sensory input from the V, IX, and X nerves, and it coordinates motor outputs from the nucleus ambiguus, involved in voluntary swallowing, and the dorsal motor nucleus of X, involved in the esophageal phase of swallowing. Axons from these motor nuclei of the X nerve innervate the muscles of swallowing.

The act of swallowing is divided into three stages: the oral stage, the pharyngeal stage, and the esophageal stage. Most neurological disorders affect the oral and pharyngeal stages. In the oral stage, the food is chewed, combined with liquids, propelled backward by the tongue (XII nerve), and then prepared as a bolus for transit into the pharynx. The nasopharynx is closed off during the oral stage by elevation of the soft palate, controlled by the X nerve.

In the pharyngeal stage, the epiglottis closes to prevent aspiration of food and liquid into the trachea, respiration is interrupted, and the pharyngeal muscles of swallowing contract in a sequential, coordinated fashion to move the bolus past the upper esophageal sphincter, and then into the esophagus. The pharyngeal stage of swallowing is largely a reflex action, and the esophageal stage is entirely involuntary.

CLINICAL PRESENTATION: SYMPTOMS AND SIGNS

Weakness of the oral muscles may produce drooling as well as difficulty propelling the food and fluids back to the pharynx, and weakness of the muscles of mastication will make it difficult to prepare the bolus of food. If the pharyngeal muscles are not functioning properly, the patient may "choke" on food or fluids, and the result may be a loud cough. In general, patients with neurogenic dysphagia complain of difficulty swallowing more with liquids than solids, since liquids require close coordination of the swallowing muscles, whereas patients with obstructions such as esophageal stricture complain more of dysphagia for solids. Occasionally, patients with pharyngeal dysphagia even regurgitate fluids up into the nose and mouth. It is important to realize, however, that aspiration into the trachea can result without any obvious choking, cough, or nasal regurgitation; such *silent aspiration* can still cause aspiration pneumonia, or more chronic problems of dehydration and malnutrition, without any complaint by the patient or caregivers of difficulty swallowing. Physicians must therefore know when to screen for swallowing difficulty in patients with neurological diseases, even when the patient does not admit to dysphagia. In rare instances, the muscles of the upper esophageal sphincter, especially the cricopharyngeus muscle, overcontract, and the patient cannot get food or fluids past the sphincter and into the esophagus. In the current literature on dysphagia, this type of stricture is rare, and surgical myotomy is rarely carried out to correct it. Esophageal motility problems are only indirectly a neurological problem, since the esophageal muscle is smooth muscle, not controlled voluntarily by the patient. Some peripheral neuropathies, such as diabetic neuropathy, can affect the contractions of the smooth muscle of the esophagus, limiting the patient's ability to swallow the bolus and have it continue down the esophagus.

DIFFERENTIAL DIAGNOSIS

The first question to be addressed is whether or not the patient has dysphagia, based on the symptoms of difficulty swallowing, choking, coughing while eating or drinking, nasal regurgitation, or the less obvious problems of recurrent aspiration pneumonia, weight loss from malnutrition, or dehydration.

The second question is whether or not the dysphagia is neurogenic. Structural problems such as esophageal stricture usually cause dysphagia for solids only, whereas most neurogenic dysphagias involve liquids. The neurologist then looks for associated symptoms and signs of neurological disorders associated with dysphagia.

Muscle diseases associated with dysphagia are usually obvious, because other muscles are weak. Most myopathies have to be at a severe stage before the bulbar muscles are affected. A few myopathies, such as oculopharyngeal dystrophy and progressive external opthalmoplegia, affect swallowing early. These patients also have a weak voice with flaccid dysarthria, and in both oculopharyngeal dystrophy and progressive external ophthalmoplegia the eyelids are ptotic, and there may be weakness of the extraocular muscles.

Neuromuscular junction disorders include myasthenia gravis, botulism, and the Lambert-Eaton myasthenic syndrome. These disorders are discussed in Chap. 35. Myasthenia usually begins with weakness in the eyelids and eye muscles, as well as the face, but dysphagia can be a relatively early sign. As with all of the other weakness symptoms in myasthenia, dysphagia worsens with repeated exertion of the swallowing muscles and improves after rest. This fatiguing can be tested at the bedside by having the patient hold the eyes elevated or the arms elevated for 60 seconds. Botulism also causes swallowing difficulty prominently, but the facial and eye muscles are usually also weak, the voice is affected, and there are autonomic signs such as dilatation of the pupils. Botulism is a medical emergency and should be diagnosed promptly. A recent, rare cause of dysphagia is muscle weakness resulting from injection of botulinum toxin (Botox) into the muscles of the neck for treatment of dystonia. These patients lack the other features of botulism. Lambert-Eaton myasthenic syndrome usually affects the limb muscles predominantly, and dysphagia is an uncommon problem in this rare disease.

The next level of the neuraxis is the peripheral nerves and the cranial nerves IX and X, involved in swallowing. Most neuropathies, as discussed in Chap. 33, affect mainly the distal parts of the limbs. When a neuropathy is severe, the bulbar muscles can be involved, but this is relatively rare in most neuropathies. A few neuropathies are more selective in their involvement. Acute inflammatory, demyelinating polyneuropathy, or Guillain-Bafre syndrome, can cause a rapid ascending paralysis that can involve muscles of breathing, muscles of swallowing and speaking, and even nerves innervating the face and eyes. Feeding a patient with Guillain-Bafre syndrome could result in aspiration pneumonia.

Disorders of the motor neuron, or anterior horn cell, can cause dysphagia. Motor neuron disease, or amyotrophic lateral sclerosis (ALS), usually begins in the arms, but occasionally the first symptoms of the disease involve the bulbar muscles, with dysphagia and dysarthria. In a clinic for unexplained dysphagia, a relatively common cause is bulbar ALS. Even in patients with more typical ALS beginning in the arms, the weakness spreads over time, and dysphagia can develop later in the illness. As in any neuro-logical disease, patients should be screened with at least a few history questions, if not a swallowing test, when dysphagia becomes a likely possibility.

Brainstem disorders can produce dysphagia via involvement of the cranial nerves IX and X or the descending corticobulbar pathways. The corticobulbar fibers can also be affected in lesions of the cerebral hemispheres. The dysphagia is most likely to be symptomatic when the lesion is bilateral. Brainstem lesions associated with dysphagia include multiple sclerosis, brainstem strokes, and tumors. In the hemispheres, stroke is a common cause of acute dysphagia. Again, strokes are most commonly associated with dysphagia when there are bilateral strokes, but a unilateral stroke on either side can result in dysphagia. Bilateral strokes with dysphagia are also associated with the syndrome of pseudobulbar palsy, a combination of dysarthria, dysphagia, and emotional lability. Studies have shown that right hemisphere lesions are more likely to lead to *silent aspiration* and development of pneumonia without any complaint of dysphagia or choking, but left hemisphere strokes can produce this picture as well. Traumatic brain injuries also affect swallowing. Neurodegenerative disorders such as Parkinson's disease, progressive supranuclear palsy, and multisystem atrophy (see Chap. 27) frequently cause dysarthria, dysphagia, and silent aspiration, especially at advanced stages of the illnesses. In Alzheimer's disease, some patients lose weight simply because they lose the desire to eat, or because the anticholinesterase medications reduce appetite, but occasionally dysphagia and aspiration occur at advanced stages of Alzheimer's disease.

LABORATORY AND RADIOLOGICAL INVESTIGATION

Diagnosis of dysphagia begins with a careful history and physical examination, including inspection of the oral cavity and pharynx, testing of the gag reflex, and sometimes even a bedside swallowing test, in which the examiner observes the patient sitting up and swallowing 3 ounces of water. Choking, gurgling, or inability to swallow the liquid are noted. The physician then asks the patient to clear his or her throat and speak, to make sure that the voice is not "wet" after the swallow. Syndromes of muscle weakness from myopathy, neuromuscular junction disease, peripheral nerve involvement, anterior horn cell, or central nervous system involvement all restrict the excursion of the soft palate and affect the gag reflex. The gag reflex is reduced in peripheral nerve and muscle diseases, increased with central nervous system disorders, but there may be a period of depression of the reflex after an acute injury such as a stroke. Fatigue of muscles may be demonstrated in myasthenia gravis.

If there is doubt about swallowing, a specific test of swallowing should be ordered. The most common test is the videofluoroscopy of swallowing or *modified barium swallow*, performed in many medical centers by speech/language pathologists and radiologists. In this procedure, a videotape is made of the swallowing structures during attempted swallowing of liquid barium, barium in a thick paste, and barium spread on crackers. The study can identify oral and pharyngeal problems, as well as penetration into the vallecula and frank aspiration of material into the trachea. Some centers use cineradiography to evaluate swallowing. Recently, a few swallowing experts have recommended screening tests using inhalation of a caustic substance such as tartaric acid, to see if the patient would manifest the appropriate choking response. Patients who fail to cough or choke are considered to be at risk of aspiration. This procedure has not been approved by Food and Drug Administration (FDA).

As mentioned earlier, it is incumbent on the neurologist to identify patients who are at risk of aspiration, malnutrition, and dehydration in the course of neurological disorders and to evaluate the patients at bedside or refer them for swallowing studies. This is especially true in stroke patients. In most stroke centers, patients are screened by either a speech/language pathologist or given the 3-ounce swallow test described above, before an oral diet is ordered. Such vigilance has greatly reduced the frequency of aspiration pneumonia after stroke. Similar vigilance should attend the management of patients with brain tumors and neurodegenerative conditions such as ALS and Parkinson's disease.

TREATMENT

As in any neurological condition, the first obligation of the neurologist is to make a diagnosis and to treat those neurological disorders that have specific medical treatments. Perhaps the best example is myasthenia gravis, where institution of anticholinesterase medications, steroids, intravenous immunoglobulin, or plasmapheresis may result in complete resolution of the swallowing difficulty.

In disorders that cannot be treated effectively, the neurologist should identify dysphagia before it results in aspiration pneumonia, malnutrition, or dehydration. The videofluoroscopy of swallowing not only serves to diagnose the swallowing problem, but it often helps the speech pathologist counsel the patient in techniques to improve swallowing and prevent aspiration. If the dysphagia is mainly for liquids, the diet can be modified to include only thickened liquids, and very dry foods such as crackers and biscuits should be avoided. Some patients benefit from a change in position, such as turning the head to the weak side. Patients are usually told to sit fully upright before attempting to swallow and to take a small bite, swallow, cough, then swallow again before proceeding to the next bite (the *supraglottic swallow* technique). Some patients benefit from using a straw for liquids, others do worse with a straw. All of these measures help to prevent aspiration pneumonia. As mentioned above, myotomy of the cricopharyngeus muscle is occasionally carried out to relieve dysphagia, but this operation is being done much more rarely than in the past. Electrical stimulation of the swallowing muscles, through the anterior neck, is being carried out in rehabilitation hospitals; evidence for the efficacy of these techniques is limited at present. For those patients who cannot swallow safely, a feeding tube is the best way to ensure preservation of hydration and nutrition. Nasogastric tubes are used only briefly, and percutaneous endoscopic gastrostomy (PEG) tubes are often preferred in patients who are likely to have dysphagia for more than a few days. Parenteral nutrition such as TPN (total parenteral nutrition) is usually reserved for those patients with anatomic problems precluding a feeding tube.

COURSE AND PROGNOSIS

The course of dysphagia parallels the prognosis of the underlying neurological condition. In stroke and traumatic brain injury, the dysphagia is usually temporary, and feeding tubes are used only until the patient regains the ability to swallow safely. In more chronic conditions such as ALS and other neurodegenerative diseases, or in patients in coma or persistent vegetative state after strokes or brain injuries, the decision to maintain the patient's nutrition with a PEG tube becomes an ethical and philosophical decision about maintaining life. This issue is discussed briefly in Chap. 37.

KEY REFERENCES

DePippo KL, Holas MA, Reding MJ, et al. Dysphagia therapy following stroke: a controlled trial. *Neurology* 1994;44:1655–1660.

Freed ML, Freed L, Chatburn RL, et al. Electrical stimulation for swallowing disorders caused by stroke. *Respir Care* 2001;46:466–74.

Garon BR, Engle M, Ormiston C. Reliability of the 3-oz water swallow test utilizing cough reflex as sole indicator of aspiration. *J Neuro Rehab* 1995;9:139–143.

Hamdy S, Rothwell JC, Singh KD, et al. The cortical topography of human swallowing musculature in health and disease. *Nature Medicine* 1996;2:1217–1224.

Horner J, Massey EW. Silent aspiration following stroke. *Neurology* 1988;38:317–319.

Kirshner HS. Causes of neurogenic dysphagia. *Dysphagia* 1989;3:184–188.

Martino R, Foley N, Bhogal S, et al. Dysphagia after stroke. Incidence, diagnosis, and pulmonary complications. *Stroke* 2005;36:2763.

Robbins J, Levine RL. Swallowing after unilateral stroke of the cerebral cortex: preliminary experience. *Dysphagia* 1988;3:11–17.

DELIRIUM AND
ENCEPHALOPATHY

INTRODUCTION

Delirium is one of the most dramatic syndromes in neurology. Delirious patients become acutely "confused", often agitated, disoriented, and unable to pay attention, form memories, or reason appropriately. Formerly, the term *delirium* was reserved for an agitated, hyperactive state, whereas the term *encephalopathy* was used for confusional states in which the level of consciousness was normal or depressed. Currently, no distinction is made between these two conditions. In fact, the following terms are all more or less synonymous: delirium, encephalopathy, acute confusional state, and toxic psychosis. A unifying definition, taken from Lipowski, is: "a transient disorder of cognition or attention, one accompanied by disturbances of the sleep-wake cycle and psychomotor behavior." Delirium, like dementia, involves multiple cognitive functions, including attention, memory, reasoning, language, and executive function. In contrast to dementia, delirium typically comes on more acutely or subacutely, and it tends to fluctuate more from hour to hour and day to day. Delirium also involves alterations in level of consciousness, either agitation and hypervigilance or drowsiness, disturbed perception (hallucinations, delusions), psychomotor abnormalities (restlessness, agitation), and autonomic nervous system hyperactivity (tachycardia, hypertension, fever, diaphoresis, tremor). All of these phenomena are relatively uncommon in dementing diseases.

Delirium is an extremely common clinical problem in the hospital. An estimated 30–50% of hospitalized elderly people become delirious, amounting to an overall incidence of about 10% of all hospitalizations. Delirium increases morbidity and mortality for any hospitalization, and the cost to society is enormous.

CLINICAL PRESENTATION: SYMPTOMS AND SIGNS

The clinical features of delirium are very distinctive. There is often a pro-drome of anxiety, restlessness, drowsiness or insomnia, and vivid dreams. As frank delirium supervenes, the patient may become either agitated or drowsy, with disruption of the normal sleep-wake cycle. Often, the confusion worsens late in the day, a phenomenon termed *sundowning* . A key to the disorder is a disruption of attention; patients become easily distracted by environmental stimuli and cannot focus on a conversation or thought process. Patients often become frankly disoriented and have difficulty forming new memories. Among language functions, the ability to write is especially sensitive to delirium. Altered perceptions are common, and many of these are the basis for the hallucinations seen in delirium; for example, an IV line may be misinterpreted as a snake. Abnormal emotional states, especially fear or anger, are common in delirium. Reduced insight and judgment are common, and some patients have paranoid ideation. As mentioned above, patients may have either increased or decreased level of consciousness, but they are likely to manifest motor restlessness or agitation, and autonomic hyperactivity, such as tachycardia, fever, sweating, tremor, hypertension, flushing, pupillary dilatation, and piloerection.

Studies of delirium have shown that there are predictable risk factors for delirium in hospitalized patients. Table 13-1 shows risk factors for delirium, adapted from two recent studies. Age is a risk factor, delirium being common in older patients. Impaired cognition, or Mini Mental State Examination (MMSE) less than 24, is a potent predictor of delirium. Presence of a fracture, use of a bladder catheter, infection, specific medications such as anticholinergic and sedative medications, and surgery are all risk factors for delirium.

Table 13-1 **Risk Factors for Delirium**

Age >80
Prior cognitive impairment, brain disease, or vision/hearing loss
Fracture on admission
Symptomatic infection
Stress, environmental changes
Neuroleptic, anticholinergic, sedative medications
Restraints, bladder catheter, surgery

DIFFERENTIAL DIAGNOSIS

Delirium must first be distinguished from syndromes of psychosis, dementia, and focal neurological abnormalities. Once a diagnosis of delirium is established, the medical cause or factors should be sought and corrected, where possible.

PSYCHOSIS

Acute psychosis, as seen in schizophrenia or bipolar affective disorder, usually occurs earlier in life than delirium, typically before age 40. Psychosis only rarely produces disorientation to time or place, as is often seen in delirium; psychotic patients may furnish abnormal thought content in answering questions, but they can almost always supply the correct date and place. For example, a psychotic patient may correctly identify the name of the hospital and the date but give a totally erroneous account of why he or she is there. Occasionally, psychotic patients provide a wrong personal identity, usually a famous person, a finding rarely seen in delirium. Likewise, the abnormal performance on tests of attention and memory seen in delirium are much less common in psychosis. Both disorders may produce hallucinations, but psychosis is more likely to involve auditory hallucinations, whereas delirium is more commonly associated with visual hallucinations. Patients with both psychosis and delirium may seem agitated or fearful, but patients with delirium are much more likely to have the autonomic disturbances of tachycardia, hypertension, and fever. In general, medical students should exercise caution in diagnosing psychosis in a patient who is frankly disoriented, has abnormal vital signs, decreased level of consciousness, or age over 40 years, without a prior history of psychosis.

DEMENTIA

Dementia, like delirium, represents a general confusional state. Dementia generally comes on much more gradually than delirium, and there is less fluctuation from day to day. In general, dementia is characterized principally by *negative* neurological signs, such as loss of attention, memory, language function, executive function, visuospatial function, and reasoning, whereas delirium is more likely to have *positive* symptoms such as agitation and autonomic hyperactivity. In fact, however, there is considerable overlap between delirium and dementia. Patients with dementia may develop acute delirium in response to metabolic stresses, medications, or even severe environmental changes. Dementia is a risk factor for the development of delirium, and the occurrence of delirium should prompt a search for causative factors.

FOCAL LESIONS

Some acute, focal lesions of the central nervous system cause a picture resembling delirium. The most common focal lesions associated with delirium are: (1) acute right temporoparietal lesions, as in strokes of the right middle cerebral artery territory; (2) unilateral or bilateral occipital lesions, often strokes in the posterior cerebral artery territory; (3) left temporoparietal lesions associated with Wernicke's aphasia; and (4) unilateral or bilateral frontal lesions.

ETIOLOGIES OF DELIRIUM

Many different medical etiologies can cause delirium. It is important for the student to form a differential diagnosis and search for a specific cause that can be treated. Table 13-2 lists some of the common causes of delirium. As mentioned above, some acute, focal lesions of the brain cause delirium. In the examples above, the diagnosis is usually straightforward, based on associated focal signs of the stroke or other process, and brain imaging studies such as computed tomography (CT) and magnetic resonance imaging (MRI) scans confirm the diagnosis. Seizures may be followed by confusion or delirium as a postictal state. Encephalitis or meningitis can cause an acute delirium; in the case of Herpes simplex encephalitis, there is often focal inflammation in the medial temporal lobes and orbitofrontal cortex.

Metabolic causes of delirium include hyper- or hyponatremia, hypercalcemia, hypo- or hypermagnesemia, and hyper- or hypoglycemia. Nutritional disorders include deficiencies of vitamins B_1, B_2 (pellagra) and B_{12}, and also general malnutrition and dehydration. Organ failure syndromes include uremia, hepatic encephalopathy, chronic respiratory insufficiency, and also hypoxemia related to pulmonary emboli, congestive heart

Table 13-2 **Etiologies of Delirium**

Metabolic/endocrine/toxic/nutritional
Drug/withdrawal
Infections: CNS, systemic
Neoplasms
Acute hydrocephalus
Trauma
Vascular: strokes, hemorrhage, vasculitis
Seizures/postictal state
Postoperative

failure, hypotension, or cardiac arrhythmia. Rare metabolic conditions such as porphyria or urea cycle abnormalities can cause delirium. Endocrine dis turbances associated with delirium include hypo- or hyperthyroidism, Addison's disease (adrenal insufficiency), hyperparathyroidism, and diabetic states such as ketoacidosis or nonketotic hyperglycemia. Many medications can induce delirium, including sedatives, tranquilizers, anticholinergics, and even antihistamines such as cimetidine. Elderly patients are more likely to develop delirium under the effects of medications, and multiple drugs used by these patients are often the combined culprits. Drugs of abuse (cocaine, amphetamines, and psychedelic drugs) can cause acute delirium. Withdrawal from alcohol or benzodiazepines, and acute alcoholic intoxication, are causes of delirium. Delirium tremens, or acute alcohol withdrawal, has long served as a model for the symptoms and signs of delirium. Chemical toxins such as insecticides, heavy metals (especially lead), and organophosphates can cause delirium. X-ray contrast agents can be associated with delirium, though the newer, ionic contrast agents are less likely to cause delirium than older contrast media.

Infections are often associated with delirium, especially central nervous system infections such as encephalitis, meningitis, or brain abscess. In elderly patients, even non-CNS infections such as urinary tract infections or aspiration pneumonia can decompensate an apparently mentally intact person into a delirious state. Families are often amazed when informed that this was the cause of the problem. Septicemias often produce acute delirium. Bacterial endocarditis with emboli to the brain is another etiology of delirium.

Neoplasms can cause delirium by a variety of mechanisms. The tumor itself may arise in an area associated with delirium, such as a frontal or medial temporal lobe. The tumor may provoke seizures, with postictal delirium. The tumor may induce a metabolic disturbance, such as hyponatremia related to the syndrome of inappropriate secretion of antidiuretic hormone. Drugs such as chemotherapeutic agents or radiation therapy can induce mental changes. Finally, the paraneoplastic syndrome of limbic encephalitis is associated with a subacute delirium or dementia; the syndrome resembles Herpes simplex encephalitis, though the time course is usually more gradual.

LABORATORY AND RADIOLOGICAL INVESTIGATION

Since the causes of delirium are so legion, the investigation of the patient must be thorough. We generally start with a detailed history, specifically with regard to past medical problems, medications (or medications that might have been stopped recently, or withdrawn from), or toxic substance exposures. A review of the patient's current medications should be a starting point. On a single week on the neurology consult service I saw a case of delirium related to withdrawal from customary use of alprazolam in an elderly lady after a total hip replacement, and another in a postoperative patient after lung resection for carcinoma whose usual dose of lorazepam was 0.5 mg, and an unwitting house officer had ordered 5 mg.

The laboratory studies needed to assess a delirious patient follow from the differential diagnosis just discussed. These are listed in Table 13-2. Routine electrolytes, renal functions, glucose, calcium and magnesium, and liver function tests detect many metabolic causes of delirium. If drugs or toxins are suspected, a urine drug screen or assay for heavy metals is appropriate. For infectious causes, a complete blood count (CBC) and differential, often urinalysis and culture, blood cultures, and chest x-ray may be diagnostic. Primary central nervous system infections such as meningitis or encephalitis require a lumbar puncture, usually preceded by a brain imaging study such as computed tomography (CT) or magnetic resonance imaging (MRI) scan. The brain imaging study will also bring out structural causes of delirium such as strokes, brain tumors, abscesses, and subdural hematomas.

TREATMENT

The principal treatment of delirium involves identification and elimination of causative factors, such as those listed above. If patients become so agitated that their health is threatened, or if they endanger others, sedative medications are necessary. The benzodiazepines have long been known to calm down patients with delirium tremens from alcohol withdrawal, and a similar effect is seen in delirium related to withdrawal from other benzodiazepines or barbiturates. Antipsychotic agents such as haloperidol have an immediate tranquilizing effect, particularly when administered parenterally, but these drugs cause extrapyramidal side effects in elderly patients, and there is also risk of autonomic changes such as hypotension. Delirium in elderly, demented patients often responds to atypical antipsychotic agents such as olanzepine, risperidone, or quetiapine (see Chap. 14), but recent warnings about the cardiovascular risk of these drugs should be taken into account. Finally, controlled studies have shown that the environment in the hospital room or intensive care unit has a major influence on the development of delirium. Maintenance of clear day-night differences in noise level and lighting, adequate sleep, use of glasses and hearing aids to avoid perceptual deprivation, and frequent orienting stimuli help reduce the incidence of delirium and also shorten hospitalizations.

COURSE AND PROGNOSIS

As compared to other hospitalized patients, delirious patients have increased mortality and longer hospital stays. A majority of patients recover from delirium, often over a period of days to weeks. Many patients recover back to their normal baselines, though there remains a risk of recurrent delirium if the patient again becomes ill or requires hospitalization or surgery. Occasionally, patients who recover from delirium are left with a mild dementia.

KEY REFERENCES

Boyer EW, Shannon W. The serotonin syndrome. *N Engl J Med* 2005;352:1112–1120.

Carney MWP, Chary TKN, Robotis P, et al. Ganser syndrome and its management. *Brit J Psychiat* 1987;151:697–700.

Daniel WF, Crovitz HF, Weiner RD. Neuropsychological aspects of disorientation. *Cortex* 1987;23:169–187.

Devinsky O, Bear D, Volpe BT. Confusional states following posterior cerebral artery infarction. *Arch Neurol* 1988;45:160–163.

Ely EW, Inouye SK, Bernard GR, et al. Delirium in mechanically ventilated patients. Validity and reliability of the confusion assessment method for the intensive care unit (CAM-ICU). *JAMA* 2001;286:2703–2710.

Ely EW, Shintani A, Truman B, et al. Delirium as a predictor of mortality in mechanically ventilated patients in the intensive care unit. *JAMA* 2004;291:1753–1762.

Ely EW, Truman B, Shintani A, et al. Monitoring sedation status over time in ICU patients. Reliability and validity of the Richmond Agitation-Sedation Scale (RASS). *JAMA* 2003;289:2983–2391.

Gootjes EC, Wijdicks EFM, McClelland RL. Postoperative stupor and coma. *Mayo Clin Proc* 2005;80:350–354.

Inouye SK. Delirium in older persons. *New Engl J Med* 2006;354:1157–65.

Inouye SK, Bogardus ST, Charpentier PA, et al. A multicomponent intervention to prevent delirium in hospitalized older patients. *JAMA* 1999;340:669–676.

Inouye SK, Charpentier PA. Precipitating factors for delirium in hospitalized elderly persons. Predictive model and interrelationship with baseline vulnerability. *JAMA* 1996;275:852–857.

Kirshner HS. Delirium and Acute Confusional States. Chapter 14 in Kirshner HS. Behavioral Neurology. Practical Science of Mind and Brain. Boston, MA: Butterworth Heinemann; 2002, p 307–324.

Kumral E, Ozturk O. Delusional state following acute stroke. *Neurology* 2004;62: 110–113.

Lawlor PG, Fainsinger RL, Bruera ED. Delirium at the end of life. Critical issues in clinical practice and research. *JAMA* 2000;284:2427–2429.

Lewis SW. Brain imaging in a case of Capgras' syndrome. *Brit J Psychiat* 1987;150:117–121.

Lipowski ZJ. Delirium (acute confusional states). *JAMA* 1987;258:1789–1792.

Marcantonio ER, Goldman L, Orav EJ, et al. The association of intraoperative factors with the development of postoperative delirium. *Am J Med* 1998;105:380–384.

Marcantonio ER, Juarez G, Goldman L, et al. The relationship of postoperative delirium with psychoactive medications. *JAMA* 1994;272:1518–1522.

Newman MF, Kirchner JL, Phillips-Bute B, et al. Longitudinal assessment of neurocognitive function after coronary artery bypass surgery. *N Engl J Med* 2001;344:395–402.

Packard RC. Delirium. *Neurologist* 2001;7:327–340.

Rummans TA, Evans JM, Krahn LE, Fleming KC. Delirium in elderly patients: evaluation and management. *Mayo Clin Proc* 1995;70:989–998.

Schor JD, Levkoff SE, Lipsitz LA, et al. Risk factors for delirium in hospitalized elderly. *JAMA* 1992;267:827–831.

DEMENTIAS

INTRODUCTION

Dementia is defined as a loss of cognitive function, usually involving memory and at least one other cognitive function, such as aphasia, apraxia, agnosia, or executive dysfunction, sufficient to cause interference with normal functioning. In contrast to delirium, dementia is defined by losses of cognitive function, more than by active phenomena such as alteration of consciousness, positive psychiatric symptoms, and autonomic dysfunction, as in delirium. Dementia is generally a more chronic process, with less variation from day to day. Recent reviews of dementia, however, have pointed out that dementia is not just a syndrome of impaired cognition, but one that also affects activities of daily living and personality, mood, and behavior.

CLINICAL PRESENTATION: SYMPTOMS AND SIGNS

We often think of dementia as a general deterioration of brain function, usually occurring in an elderly person. In fact, like all neurodegenerative diseases, dementias are very selective in the neuronal populations that degenerate, and the symptoms and signs are likewise specific. The prototype of a dementing illness is Alzheimer's disease, which has a predilection for neurons of the association cortex, the hippocampus and neighboring structures, and the deep frontal nuclei, such as the nucleus basalis of Meynert. The resulting symptoms and signs almost always involve short-term memory; at first, more remote memory and general information are preserved. If short-term memory is the only deficit, and the patient is not yet disabled, the diagnosis is called *mild cognitive impairment*. Such patients may progress to full-blown dementia over a period of a few years, but some remain nondisabled for many years. As dementia worsens, however, other deficits ensue. Insight and judgment are usually affected early. Many patients have language deficits, especially loss of recall of names. Some patients have apraxia, involving loss of the ability to use familiar tools and appliances. Some have deficiencies in right hemisphere functioning such as difficulty remembering

Table 14-1 **Warning Signs of Early Dementia**

Memory loss that affects job skills
Difficulty performing familiar tasks
Problems with language
Disorientation to time and place
Decreased judgment
Problems with abstract thinking
Misplacing objects
Changes in mood or behavior
Changes in personality
Loss of initiative

Source: Adapted from AAN Practice Guideline, 2001.

familiar routes or recognizing family members. Almost all have impaired "executive functions," or loss of the ability to plan multistep tasks and organize goal-directed behaviors. Primary motor and sensory areas of the brain are not affected by most dementing illnesses, such that patients usually have normal strength, coordination, gait, and sensation. An exception to the rule that sensory functions are preserved is the early loss of smell in many patients with Alzheimer's disease.

The American Academy of Neurology has published a practice guideline concerning the early diagnosis of dementia. This guideline emphasizes early warning symptoms and signs; these are shown, in slightly adapted form, in Table 14-1. Note that many of the items involve memory loss; one item each has to do with language and praxis, and the last three items reflect abnormal mood, behavior, and personality.

DIFFERENTIAL DIAGNOSIS

First, dementia must be distinguished from other conditions that mimic it. These include depression, delirium, and focal neurological lesions.

DEPRESSION

Depression can sometimes look like dementia, in that depressed patients often pay poor attention, fail to remember what they are told, and withdraw into themselves, with less social interaction. In the past, emphasis was placed on *depressive pseudodementia*. Currently, however, depression is rather considered a contributing factor in the disability of a demented patient, and a treatable factor at that. Patients with depression have a true, not a *pseudo* memory loss. In addition, patients in the earliest stages of dementias such as Alzheimer's disease often have enough insight to suffer a reactive depression, and treatment of the mood disorder may improve the patients' functioning.

DELIRIUM

Delirium is another syndrome resembling dementia. As discussed in Chap. 13, delirium involves impaired cognitive functions, like dementia, but delirium is usually more acute in onset, more variable from hour to hour and day to day. In addition, positive psychiatric symptoms such as delusions and hallucinations are more common in delirium than in dementia, and alteration of consciousness and autonomic dysfunction are also more common in delirium. The distinction between delirium and dementia is not absolute; the two overlap. Dementia is a risk factor for the development of delirium, and a demented patient may become delirious with minor factors such as new drugs, infections including urinary tract infections, and even changes in the environment when a patient is hospitalized or moved to a nursing facility. Like depression, delirium can be considered a treatable factor in dementia, and the cause of the delirium should be assiduously sought.

FOCAL LESIONS

Focal brain lesions can also mimic dementia, especially those that cause increased intracranial pressure or hydrocephalus, such as brain tumors or subdural hematomas. Aphasia related to left hemisphere lesions may make it hard to test other cognitive functions. Lesions in the area of the left angular gyrus, in the parietal lobe, may mimic dementia by producing deficits in naming, reading, writing, constructional ability, and calculations. Frontal lobe lesions may affect cognitive function, behavior, and emotional state in ways resembling dementia.

There are many dementing illnesses. Some of the more common ones are listed in Table 14-2.

In this chapter, we shall describe features of some of the specific dementias other than Alzheimer's disease, which will be discussed in Chap. 26, and Parkinson's disease and related disorders, presented in Chap. 27. Perhaps the most important concept is the identification of "treatable dementias." This should be the first goal of diagnosis, since the dementia may be reversed with proper treatment, or at least further progression can be prevented. The principal, treatable causes of dementia are listed in Table 14-3.

The metabolic and toxic syndromes listed in Table 14-2 generally present more as delirium than dementia, with a more acute course, more disturbance

Table 14-2 **Dementing Diseases (Medical)**

1. **Metabolic, nutritional, endocrine, toxic disorders**
   a. Metabolic disorders
      1. Hyponatremia, hypocalcemia
      2. Renal, hepatic, pulmonary failure, dialysis dementia
   b. Nutritional disorders (pernicious anemia, pellagra, thiamine deficiency)
   c. Endocrinopathies (hypothyroidism, hyperthyroidism, Hashimoto's encephalopathy, Cushing's, hyperparathyroidism)
   d. Toxic disorders
      1. Heavy metals, chemicals
      2. Drug encephalopathies, polypharmacy
      3. Alcoholism
      4. Marchiafava-Bignami syndrome
2. **Infections**
   a. Neurosyphilis
   b. Chronic meningitis (bacterial, fungal, brucella, TB, sarcoidosis)
   c. Parasitic diseases, e.g., cysticercosis
   d. Viral encephalitis
   e. Subacute sclerosing panencephalitis (SSPE)
   f. Progressive multifocal leukoencephalopathy (PML)
   g. Creutzfeldt-Jakob disease
   h. Acquired immunodeficiency syndrome (AIDS)
3. **Vascular diseases**
   a. Multiinfarct dementia, large infarcts, lacunar state
   b. Binswanger's disease
   c. Cholesterol emboli
   d. Collagen vascular diseases
   e. Arteriovenous malformation
   f. Subacute diencephalic angioencephalopathy
4. **Neoplasms**
   a. Mass lesions, increased intracranial pressure, hydrocephalus
   b. Multiple metastases
   c. Meningeal carcinomatosis
   d. Chemotherapy, radiation effects
5. **Normal pressure hydrocephalus**
6. **Neurodegenerative diseases**
   a. Alzheimer's disease
   b. Pick's disease and frontotemporal dementia
   c. Parkinson's disease and Lewy body dementia
   d. Other rare dementing illnesses

Table 14-3 **Treatable Causes of Dementia**

Diseases simulating dementia
Depression
Mass lesion
  Tumor
  Subdural hematoma
  Abscess
Delirium
  Metabolic encephalopathy
  Toxic or drug-induced encephalopathy
  Miscellaneous (see Chap. 13)
Miscellaneous treatable dementing diseases
  Vitamin B_{12} deficiency
  Endocrinopathies
    Hypothyroidism
    Hyperthyroidism
    Cushing's syndrome
    Hyperparathyroidism
Infections
  Chronic meningitis
  Syphilis
  Cysticercosis
Normal pressure hydrocephalus

of the level of consciousness, and more association with active psychiatric and autonomic changes than most dementias, as described in Chap. 13. Occasionally, they present slowly enough to mimic a dementing illness, and for this reason screening laboratory tests should always be carried out as part of the initial diagnosis of dementia.

Alcoholism is of special interest because it has been a rich source of neurological syndromes. Acute alcoholic intoxication produces an encephalopathy, usually associated with ataxia and slurred speech. Alcohol withdrawal produces the classic encephalopathy, delirium tremens, with tremor, confusion, and hallucinations, as well as autonomic changes. Chronic alcohol use is associated with brain atrophy, and perhaps with dementia. Perhaps the most striking chronic syndrome related to alcoholism, however, is the Wernicke-Korsakoff syndrome, related to thiamine deficiency. This syndrome can present with acute symptoms of nystagmus or extraocular muscle palsies, ataxia, and severe amnesia, or loss of short-term memory function, sometimes associated with confabulation, or "making up" answers to questions. The Wernicke-Korsakoff syndrome can result in a permanent loss of short-term memory, though technically the patient is not demented, since mental operations other than memory may remain normal.

The infectious causes of dementia, listed in Table 14-2, can include meningitis, encephalitis, and brain abscess. A dementing disease only recently placed in the infectious category is Creutzfeldt-Jakob disease. This is a rare disorder, with incidence figures of 1–2 per million people, world-wide. The disease often begins with cognitive loss, but other presentations are well documented, including ataxia, myoclonus, seizures, or blindness. The disease progresses rapidly, with most patients living less than 6 months from the first symptom. Myoclonic jerks, seizures, and periodic discharges on electroencephalogram (EEG) are characteristic, though none of these symptoms occurs in all patients or at all stages of the disease. Computed tomography (CT) scans have been of little help, but abnormal signal in the deep nuclei on magnetic resonance imaging (MRI) has recently been described, including bright signal on diffusion weighted imaging (DWI) resembling stroke. A spinal fluid protein, termed the 14-3-3 protein, may be helpful in some cases. The disease has no known treatment and is uniformly fatal. What was thought to be a neurodegenerative disease has been shown definitively to be an infectious disorder, carried by a unique pathogen called a *prion*, or proteinaceous infectious particle. The disease can be spread by tissue from a patient, as in corneal transplants, growth hormone made from ground up pituitary gland, dural transplants, or even via instruments such as depth electrodes. This contagious risk has led to great fear of the disease, though the agents do not appear to spread except by direct tissue exposure, and contamination can be inactivated by use of simple bleach (Chlorox). Other cases appear to be hereditary.

Vascular dementia

Vascular dementia is a complex topic. Strokes destroy brain tissue, and the presence of even single strokes, let alone multiple ones, can lead to dementia. Several subtypes of vascular dementia have been described (Table 14-2 lists only a few of the causes). In general, the patient with vascular dementia should have a history of stroke-like acute events, or step-wise rather than gradual deterioration of mental function. The presence of stroke risk factors such as hypertension, diabetes, and hyperlipidemia, the finding of focal neurological deficits on exam, and, perhaps most importantly, evidence of infarctions on a brain imaging study, support the diagnosis of vascular dementia. An infarct means a dark area on a CT brain scan or T1-weighted MRI; the T2-bright *deep white matter ischemic disease* seen on many MRI scans does not automatically qualify the patient as having a vascular dementia. Many patients have a combination of strokes and Alzheimer's disease; this combination is difficult to distinguish from pure vascular dementia. Several diagnostic scales have been proposed to diagnose vascular dementia, a few of which are cited in the references at the end of this chapter.

Brain tumors

Neoplasms, like strokes, can cause dementia by local tissue destruction, edema and effects at a distance, secondary infections, "remote effects of cancer" (referred to as *paraneoplastic syndromes*), and also via treatment effects (radiation damage, leukoencephalopathy from some chemotherapeutic agents). The disease *limbic encephalitis* is a paraneoplastic syndrome often presenting with acute delirium or dementia, with changes in the medial temporal lobes on MRI resembling those of Herpes simplex encephalitis.

Normal pressure hydrocephalus

Normal pressure hydrocephalus (NPH), first described by Hakim and Adams in the 1960s, presents as a triad of mental slowing or dementia, gait disturbance, and urinary incontinence. The patient is initially just slow mentally, but over time a true dementia ensues. The gait disorder often appears as if the patient has just forgotten how to walk; the patient stands, with the feet appearing glued to the ground, or with an initial hesitancy and initiation of very small, slow steps. The diagnosis depends on the clinical triad of cognitive dysfunction, gait difficulty, and urinary incontinence, together with the presence of enlarged ventricles on brain imaging studies, out of proportion to any cortical atrophy or enlargement of the cortical subarachnoid space. Some neurologists perform a diagnostic lumbar puncture to measure the opening pressure, and also to remove a large volume of spinal fluid and see if this brings about any temporary improvement. This trial of cerebrospinal fluid (CSF) drainage is of debatable usefulness, as are other proposed tests such as artificial spinal fluid infusion tests or isotope cisternograms. Figure 14-1 shows an MRI scan of a patient with NPH.

The key issue is whether patients with NPH will improve with a ventriculoperitoneal shunt, to drain CSF out of the ventricles and into the abdomen, thereby reducing the pressure within the ventricles. Many published series have indicated success rates in the 50–60% range, rarely higher. Currently, shunt manufacturers are advertising their products to the public, and interest in NPH as a treatable cause of dementia is at a high point.

Neurodegenerative dementias

The most common dementing illness is Alzheimer's disease, which will be considered in Chap. 26. Related disorders such as frontotemporal dementia and Pick's disease will be discussed there as well. Another family of neurodegenerative disorders involves the combination of movement disorders and cognitive changes, including Parkinson's disease with dementia, Lewy body dementia, corticobasal degeneration, progressive supranuclear palsy, multisystem atrophy, Huntington's disease, and Wilson's disease. These disorders will be discussed in Chap. 27.

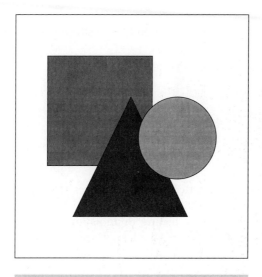

Figure 14-1   **MRI image of a patient with NPH** The scan shows enlarged ventricles, out of proportion to cortical atrophy. The patient had a good response to ventriculoperitoneal shunting.

LABORATORY AND RADIOLOGICAL INVESTIGATION

When considering the myriad of dementing diseases discussed in this chapter, the physician must consider the common clinical syndromes of dementia. The first step, of course, is the verification of dementia, as opposed to the differential diagnoses of delirium, depression, or focal brain lesion. A careful history and physical examination are essential, including a bedside mental status examination such as the Mini Mental State Examination (MMSE), preferably with clock drawing in addition. In doubtful cases, more detailed neuropsychological testing is advisable. A careful history of medical symptoms and diseases, medications, and toxic exposures is important.

In 2001, the American Academy of Neurology issued a practice guideline on the diagnosis of dementia, including a list of early warning signs (Table 14-1), and a list of recommended laboratory tests (Table 14-4).

Laboratory screening should always include routine blood testing including complete blood count, basic metabolic profile, liver function tests, thyroid function tests, vitamin B_{12} level, sedimentation rate, and if there is any clinical suspicion, a serological test for syphilis or HIV. Genetic tests such as apolipoprotein E4 genotyping and Tau protein levels in spinal fluid

Table 14-4 **Laboratory Tests Required for the Diagnosis of Dementia**

CBC, electrolytes, glucose, BUN/creat
LFT's, TFT's, ESR
B_{12} level
Depression screening
CT or MRI scan

are not routinely recommended. These can ethically be performed in a symptomatic patient for help with diagnosis, but they are rarely definitive. Most neurologists feel that genetic testing in an asymptomatic individual at risk for Alzheimer's disease is not justified, since there is no treatment at present. Likewise, a spinal tap is indicated only when the physician suspects a chronic infection such as meningitis, or the patient is being evaluated for normal pressure hydrocephalus (see above). A brain imaging test, CT or MRI scan, is always indicated in the diagnosis of dementia, not so much because it is helpful in diagnosing Alzheimer's disease, but because it serves to exclude other more treatable entities such as subdural hematoma, brain tumor, normal pressure hydrocephalus, and also to detect the presence of strokes. MRI scanning can sometimes be misleading in its sensitivity to deep white matter ischemic lesions, which do not exclude the diagnosis of Alzheimer's disease. Finally, functional brain imaging with single photon emission computed tomography (SPECT) or positron emission tomography (PET) scanning can be helpful, especially in difficult diagnostic cases. PET scanning for uptake of flurodeoxyglucose (FDG-PET) indicates areas of hypometabolism, often in the absence of major structural change on a CT or MRI scan. The most characteristic pattern in early Alzheimer's disease is a biparietal hypometabolism, later with addition of frontal and temporal hypometabolism. Fig. 14-2 shows a fairly typical PET scan from a patient with mild Alzheimer's disease (AD), showing the reduced metabolism in both parietal lobes. Other dementing diseases, such as frontotemporal dementia (see Chap. 26) typically show more focal areas of hypometabolism in the frontal or temporal lobes on one or both sides, in the absence of the characteristic biparietal changes seen in AD.

The difficult issues of cerebrovascular disease and dementia are best clarified by clinical history and examination, including the Hachinski index, a clinical scoring system for separating vascular dementia from Alzheimer's disease (Hachinksi et al. 1975), and examination of the CT or MRI scan for evidence of infarcts. The *subcortical* dementias are best evaluated clinically, by the combination of motor and cognitive changes. Normal pressure hydrocephalus is diagnosed by the clinical triad of dementia, gait disorder, and

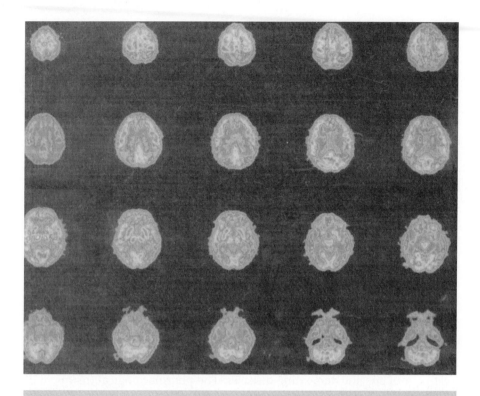

Figure 14-2 **PET scan from a patient with early Alzheimer's disease** Note the reduced glucose metabolism in both parietal lobes.

urinary incontinence, with confirmation of ventricular enlargement out of proportion to cortical atrophy on neuroradiological studies. Finally, the primary degenerative dementias, Alzheimer's and Pick's diseases, are diagnosed presumptively by the typical clinical evolution, absence of features of the other diseases, and normal laboratory tests except for the neuroradiological finding of cerebral atrophy. PET scanning is helpful in distinguishing these two degenerative dementias, showing the differential lobar involvement of biparietal hypometabolism in AD and frontal or temporal atrophy in Pick's disease or frontotemporal dementia. The National Institute of Neurological and Communicative Diseases and Stroke/Alzheimer's Disease and Related Disorders Associations (NINCDS/ADRDA) criteria for the diagnosis of presumed Alzheimer's are discussed in Chap. 26. Alzheimer's disease currently accounts for over half of the diagnosed cases of dementia, and mixed Alzheimer's disease and vascular dementia is the next most common type.

TREATMENT

The first goal of diagnosis of dementia is the identification of treatable causes, or treatable factors. Occasionally, a patient is diagnosed with a metabolic disorder such as hypothyroidism or vitamin B_{12} deficiency, and treatment of this disorder "cures" the dementia. Infections such as chronic fungal meningitis can be treated with antimicrobial agents. Patients with brain tumors such as large meningiomas can greatly benefit from surgery. Patients with normal pressure hydrocephalus can improve after shunting. Subdural hematomas can be drained. Unfortunately, the identification of a treatable cause of dementia occurs in a small minority of patients.

Depression is a major confounding factor in dementia. Rarely, a depressed patient may have *pseudodementia*, meaning that the cognitive dysfunction is cured by the treatment of depression. More often, patients with early dementia have enough insight to be depressed, and their cognitive function can improve somewhat, though not to normal, with antidepressant drug treatment. In general, I recommend a trial of antidepressant therapy if there is any reasonable suspicion of depression as a factor in the dementia. Further discussion of the behavioral and psychiatric management of patients with dementia will be presented in Chap. 26.

Once the treatable causes of dementia have been eliminated, and the issue of depression has been addressed, what remains is the very limited treatment of specific dementing diseases. The pharmacological treatment of Alzheimer's disease and frontotemporal dementia will be considered in Chap. 26. The dementia associated with Parkinson's disease and related syndromes is discussed in Chap. 27.

COURSE AND PROGNOSIS

The course of a dementing illness depends, of course, on the specific diagnosis. The treatable dementias may improve or resolve after treatment. Most other dementias are gradually progressive, at varying rates, to the point of total dependency. In the end, the patient depends on caregivers for administration of medications, even simple activities of daily living such as dressing, bathing, grooming, and even eating. Behavior changes also become more common in advanced dementias. End of life issues, such as whether to support nutrition with feeding tubes, often become relevant in late stages of dementing illnesses.

KEY REFERENCES

Consensus Conference. Differential diagnosis of dementing diseases. *JAMA* 1987;258:3411–3416.

Cummings JL. Alzheimer's disease. *N Engl J Med* 2004;351:56–67.

Erkinjuntti T, Sulkava R, Kovanen J, et al. Suspected dementia: evaluation of 323 consecutive referrals. *Acta Neurol Scand* 1987;76:359–364.

Hachinski VC, Iliff LD, Zilkha E, et al. Cerebral blood flow in dementia. Arch Neurol 1975;32:632–637. (This article includes the Hachinski ischemic score).

Kirshner HS. Mild cognitive impairment: To treat or not to treat. *Curr Neurol Neurosci Rep* 2005;5:455–457.

Knopman DS, Boeve BF, Petersen RC. Essentials of the proper diagnoses of mild cognitive impairment, dementia, and major subtypes of dementia. *Mayo Clin Proc* 2003;78:1290–1308.

Knopman DS, DeKosky ST, Cummings JL, et al. Practice parameter: diagnosis of dementia (an evidence-based review). *Neurology* 2001;56:1143–1153.

Larson EB, Reifler BV, Sumi SM, et al. Diagnostic tests in the evaluation of dementia. *Arch Intern Med* 1986;146:1917–1922.

Mayeux R, Stern Y, Rosen J, et al. Is subcortical dementia a recognizable clinical entity? *Ann Neurol* 1983;14:278–283.

Piccini C, Bracco L, Amaducci L. Treatable and reversible dementias: an update. *J Neurol Sci* 1998;153:172–81.

Prusiner SB. Shattuck lecture—neurodegenerative diseases and prions. *New Engl J Med* 2001;344:1516–1526.

Quinn J, Kaye J. The neurology of aging. *Neurologist* 2001;7:98–112.

APHASIA

INTRODUCTION

Aphasia is defined as an acquired loss of language function. Aphasias are common, occurring in about 20% of strokes, but also in other focal neurological disorders, such as traumatic brain injury, brain tumors, brain abscesses, and even in neurodegenerative diseases such as Alzheimer's disease. Even more important than its incidence, however, is the importance of language as a major factor in a person's quality of life. Language communication is a principal part of what makes us human, and what separates humans from lower animals. Historically, aphasia was also the first syndrome of focal cortical dysfunction to be localized in the brain, and it therefore played a major role in the development of our understanding of cerebral localization and brain function.

CLINICAL PRESENTATION: SYMPTOMS AND SIGNS

Aphasias can be categorized into several types based on the bedside language examination, sometimes supplemented by information about the localization of the lesion. There are eight classical aphasia syndromes. The aphasia syndromes and their features are shown in Table 15-1.

Broca's aphasia

Broca's aphasia is syndrome of nonfluent speech, with effortful speech productions, very short phrase length, and impaired repetition. Naming is also impaired, with long pauses for word finding, but patients do respond to cues such as the initial sound or phoneme of the correct word. Auditory comprehension is usually functional for simple communication such as following simple commands or engaging in conversations with friends and family members, but on more detailed testing there are deficits in the comprehension of complex syntax. Reading aloud is hesitant, and reading for meaning is often more impaired than auditory comprehension. Writing is affected at

Table 15-1 **Features of the Aphasias**

Feature	Broca	Wernicke	Global	Cond	Anomic	TCM	TCS	MTC
Speech	Non-fluent	Fluent, paraphasic	Non-fluent	Fluent	Fluent	Non-fluent	Fluent	Non-fluent
Naming	Poor	Paraphasic	Poor	Varies	Poor	Varies	Paraphasic	Poor
Repetition	Poor	Poor	Poor	Poor	Good	Good	Good	Good
Comp	Good	Poor	Poor	Good	Good	Good	Poor	Poor
Reading	Varies	Poor	Poor	Good	Good	Good	Poor	Poor
Writing	Poor	Paragraphic	Poor	Good	Good	Non-fluent	Paragraphic	Poor

least as severely as spontaneous speech. Very central to the language disorder of Broca's aphasia is a difficulty with syntax, on both the expressive and receptive sides of language. The loss of syntax in expressive speech is called *agrammatism*, and the speech productions are often referred to as *telegraphic*, meaning that the major nouns are present, but few if any syntactic words in-between. An example would be "Saturday, fishing, son", spoken instead of "on Saturday, I am going fishing with my son".

The lesion localization in Broca's aphasia usually involves the left inferior frontal cortex, anterior to the motor strip. Patients with lesions restricted to this area usually recover well, whereas patients with lasting Broca's aphasia usually have larger frontoparietal lesions. Figure 15-1 shows a magnetic resonance imaging (MRI) scan from a patient with Broca's aphasia.

Wernicke's aphasia

Wernicke's aphasia is a syndrome of fluent speech, with paraphasic substitutions (incorrect or nonexistent sounds or words), such that spoken productions may be totally unintelligible. In milder cases, the listener may have an idea where the sentence is going, but it goes off track in mid expression. Naming is also impaired; unlike Broca's aphasics, who struggle to get the word and benefit from cues, patients with Wernicke's aphasia often utter completely unrelated words, or nonexistent words. Repetition is usually impaired as well, and sometimes it is hard to get the patient's cooperation for this task. Auditory comprehension is impaired, partially or completely. Reading is usually impaired in a similar way to auditory comprehension. Occasional patients may read better than they comprehend spoken language, or vice versa. This difference in language modalities may be important in establishing communication with the patient, perhaps by writing messages to the patient rather than saying them. Writing in patients with Wernicke's

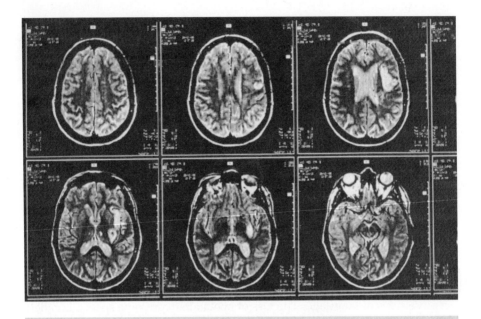

Figure 15-1 ***MRI scan from a patient with Broca's aphasia*** Lesion in left frontal cortex and subcortical white matter and insula. Patient had Broca's aphasia and apraxia of speech, recovered well over several weeks.

aphasia is usually well formed, but it is nonsensical, like their speech, and in addition spelling errors are apparent.

   Wernicke's aphasia is usually associated with a lesion of the left superior temporal region, sometimes extending into the left inferior parietal lobule. Figure 15-2 shows an MRI from a patient with an embolic stroke and Wernicke's aphasia.

Conduction aphasia

Conduction aphasia is a syndrome in which spontaneous speech is relatively fluent, though many patients produce sound substitutions (*literal paraphasic errors*, such as "ben" for "pen"), giving the speech a more hesitant, jerky quality than that of Wernicke's aphasia. Naming performance is variable, impaired in some patients. Auditory comprehension is preserved. The key feature of conduction aphasia is the severe impairment of repetition. Patients can produce long utterances but sometimes cannot repeat a single, multisyllabic word. Reading and writing are variably impaired; reading aloud and copying may seem to share the same deficiency as spoken repetition.

   The lesions of conduction aphasia classically spare both the frontal lobe Broca's area and the temporal lobe Wernicke's area, but disrupt connections

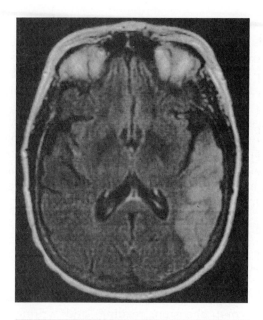

Figure 15-2 **MRI** (FLAIR sequence) showing L temporal infarction in a patient with acute Wernicke's aphasia after a cerebral embolus.

between the two. In case series, many cases of conduction aphasia have lesions in the left inferior parietal region, a few in the temporal lobe but sparing much of Wernicke's area. By the classic *disconnection syndrome* model first proposed by Wernicke, conduction aphasia represents a disconnection between an intact Wernicke's area, which subserves normal comprehension, and an intact Broca's area, which subserves fluent expression. Repetition requires the transmission of language information that has been decoded in Wernicke's area to Broca's area for repetition, via a white matter tract called the *arcuate fasciculus*. Other authorities have pointed out that the inability to keep a string of language symbols in the immediate memory stream could also explain the impaired repetition of conduction aphasia. The inferior parietal cortex is important in sequencing syllables in both expressive and receptive language functioning, and damage to this area may underlie some of the phenomena of conduction aphasia.

Conduction aphasia is less common than either Broca's or Wernicke's aphasia, representing less than 10% of aphasia cases. It has been theoretically important, however, in our understanding of language representation in the brain.

Global aphasia

Global aphasia is a *total aphasia*, in which speech is nonfluent, as in Broca's aphasia, but comprehension is also impaired, as in Wernicke's aphasia. All of the other bedside language functions, naming, reading, and writing, are also severely impaired. The patient is basically unable to communicate verbally at all.

The lesions associated with global aphasia are usually large, comprising much of the left frontal, temporal, and parietal lobes. Most patients also have dense right hemiparesis, right hemisensory loss, and often right hemianopsia. Very occasionally, a large lesion such as a stroke may affect both Broca's and Wernicke's area but spare the motor strip, producing global aphasia without hemiparesis.

Anomic aphasia

Anomic aphasia is a loss of ability to come up with specific names. The patient will pause, seeking to find a word, or will produce a circumduction (asked to name a key, the patient might respond, "You know, the thing you use to start your car"). Most patients have fluent speech and preserved repetition, auditory comprehension, reading, and writing (except for the inability to write names). This syndrome occurs to some extent in normal aging, but with some left hemisphere disorders the loss of naming ability is severe.

The lesions of anomic aphasia are more variable than those of the other aphasia syndromes. Lesions of the deep temporal lobe or parietal lobe may cause anomic aphasia, but anomia can also be the last stage of recovery in patients with aphasia related to frontal, temporal, or parietal lesions. Anomic aphasia is also seen in acute confusional states and in dementing illnesses such as Alzheimer's disease.

Transcortical aphasias

The last three of the eight traditional aphasia syndromes are transcortical motor, transcortical sensory, and mixed transcortical aphasia. These transcortical aphasias all feature preserved repetition or even an increased tendency to repeat (*echolalia*). The name *transcortical* derives from the concept that these aphasias result not from direct damage to the perisylvian language cortex, but rather from disruption of input from other areas of the association cortex into the language cortex.

Transcortical motor aphasia (TCMA) resembles Broca's aphasia, except that repetition is intact. The Russian neuropsychiatrist Luria called this variety of aphasia *dynamic aphasia*, implying that these patients have simply lost the dynamism to speak. Patients with TCMA will often speak a word or two, sometimes after a delay, and sometimes in a whispered voice. They may answer questions limited to one word answers, but may just remain silent when asked a question requiring a longer answer. By contrast, they may repeat long phrases or sentences without difficulty. Such patients can often produce names, comprehend sentences, read, and even write.

The lesions of transcortical motor aphasia usually involve the left frontal lobe, either anterior or deep to Broca's area, or in the medial frontal cortex, in the vicinity of the supplementary motor area.

Transcortical sensory aphasia resembles Wernicke's aphasia, except that repetition is intact. The patient speaks fluently, but with paraphasic errors, and comprehension is severely impaired.

Transcortical sensory aphasia may be seen with lesions near the junction of the temporal, parietal, and occipital lobes, or it may be seen in dementing conditions. It is an uncommon condition.

Mixed transcortical aphasia, also called the syndrome of isolation of the speech area, resembles global aphasia except for the ability to repeat, often excessively. There is no communication in the form of meaningful spoken expression, naming, comprehension, reading, or writing.

This syndrome has been described with lesions damaging much of the frontoparietal association cortex, as in large watershed infarctions associated with hypoxia. It has also been described later in the course of dementing illnesses such as Alzheimer's disease.

The eight classical aphasia syndromes, just discussed, do not include all of the clinically important language syndromes. Other aphasias have been described, and some of the more common ones will be discussed briefly.

Subcortical aphasias

Subcortical aphasias are named for their lesion localization rather than their language features, so the diagnosis cannot be made reliably without a brain imaging study. There are, however, some relatively specific patterns of language disorder with subcortical lesions. The *anterior subcortical aphasia syndrome* usually involves lesions of the head of the caudate nucleus, anterior limb of the internal capsule, and anterior putamen. The patient has a nonfluent aphasia resembling Broca's aphasia, but usually with more dysarthria and less syntactic comprehension disturbance. *Thalamic aphasia*, associated with lesions of the dominant thalamus, is a fluent aphasia somewhat resembling Wernicke's aphasia, but with better comprehension. Another feature of thalamic aphasia is a tendency for the patient to speak intelligibly when alert, but to sink into unintelligible jargon when drowsy. Other less common subcortical aphasia syndromes have been described.

Aphemia

Aphemia is a syndrome of muteness or extremely nonfluent speech, in a patient with no other language deficit. The patient can comprehend spoken language, read, and even write. This syndrome resembles a motor speech disorder rather than a true language disorder, hence there is some question that it represents a true aphasia. The lesion usually lies in the cortex just posterior to Broca's area, often involving the primary motor cortex for the face.

Pure word deafness

Pure word deafness is a syndrome in which patients act deaf, except that they can hear pure tones and recognize and identify nonverbal sounds, such as animal noises or honking horns. They have a selective inability to understand spoken words. Repetition is also impaired, but naming, reading, and writing are normal. Spontaneous speech is fluent, but most cases have some degree of paraphasic substitutions. The lesions of pure word deafness are often bilateral, affecting the auditory cortex in both temporal lobes. Occasional cases have been described with unilateral, left temporal lesions.

Alexias

Alexia refers to an acquired disorder of reading. Many patients with aphasia also have reading difficulty, a phenomenon sometimes called *aphasic alexia*, but two classical syndromes involve either reading or reading and writing out of proportion to other deficits. Linguistic analyses have defined several variants of alexia, but these linguistic classifications have not proved useful in terms of neurological diagnosis and treatment, with the exception of the two classical alexia syndromes discussed below. Deep alexia refers to reading in which only very common nouns and verbs are recognized; these patients usually have severe aphasia. Phonological alexia refers to the ability to read words aloud, but again only familiar nouns and verbs are understood. Surface alexia refers to patients who can read laboriously, converting graphemes (written syllables) into phonemes (spoken syllables), but they cannot recognize a word for its meaning.

ALEXIA WITH AGRAPHIA

Alexia with agraphia is a syndrome in which patients who formerly were able to read and write become effectively illiterate. Speech is fluent, though there may be some paraphasic substitutions. Naming may be impaired, but repetition and auditory comprehension are preserved. Both reading and writing are essentially nonfunctional; in most cases, spelling is severely affected. The lesion in this syndrome is usually in the left parietal lobe, especially the inferior parietal lobule comprising the supramarginal and angular gyri.

ALEXIA WITHOUT AGRAPHIA

Alexia without agraphia, or pure alexia, is a syndrome in which patients cannot read, but they can write; in fact, some patients can write a sentence, then not be able to read it after a short delay. Spontaneous speech is typically normal, as is auditory comprehension and repetition. Naming is intact, except that some patients have difficulty naming colors, a phenomenon termed *color anomia* or *color agnosia*. These patients have not lost the concept of color names;

they can name colors in the abstract, such as the color of a banana or a cardinal, but they cannot identify the color of an object by sight. They are not color blind, because they can match objects of similar color. The deficit is a failure to identify a perceived color with its name. Other features of the pure alexia syndrome include the presence of a right visual field defect, hemianopsia or quadrantanopsia, in most cases, and also short-term memory difficulty.

The lesion in pure alexia involves the left occipital lobe, most commonly a stroke in the left posterior cerebral artery territory. This territory also includes the hippocampus and related structures in the left medial temporal lobe, explaining the memory difficulty, and the splenium of the corpus callosum. The callosal lesion prevents visual information from the right occipital lobe from being transferred to the left hemisphere language centers. This "disconnection" mechanism is thought to explain the loss of reading, despite the fact that the patient can see letters in the left visual field, and also the color naming difficulty. Figure 15-3 shows an MRI scan from a patient with a left posterior cerebral artery territory infarction and the syndrome of pure alexia without agraphia.

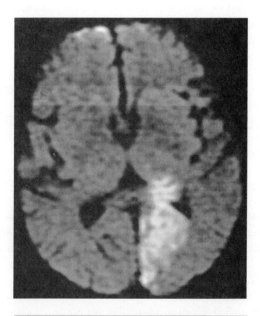

Figure 15-3 **MRI, diffusion-weighted, from a patient with pure alexia without agraphia** MRI shows infarction of the left posterior cerebral artery territory, with infarction in the left, medial occipital lobe and the splenium of the corpus callosum.

Agraphias

Agraphias are acquired disorders of writing. Agraphia, like alexia, can be a part of any aphasic syndrome (*aphasic agraphia*). Occasionally, agraphia occurs in relative isolation. Classically, the lesion localization in pure agraphia is in the left frontal lobe, above Broca's area. Agraphias, like alexias, have been divided into several linguistic categories; these are beyond the scope of this book and have not been shown to be of practical use in neurological diagnosis and treatment.

DIFFERENTIAL DIAGNOSIS

The classification of language deficits helps to localize the lesion, but not to diagnose the etiology of the disorder. As in the rest of neurology, clues to the etiologic diagnosis are best found in the history. Aphasia of abrupt onset usually represents a stroke, though occasionally aphasia can come on rapidly in the aftermath of a seizure (Todd's paralysis), traumatic brain injury, a brain tumor, or even an inflammatory condition. In stroke, aphasia can occur as a result of ischemia related to internal carotid occlusion, an embolus to the middle cerebral artery, or a hemorrhage in the left basal ganglia, with pressure on the overlying language cortex.

In ischemic stroke, most aphasia syndromes lie within the middle cerebral artery (MCA) territory; a complete MCA stem occlusion results in global aphasia, a superior branch occlusion results in Broca's aphasia, and an inferior branch occlusion results in a Wernicke's or conduction aphasia. Only a few aphasia syndromes do not reflect MCA territory ischemia. The syndrome of transcortical motor aphasia generally reflects ischemia in the left anterior cerebral artery territory, and the syndrome of pure alexia without agraphia reflects ischemia in the left posterior cerebral artery territory. Deep, subcortical lesions produce aphasia only if they are fairly large; a typical small vessel, lacunar stroke does not result in aphasia.

Other than stroke, aphasia can be produced by traumatic brain injury, brain abscess, meningoencephalitis, and, more rarely, inflammatory disorders such as multiple sclerosis. Herpes simplex encephalitis is notorious for producing aphasia when it involves the left temporal lobe, usually in the setting of a febrile illness, confusion, and seizures.

Aphasia can be a part of a more general cognitive deficit in neurodegenerative disorders and dementia. Here the subacute or chronic, slowly progressive course, together with the association with other cognitive and elementary neurological symptoms and signs, are helpful in diagnosis. The most specific aphasia syndrome in dementing illness is the syndrome termed *primary progressive aphasia* by Mesulam. In this disorder, patients generally manifest a progressive, nonfluent aphasia, often resembling Broca's aphasia, but gradually worsening over time. The syndrome falls within the category of *frontotemporal dementia,* first described by British authors, which can present with frontal lobe behavioral changes, or with nonfluent language degeneration. Frontotemporal dementia will be discussed in more detail in Chap. 26. A variant of primary progressive aphasia is *semantic dementia,* in which the patient first loses the ability to recall names, and then over times loses the meaning of words spoken to him or her. The pathology underlying semantic dementia can be either frontotemporal dementia or Alzheimer's disease (AD). Finally, Alzheimer's disease itself produces aphasia, among other cognitive deficits such as memory loss, executive dysfunction, apraxia, agnosia, and others. In Alzheimer's disease, recall of proper names is lost first, then discourse becomes simplified and impoverished, and in later stages, ability to read, write, and even understand spoken language become affected. Simple mechanics of speech, including spontaneous speech, repetition, and reading aloud, remain intact until late stages of the disease. These changes occur, of course, amidst the other cognitive deficits that usually make the diagnosis obvious. Occasionally, relatively isolated aphasic deficits initiate the cognitive decline of AD, but other cognitive deficits develop over time.

LABORATORY AND RADIOLOGICAL INVESTIGATION

The principal diagnostic tests used in diagnosis of aphasia are detailed testing batteries administered by speech/language pathologists or neuropsychologists, and brain imaging studies, usually computed tomography (CT) or MRI scans. The localizations given in this chapter for the specific aphasia syndromes came originally from pathological mapping of the lesions at autopsy, but in recent years they have been refined by the simultaneous mapping of the lesion in life with CT or MRI scans. An electroencephalogram (EEG) can occasionally be helpful in diagnosing seizure foci, and EEG mapping in patients being evaluated for epilepsy surgery has further defined the correlations between specific brain areas and language function. Recently, functional brain imaging modalities such as positron emission tomography (PET) scanning and functional MRI (fMRI) have also helped to identify areas of the brain that become activated during specific language tasks, both in normals and in patients with aphasia secondary to strokes or other brain disorders. These studies are refining our understanding of the relationships of language functions and specific areas of the brain.

TREATMENT

The treatment of an aphasic patient has two aspects. First, the medical cause of the aphasia and the appropriate treatment must be addressed. For example, if the aphasia is related to a stroke, acute treatments and secondary preventive managements should be initiated. If the cause is seizures, antiepileptic therapy and definition of the causative lesion are paramount. The second aspect is the treatment of the aphasia itself. In most cases, this is carried out via a trained, speech-language pathologist, or *speech therapist*. A number of studies have indicated that treatment of aphasia is effective, especially in helping the patient communicate with friends and family members. Physicians oversee speech therapy and other rehabilitative efforts. Occasionally, drugs such as stimulants or dopaminergic agents are prescribed along with speech therapy, but this area of treatment is in an early stage of development.

COURSE AND PROGNOSIS

If the cause of aphasia is an acute lesion such as a stroke or traumatic brain injury, the course is usually one of gradual improvement, and the prognosis is good. Aphasias tend to change not only in severity, but also in the type of aphasia. Global aphasia tends to evolve towards Broca's aphasia, and Wernicke's and conduction aphasias tend to evolve towards anomic aphasia. Anomia is often the most prominent residual deficit after recovery in all of the aphasic syndromes.

KEY REFERENCES

Alexander MP, Naeser MA, Palumbo C. Broca's area aphasias: aphasia after lesions including the frontal operculum. *Neurology* 1990;40:353–362.

Alexander MP, Naeser MA, Palumbo CL. Correlations of sub-cortical CT lesion sites and aphasia profiles. *Brain* 1987;110:961–991.

Appell J, Kertesz A, Fisman M. A study of language functioning in Alzheimer's patients. *Brain Lang* 1982;22:23–30.

Boatman D, Gordon B, Hart J, et al. Transcortical sensory aphasia: revisited and revised. *Brain* 2000;123:1634–1642.

Catani M, Jones DK, ffytche DH. Perisylvian language networks of the human brain. *Ann Neurol* 2005;57:8–16.

Damasio AR. Aphasia. *N Engl J Med* 1992;326:531–539.

Damasio H, Damasio AR. The anatomical basis of conduction aphasia. *Brain* 1980;103:337–350.

Freedman M, Alexander MP, Naeser MA. Anatomic basis of transcortical motor aphasia. *Neurology* 1984;34:409–417.

Kirshner HS. *Behavioral Neurology: Practical Science of Mind and Brain*. Boston, MA: Butterworth Heinemann; 2002.

Kirshner HS. *Handbook of Neurological Speech and Language Disorders*. New York: Marcel Dekker, Inc.; 1995.

Kirshner HS, Casey PF, Henson J, et al. Behavioral features and lesion localization in Wernicke's aphasia. *Aphasiology* 1989;3:169–176.

Kirshner HS, Tanridag O, Thurman L, et al. Progressive aphasia without dementia: two cases with focal spongiform degeneration. *Ann Neurol* 1987;22:527–532.

Kreisler A, Godefroy O, Delmaire C, et al. The anatomy of aphasia revisited. *Neurology* 2000;54:1117–1123.

Mesulam M-M. *Principles of Behavioral and Cognitive Neurology.* 2nd Ed. Oxford: Oxford University Press; 2000.

Mesulam M-M. Primary progressive aphasia—a language-based dementia. *N Engl J Med* 2003;349:1535–1542.

Wertz RT, Weiss DG, Aten J, et al. Comparison of clinic, home, and deferred language treatment for aphasia: a Veterans Administration cooperative study. *Arch Neurol* 1986;43:653–658.

HEADACHE

INTRODUCTION

Headache is one of the most common afflictions of mankind, as well as among the most frequent causes of lost work and visits to physicians. An important part of the knowledge base of any medical student or physician should be the ability to diagnose and treat headache syndromes and to determine which ones are serious.

Any discussion of headache must begin with consideration of the pain-sensitive structures in the head. It may surprise many medical students to learn that the brain itself is not sensitive to pain; neurosurgeons can operate on awake patients, place and move depth electrodes, even cut tissue with a scalpel, and the patient does not experience any discomfort. The blood vessels and meninges covering the brain contain pain-sensitive nerve endings, so lesions in the brain associated with increased intracranial pressure do cause headache. Patients seem to know this, because they frequently worry that they have a brain tumor when bothered by headaches, but in fact brain tumors present more commonly with neurological deficits or with seizures than with headaches. Other pain-sensitive structures within the cranium include the paranasal sinuses, the eyes, the teeth, gums, and the temporo-mandibular joints, and indirectly the cervical spine. Consideration should be given to these sources of pain before the physician diagnoses a primary headache syndrome such as migraine or tension headache.

CLINICAL PRESENTATION: SYMPTOMS AND SIGNS

Headaches are characterized by their location on the head, their severity (often expressed as pain on a scale of 1 to 10), their character (aching, stabbing, throbbing), and associated symptoms, such as stiff neck, fever, photophobia, phonophobia, nausea and/or vomiting, visual disturbance, and associated neurological symptoms such as numbness, tingling, weakness, confusion, or speech difficulty. Every headache history should include these features.

Table 16-1 **Features of Headache Requiring Work-up**

First occurrence, especially with abrupt onset
Worst severity, especially with increased headache on coughing or straining
Focal neurological symptoms
Focal neurological signs
Fever
Stiff neck

In general, a headache is considered potentially serious if it is the worst headache of a person's life, if it is a new phenomenon (no prior headache history), or if it is associated with fever, stiff neck, vomiting, or focal neurological symptoms and signs. The presence of any of these symptoms and signs should dictate immediate evaluation of the headache, with in most cases an emergency brain imaging study such as a computed tomography (CT) or magnetic resonance imaging (MRI) scan. Table 16-1 lists headache features suggesting a serious cause and a need for urgent evaluation.

DIFFERENTIAL DIAGNOSIS

We shall discuss common, specific types and causes of headaches, beginning with the more serious and important to diagnose quickly, and then continuing with a discussion of the more common headache syndromes.

Subarachnoid hemorrhage

Subarachnoid hemorrhage is usually related to a ruptured aneurysm. The diagnosis and treatment of subarachnoid hemorrhage is discussed in Chaps. 23 and 24. Briefly, a ruptured aneurysm usually presents with a sudden headache, often the worst of a person's life, sometimes associated with brief loss of consciousness at onset, and often accompanied by stiff neck. A patient with this type of headache should be advised to go directly to an emergency department and should receive a CT scan. Even if this is negative, a lumbar puncture is often indicated to exclude a small subarachnoid hemorrhage.

CNS infections (meningitis and encephalitis)

Headache accompanied by fever, especially in the presence of stiff neck, should raise suspicion of meningitis or encephalitis. As with subarachnoid hemorrhage, patients with this presentation should go directly to a hospital and receive emergent brain imaging, as well as a lumbar puncture. In the case of bacterial meningitis, institution of antibiotic therapy promptly may be lifesaving. There has been a long debate as to the safety of immediate lumbar puncture, before a CT scan, in a patient with fever and stiff neck. If such a patient is alert and has no papilledema on funduscopic examination, this is probably safe. In most hospitals, however, immediate antibiotic coverage, followed by prompt CT imaging and then a lumbar puncture, has been adopted as the safest and best approach. Certainly the administration of antibiotics should not be delayed more than a few minutes by the need to obtain brain imaging and spinal fluid. Antibiotic regimens must be broad spectrum and usually include a cephalosporin such as ceftriaxone and often a drug with gram negative coverage as well, such as gentamicin. Fungal and tuberculous meningitis are much like bacterial meningitis in their presentations, except that the illness may be more subacute or even chronic. Viral meningitis is usually a benign syndrome with headache, fever, and stiff neck, but no abnormality of mental status and no focal neurological signs. Encephalitis, on the other hand, usually features confusion or delirium at presentation, along with headache and fever, and often seizures and focal neurological symptoms and signs.

Brain abscess can also cause headache, but the main resemblance is to brain tumor, as discussed later in this chapter. Abscesses develop slowly and often present with focal deficits. Headache and fever are present in only about half of the cases. Many patients appear ill and have experienced weight loss, as well as general malaise and subtle, focal neurological symptoms and signs. Diagnosis is with CT or MRI scan and requires a high index of suspicion. Epidural abscess can be very subtle in its presentation, much like subdural hematoma.

Headache and cerebrovascular disease

Headache can occasionally be a harbinger of stroke, either hemorrhagic or ischemic. Hemorrhages can occur into the epidural, subdural, subarachnoid, and intracerebral spaces. Epidural and subdural hemorrhages are usually the result of trauma. Epidural hemorrhages generally occur very acutely after head trauma, classically with a brief lucid period following the injury, but then a rapid slide into unconsciousness. Not every patient with epidural hematoma, however, follows this pattern, so any rapid decline after a traumatic brain injury should be considered a possible sign of an expanding hematoma. Headache may be a feature in the early hours. Prompt recognition of these hemorrhages is crucial, since the treatment is virtually always emergency surgery, unless the hemorrhage is very small. Subdural hematomas may occur acutely after head trauma, especially in younger patients, or may be delayed, in which case the patient may not even recall the original trauma. Subdural hematomas often occur in elderly patients with brain atrophy, and the trauma itself may be trivial. The patient usually presents with drowsiness, sometimes headache, and subtle, focal neurological symptoms and signs. The diagnosis is made by a CT or MRI scan. Physicians need to have a high index of suspicion for subdural hematomas in elderly patients with mental deterioration. The treatment is again usually surgical, though patients with small subdural hematomas may be followed conservatively. Subarachnoid hemorrhage was discussed earlier in this chapter. Headache is generally a much more prominent feature of subarachnoid hemorrhage than of the other hemorrhages. Finally, intracerebral hemorrhage usually presents like a stroke, with the development of a focal neurological deficit in an awake patient. Headache may be a feature, since hemorrhages do stretch the meninges and cause increased intracranial pressure. Rarely, a hemorrhage will be in a "silent" part of the brain, such as a frontal pole, or the right temporal lobe, or directly into the ventricular system. In these instances, focal signs may be subtle or absent, and the patient may present just with headache and drowsiness. One sign of intracerebral hemorrhage is the associated hypertension that commonly occurs. Again, a CT scan is diagnostic. Management of intracerebral hemorrhage is discussed in Chaps. 23 and 24.

Ischemic strokes also cause headache via brain edema, mass effect, stretching of the meninges, and increased intracranial pressure. In general, headache is a presenting symptom in about half of patients with intracerebral hemorrhage, and in about a fourth of those with ischemic stroke. The diagnosis of ischemic stroke is usually made more by the focal symptoms and signs than by the presence of headache. Some types of stroke, such as cerebral venous sinus thrombosis or vasculitis, cause particularly prominent headaches.

Venous sinus thrombosis is a relatively rare cause of stroke, but a diagnosis that is prominently associated with headache. In the preantibiotic era, patients with untreated ear infections developed mastoiditis, followed by thrombosis of the lateral venous sinus, a condition sometimes called *otitic hydrocephalus*. In the current era, venous sinus thrombosis is usually associated with a hypercoagulable state, pregnancy or the puerperium, or occasionally in a very dehydrated, elderly patient. The symptoms typically begin with headache, often resembling closely the syndrome of idiopathic intracranial hypertension or *pseudotumor cerebri* (see below). Serious consequences can develop in patients with cerebral venous thrombosis, however, such as cerebral hemorrhage, venous infarction, or seizures. The patient may have symptoms and signs of increased intracranial pressure, including papilledema. Prompt diagnosis is imperative. The diagnosis is usually made by a magnetic resonance scan with venography (MRV), but occasionally the thrombosis of the superior sagittal sinus can be detected on a contrasted CT or MRI scan, where the sagittal sinus is imaged in cross section as it descends at the back of the brain. Catheter angiography or CT angiography can also be done to confirm the diagnosis. If the thrombosis is caused by an infection, intravenous antibiotics are mandatory. Two small, randomized trials have supported anticoagulation of patients with cerebral venous sinus thrombosis, and this treatment is supported by a broad consensus of opinion. Some authorities advocate direct intravascular thrombolysis for cases refractory to anticoagulation.

In vasculitis, the involvement of pain endings in vessels presumably mediates the headaches, and the diagnosis is usually suspected when a relatively young patient experiences multifocal cerebral infarctions and prominent headaches. Cerebral vasculitis can either be a part of a systemic vasculitis disease or isolated to the central nervous system. In the systemic vasculitis syndromes, screening with blood tests such as the sedimentation rate, antinuclear antibody, and antineutrophil cytoplasmic antibody (ANCA) can help in diagnosis. In primary central nervous system (CNS) vasculitis, however, these tests are usually normal. The diagnosis must be suspected on clinical grounds and confirmed by an MRI scan, usually showing multifocal infarctions, and ultimately by a brain and meningeal biopsy, confirming inflammatory cells within vessel walls. Treatment is complex and includes corticosteroids and immunosuppressive agents such as cyclophosphamide.

A specific vasculitis syndrome associated with headaches in older people is giant cell arteritis, also called temporal arteritis. The disorder is named for the arteritis occurring in the superficial temporal artery, sometimes associated with palpable thickening of the artery. The disorder can present either with diffuse aches and pains (polymyalgia rheumatica) or with sudden loss of vision in one eye, the hallmark of temporal arteritis. This disease can cause blindness as well as severe headaches, and occasionally stroke syndromes. The disease is rare before the age of 50 and increases in incidence with increasing age. The diagnosis can be suspected on the basis of an elevated sedimentation rate or C-reactive protein, but biopsy of the superficial temporal artery is required for definitive diagnosis. The treatment is oral corticosteroids, often over a period of months or even a year or two. Side effects in elderly patients can be a severe problem, so definitive diagnosis by biopsy is strongly recommended.

Idiopathic intracranial hypertension

Closely related to the symptoms of cerebral venous sinus thrombosis is the idiopathic condition called *pseudotumor cerebri* or benign intracranial hypertension, recently renamed *idiopathic intracranial hypertension* or IIH. This condition usually occurs in young people, women more than men, and there is an association with obesity. A number of other conditions have been associated with IIH, including iron deficiency anemia, steroid use or withdrawal from steroids, and many medications, including tetracycline. A list of these associated disorders and drugs is shown in Table 16-2. The typical patient presents with headaches, daily in occurrence, and often papilledema, yet a head CT or MRI scan is usually normal (hence the term *pseudotumor*). The neurological examination is normal, except for papilledema, and sometimes an enlarged blind spot on careful visual field testing. The exact cause of the syndrome of IIH is unknown, though a defect in the reabsorption of

Table 16-2 **Causes of Idiopathic Intracranial Hypertension**

Corticosteroids or withdrawal from corticosteroids
Vitamin A in large doses
Hypercapnea, obstructive sleep apnea
Guillain-Barré syndrome (secondary to high CSF protein)
Uremia
Drugs
   Cimetidine
   Isoretinoin
   Minocycline, tetracyclines
   Nalidixic acid
   Prednisone, prednisolone, methylprednisolone
   Tamoxifen
   Trimethoprim-sulfamethoxazole

cerebrospinal fluid (CSF) is suspected. Lumbar puncture yields a very high opening pressure but normal CSF cell counts, chemistries, and cultures. Drainage of spinal fluid via a spinal tap may bring immediate relief.

The treatment of idiopathic intracranial hypertension usually involves serial lumbar punctures, drugs like the carbonic anhydrase inhibitor acetazolamide (Diamox) to reduce CSF formation, or occasionally CSF drainage procedures such as ventriculoatrial or lumbar-peritoneal shunts. Surgical fenestration of the optic sheath produces a temporary outlet for CSF with lesser risk, but it is often not definitive. Patients with IIH must be followed closely, since the increased pressure leads to enlargement of the physiological blind spot, followed by progressive loss of vision. Some patients have sudden, bilateral visual obscurations, associated with periods of greatly increased intracranial pressure. These episodes may warn of blindness. It is this potential for loss of vision that has caused authorities to abandon the name *benign intracranial hypertension*.

Hydrocephalus

Hydrocephalus is a disorder in which the cerebral ventricles enlarge. The cause may be an obstruction in the CSF pathway (*obstructive hydrocephalus)* or a *communicating hydrocephalus*, in which there is no obstruction. The elevated pressure in the ventricles puts traction on the meninges, and headache supervenes. The headache is generally worse when the enlarged ventricles develop more rapidly. The most serious example is acute obstruction of the ventricular system, for example by a colloid cyst of the III ventricle. Such lesions can cause acute headache, sudden collapse, and death.

Other symptoms of hydrocephalus include confusion, drowsiness, gait difficulty, and urinary incontinence. When hydrocephalus develops gradually, headache may be absent, and the patient may present with the triad of gait difficulty, dementia, and urinary incontinence. *Normal pressure hydrocephalus* means hydrocephalus with normal CSF pressure on lumbar puncture. This condition, discussed in Chap. 14, is associated with a triad of dementia, gait difficulty, and urinary incontinence.

Low pressure headaches

Headaches can also occur in the setting of reduced CSF pressure. The most common cause of low-pressure headache is the post-lumbar puncture, or *spinal headache*. The characteristics of a *spinal* headache are precipitation of the headache when standing or walking, relief with lying down, and a dull, bilateral, usually posterior distribution of the headache, which worsens progressively the longer the patient remains upright. The headache presumably relates to low pressure brought about by leakage of CSF from the puncture site. The headache can be treated by bed rest, drinking extra fluids, possibly by caffeine or tea, and in refractory cases by placement of a *blood patch*, an epidural injection of the patient's own blood to stop the leak. Low pressure headaches occasionally occur spontaneously, in the absence of a spinal tap. Some cases are related to a dural tear with a CSF leak. One sign associated with chronic low pressure headache is thickening of the meninges on MRI brain imaging. Investigation of the location of the CSF leak can be carried out by injection of a radionuclide into the spinal fluid and the isotope scanning over the head and spine.

Brain tumors

Headaches can occasionally be a harbinger of a brain tumor, brain abscess, or other space-occupying lesion. As mentioned above, brain tumors much more commonly present with focal deficits or seizures than with headache. While many patients do endorse headaches, they are often dull in character, not terribly severe, often occurring on awakening and then gradually improving. Brain tumors are discussed in Chap. 36. A very similar presentation can be seen with brain abscess, except that fever is more likely to be associated with focal neurological signs, along with headache.

Sinusitis

Sinusitis is a much-touted cause of headache, perhaps the most common diagnosis of patients themselves regarding their own headaches. Sinusitis is usually associated with fever, nasal discharge and stuffiness, and a pressure sensation directly over the paranasal sinuses, in the frontal region, cheeks, nose, ears, or teeth. Diagnosis can be made with x-rays or CT of the sinuses, and treatment involves antibiotics, decongestants, antihistamines, and occasionally surgical drainage of the sinuses. Resolution of the headache following treatment may confirm the diagnosis of sinus headache. Sphenoid sinusitis is the most potentially serious of the bacterial sinusitis syndromes, since it can be associated with meningitis. Fungal sinusitis, as in the syndrome of mucormycosis seen in diabetic patients, can be serious and refractory to treatment.

Whereas sinusitis ranks very high among patients' self diagnoses of their headaches, confirmed sinusitis as a cause of headache is much less frequent. Even physicians tend to overdiagnose sinus headaches. Migraine and cluster headaches often present with pressure and pain in the general area of the orbits and sinuses, and these syndromes are considerably more common than sinus headaches. Cluster headaches often are associated with autonomic symptoms such as sinus congestion and tearing of the eyes, and even migraine may occasionally cause such symptoms. As we shall see later in Chap. 30 migraine is much more common than sinus headache, and the treatments differ greatly.

Temporomandibular joint arthritis headache

Temporomandibular joint (TMJ) arthritis is another somewhat faddish headache diagnosis. Patients with a palpable click in the TMJ may indeed develop aching in the side of the head with prolonged chewing, but TMJ clicking is also present in many individuals who do not complain of headache. Like sinusitis, TMJ headache is overdiagnosed both by patients themselves and by physicians. The diagnosis should be reserved for patients with typical headaches associated in locations adjacent to the TMJ and worsened by chewing. Treatment involves bite blocks, nonsteroidal anti-inflammatory drugs, and occasionally TMJ surgery.

Cervicogenic headaches

Cervical spondylosis is a common cause of dull, aching, posterior headaches in older patients. The physician should look for symptoms and signs of associated cervical nerve root or spinal cord involvement, which may be of more serious importance to the patient. The headache associated with cervical spondylosis can be treated with muscle relaxants, nonsteroidal anti-inflammatory drugs, and therapy techniques such as massage or cervical traction. Imaging with MRI may be indicated.

Occasional younger patients have *cervicogenic* headaches, also beginning in the back of the head and neck, but often then becoming more generalized, throbbing, and associated with nausea, photophobia, and phonophobia. Many such headaches may be migraine variants, perhaps with a cervical triggering factor.

One other, rare cause of headache is traction on the dura in the posterior fossa by a congenital malformation such as the Arnold-Chiari syndrome. This is a congenital problem, but some patients live into adulthood before they become symptomatic with headache, neck pain, and gait ataxia. The Chiari malformation can also be associated with hydrocephalus, which can cause headache. The diagnosis is easily made on the midline sagittal image of an MRI scan. The treatment involves surgical decompression.

Benign Headache Syndromes

Migraine and cluster headache, as well as the overlapping syndromes of chronic daily headache, analgesic rebound headache, and tension headache are discussed in Chap. 30.

LABORATORY AND RADIOLOGICAL INVESTIGATION

Laboratory testing will obviously vary with the specific headache syndrome being evaluated. The most difficult issue is knowing when to obtain a brain imaging study. In making this decision, the physician must consider first the most serious and potentially treatable headache diagnoses. A sudden onset headache, especially if it is the first such headache or the worst such headache the patient has ever experienced, should always earn the patient a CT scan, and possibly a lumbar puncture, even if the CT is negative. If the patient has focal neurological signs, papilledema, or depressed level of consciousness along with headache, again a CT or MRI scan is indicated. If fever or stiff neck suggest meningitis, a lumbar puncture is indicated, but most experts recommend imaging first with CT scan, and coverage with immediate antibiotics if a delay in the lumbar puncture is expected. Brain imaging will also be helpful in the diagnosis of mass lesions such as brain tumors or abscesses, subdural and epidural hematomas, and hydrocephalus. Benign intracranial hypertension must be diagnosed by measurement of CSF pressure via a lumbar puncture, but again a brain imaging study must always be performed first. If sinusitis is suspected, CT or MRI of the sinuses will aid in diagnosis. For temporal arteritis, a sedimentation rate or C- reactive protein will be helpful, but a temporal artery biopsy may ultimately be necessary.

TREATMENT

The treatment of a headache syndrome depends critically on the specific headache diagnosis. Most of the major therapies are mentioned above. Treatment of migraine, cluster headache, and chronic daily headache is discussed in Chap. 30.

KEY REFERENCES

General

Goadsby PJ. The pharmacology of headache. *Prog Neurobiol* 2000;62:509–525.

Kaniecki R. Headache assessment and management. *JAMA* 2003;289:1430–1433.

Kirshner HS. Management of headache. In: *Contemporary Issues in Chronic Pain Management. Chapter 13.* In: Parris WCV, ed. Boston, MA

Schwartz BS, Stewart WF, Simon D, et al. Epidemiology of tension-type headache. *JAMA* 1998;279:381–383.

Subarachnoid hemorrhage

Jakobsson K-E, Saveland H, Hillman J, et al. Warning leak and management outcome in aneurismal subarachnoid hemorrhage. *J Neurosurg* 1996;85:995–999.

Kowalski RG, Claassen J, Kreiter KT, et al. Initial misdiagnosis and outcome after subarachnoid hemorrhage. *JAMA* 2004;291:866–869.

Vermeulen M. Subarachnoid hemorrhage: diagnosis and treatment. *J Neurol* 1996;243:496–501.

Stroke

Arboix A, Massons J, Oliveres M, et al. Headache in acute cerebrovascular disease: a prospective clinical study in 240 patients. *Cephalalgia* 1994;14:37–40.

Kawamura J, Meyer JS. Headaches due to cerebrovascular disease. *Med Clin NA* 1991;75:617–630.

Welch KMA, Levine SR. Migraine-related stroke in the context of the International Headache Society classification of head pain. *Arch Neurol* 1990;47:458–462.

Infections

Bonadio WA, Mannenbach M, Krippendorf R. Bacterial meningitis in older children. *Am J Dis Children* 1990;144:463–465.

Chun CH, Johnson JD, Hofstetter M, et al. Brain abscess. A study of 45 consecutive cases. *Medicine* 1986;65:415–431.

Lew D, Southwick FS, Montgomery WW, et al. Sphenoid sinusitis. A review of 30 cases. *N Engl J Med* 1983;309:1149–1154.

Smith JE, Aksamit AJ. Outcome of chronic idiopathic meningitis. *Mayo Clin Proc* 1994;69:548–556.

Temporal arteritis, other vasculitis syndromes

Caselli RJ, Hunder GG. Giant cell (temporal) arteritis. *Neurol Clin* 1997;15:893–902.

Gonzalez-Gay MA, Barros S, Lopez-Diaz MJ, et al. Giant cell arteritis: disease patterns of clinical presentation in a series of 240 patients. *Medicine* 2005;84:269–276.

Greenan TJ, Grossman RI, Goldberg HI. Cerebral vasculitis: MR imaging and angiographic correlation. *Radiology* 1992;182:65–72.

Koo EH, Massey EW. Granulomatous angiitis of the central nervous system: proean manifestations and response to treatment. *N Neurol Neurosurg Psychiat* 1988;51:1126–1133.

Launes J, Iivanainen M, Erkinjuntti T, et al. Isolated angiitis of the central nervous system. *Acta Neurol Scand* 1986;74:108–114.

MacLaren K, Gillespie J, Shrestha S, et al. Primary angiitis of the central nervous system: emerging variants. *QJM* 2005;98:643–654.

Moore PM. Central nervous system vasculitis. *Curr Opin Neurol* 1998;11:241–246.

Moore PM, Cupps TR. Neurological complications of vasculitis. *Ann Neurol* 1983;14:155–167.

Smetana GW, Shmerling RH. Does this patient have temporal arteritis? *JAMA* 2002; 287:92–101.

Stone JH. Polyarteritis nodosa. *JAMA* 2002;288:1632–1639.

Younge BR, Cook BE Jr, Bartley GB, et al. Initiation of glucocorticoid therapy: before or after temporal artery biopsy? *Mayo Clin Proc* 2004;79:483–491.

Weyand CM, Goronzy JJ. Giant-cell arteritis and polymyalgia rheumatica. *Ann Intern Med* 2003;139:505–515.

Weyand CM, Goronzy JJ. Medium- and large-vessel vasculitis. *N Engl J Med* 2003;349: 160–168.

Idiopathic intracranial hypertension

Binder DK, Horton JC, Lawton MT, et al. Idiopathic intracranial hypertension. *Neurosurgery* 2004;54:538–552.

Digre KB, Corbett JJ. Idiopathic intracranial hypertension (pseudotumor cerebri): a reappraisal. *Neurologist* 2001;7:2–67.

Radhakrishnan K, Ahlskog JE, Garrity JA, et al. Idiopathic intracranial hypertension. *Mayo Clin Proc* 1994;69:169–180.

Other mechanisms of headache

Bovim G, Sand T. Cervicogenic headache, migraine without aura and tension-type headache. Diagnostic blockade of greater occipital and supra-orbital nerves. *Pain* 1992;51:43–48.

Cady RK, Dodick DW, Levine HL, et al. Sinus headache: a neurology, otolaryngology, allergy, and primary care consensus on diagnosis and treatment. *Mayo Clin Proc* 2005;80:908–916.

Kuntz KM, Kokmen E, Miller P, et al. Post lumbar puncture headaches: experience in 501 consecutive procedures. *Neurology* 1992;42:1884–1887.

Mokri B. Spontaneous cerebrospinal fluid leaks: from intracranial hypotension to cerebrospinal fluid hypovolemia—evolution of a concept. *Mayo Clin Proc* 1999;74:1113–1123.

Mokri B, Piepgras DG, Miller GM. Syndrome of orthostatic headaches and diffuse pachymeningeal gadolinium enhancement. *Mayo Clin Proc* 1997;72:400–413.

Reik L, Hale M. The temporomandibular joint pain-dysfunction syndrome: a frequent cause of headache. *Headache* 1981;21:151–156.

FOCAL PAIN SYNDROMES

INTRODUCTION

One of the most common symptoms a neurologist is called upon to diagnose and treat is pain. Pain may be divided by location, focal or generalized, or by location in the body. Pain syndromes of a more generalized type, such as those seen with peripheral neuropathy, are discussed in Chap. 33.

In this chapter, we shall consider four general types of pain: facial pain, neck pain, low back pain, and neuropathic (dysesthetic) pain. Along with headache, these comprise the most common of the focal pain syndromes.

Facial pain

Many causes must be considered for facial pain. First, intraocular problems such as glaucoma, orbital pseudotumor, or detached retina cause pain in the region of the eye, forehead, and cheek. Other conditions affecting the orbit such as carotid-cavernous fistula or dural arteriovenous (AV) malformation can also present with periorbital pain.

In the cheek area, sinusitis or tumors of the paranasal sinuses present with both facial pain and headache. In the maxillary or mandibular area of the face, sinusitis and dental problems such as tooth abscesses and temporo-mandibular joint dysfunction also cause focal pain, as discussed in Chap. 16.

A very characteristic facial pain syndrome is trigeminal neuralgia. This syndrome involves very sharp, sudden paroxysms of pain, in one or more of the divisions of the trigeminal nerve territory, usually just on one side of the face. The pain may be triggered by a touch or temperature sensation on the face or inside the mouth; sometimes hot or cold foods, or the simple act of chewing, will induce the pain. Patients say that the pain is the most severe, intolerable pain they have ever experienced. It may occur several times per day, and it may occur day after day, or it can go into temporary remissions of weeks, months, or years. The disorder can occur in either gender at any age, but it is more common in older people, and in women more than men.

The cause of trigeminal neuralgia is unknown. One theory holds that an artery or branch pulsates against the nerve, just before it enters the brainstem in the pons. A neurosurgical procedure, called the Jannetta procedure or *microvascular decompression*, involves dissection of the nerve and separation of the nerve from any adjacent blood vessels, via a posterior fossa operation.

The treatment of trigeminal neuralgia usually involves trials of medications first, with surgical procedures reserved for very refractory or severe cases. The medication with the best results in trigeminal neuralgia is carbamazepine (Tegretol), usually begun at a low dose of 100 mg bid and increased as tolerated. A related drug, oxcarbazepine (Trileptal) also appears to be effective in trigeminal neuralgia. Other antiepileptic drugs also seem to relieve neuropathic pain. These include gabapentin (Neurontin), pregabilin (Lyrica), topiramate (Topamax), and levetiracetam (Keppra). These drugs are usually less effective than carbamazepine in trigeminal neuralgia. The antispasticity drug baclofen has also been used in trigeminal neuralgia, again with lesser efficacy as compared to carbamazepine. For patients requiring surgery, the posterior fossa exploration and *microvascular decompression* has been the most successful, with remission rates of approximately 80%. A less invasive procedure, radiofrequency rhizotomy of the trigeminal root and ganglion, can be accomplished via placement of a spinal needle under the zygomatic arch and into the ganglion. This procedure often leaves some sensory loss in the area of the face affected, and the pain can recur months or years after the procedure. The remaining treatment for trigeminal neuralgia is radiosurgery, such as the gamma knife or cold photon knife, applied to the trigeminal ganglion. This procedure has not been tested as well as microvascular decompression and radiofrequency rhizotomy.

Patients with chronic facial pain of less acute, lancinating variety are often classified under the term *atypical facial pain*. Some such patients also have numbness on the affected side of the face. Appropriate diagnostic procedures such as MRI scanning are needed to exclude a structural lesion that would affect the trigeminal nerve or its central connections in the brainstem. The treatment of atypical facial pain is problematic. Surgery has not been shown effective, and medical treatments for neuropathic pain (see below) are the treatments of choice, but often with limited efficacy.

Neck pain

The most common type of pain affecting the neck is cervical spondylosis and radiculopathy. This is a very common condition, with incidence figures of 60–100/100,000 people annually, though the prevalence of this disorder is undoubtedly much higher. In young people with trauma, the cause may be an acute disk bulge impinging on an exiting nerve root, but in older people and those without antecedent trauma the leading cause is *cervical spondylosis*. Cervical spondylosis involves degenerative changes in the uncovertebral joints anteriorly and the zygoapophyseal joints posteriorly, especially when the dorsal root ganglion of the exiting root is compressed or inflamed.

The diagnosis of cervical radiculopathy is made by a careful history, physical examination, and imaging studies such as the MRI scan of the cervical spine. There is typically a combination of local neck pain and radiating pain going down the arm, in addition to which there may be physical evidence of a nerve root lesion in terms of focal weakness of arm or hand muscles, loss of a tendon reflex, or focal sensory loss in a nerve root distribution. In general, a disk bulge at a specific interspace, such as C5-6, involves the nerve root numbered at the lower level, such as C6. The typical nerve root syndromes were shown in Table 2-1 in Chap. 2.

In the cervical spine, a critical issue is whether the syndrome reflects exclusively nerve root impingement, or whether the spinal cord is involved. Subtle evidence of myelopathy can include symptoms of bladder urgency, mild weakness and spasticity in the legs, and difficulty walking. The diagnosis of cervical myelopathy is much more critical than that of uncomplicated cervical radiculopathy, because of the risk of irreversible spinal cord damage.

Most patients with cervical radiculopathy have cervical disk disease or spondylosis, degenerative joint disease of the cervical spine, as the cause. Occasionally a more serious condition such as epidural abscess, diskitis, or a tumor can present with similar symptoms. Clues to these more serious diagnoses include fever, unexplained weight loss, known history of a neoplasm, an immunosuppressed state, or a history of intravenous drug abuse.

The definitive diagnosis of cervical radiculopathy usually involves an MRI scan of the cervical spine. Figure 17-1 shows a sagittal, T2-weighted scan through the cervical spine. Occasionally, a computed tomography (CT) myelogram is necessary for diagnosis. CT imaging without intrathecal contrast is much less useful. Confirmation of nerve damage in a radicular distribution can also be achieved with electromyography.

The natural course of cervical radiculopathy is quite variable. Many patients can be treated conservatively through a bout of radicular pain, and then the disorder will remain in remission for months or years. Other patients develop intractable pain or symptoms of myelopathy, at which point surgery becomes necessary. It is also of interest that studies of MRI in middle-aged and elderly people have shown that many have disc bulges, nerve root compression, and even apparent spinal cord impingement, without any more than minor symptoms.

The treatment of cervical radiculopathy is divided into conservative versus surgical approaches. Conservative treatment consists of first rest and later exercises, immobilization with soft or hard collars, cervical traction devices, and pain medications, including narcotic analgesics, anti-inflammatory agents, and sometimes muscle relaxants. Short courses of corticosteroids such as prednisone sometimes settle down the inflammation and pain. Injections to relieve pain, such as epidural steroid injections, are also recommended by some practitioners. In general, physical therapy techniques or cervical traction should not be initiated before the cervical spine is imaged, since an

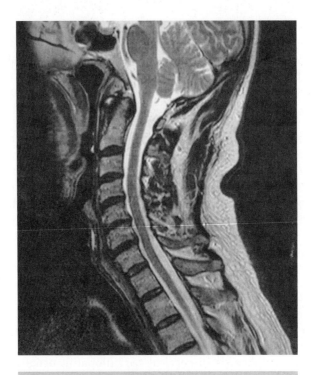

*Figure 17-1 **Cervical spine MRI.*** This 56-year-old
man presented with sharp neck pain and radiation
down the left arm, with numbness in a C6 distribution.
The sagittal T-2 weighted MR image shows protrusion
of the C5-6 disk, and to a lesser extent, C6–7.

incipient spinal cord compression could be worsened by such maneuvers.
Chiropractic manipulation can be even more risky in this situation.
Surprisingly, virtually none of these treatments has been subjected to randomized clinical trials. Surgical treatment is mainly directed at patients with
cervical spinal cord compression or intractable radicular pain and related
motor and sensory deficits, persisting at least 6 weeks. In the past, posterior
cervical laminectomy was the procedure of choice, but currently anterior cervical diskectomy and fusion is favored because of the shorter hospital stay
and quicker recovery associated with this procedure. Bony fusion procedures
or anterior spinal plates are often needed, especially if the surgery involves
more than one disk space. Surgical series have generally shown high per-
centages of pain relief, in the vicinity of 75%. In general, patients treated surgically do better than conservatively managed patients for the first 6-12
months, but in one study there were no differences after 2 years.

Another common cause of neck pain is the cervical strain injury, or *whiplash*. As compared to the symptoms of cervical radiculopathy, these patients often have very diffuse neck pain and stiffness, often without definite radicular symptoms, or with very widespread pain in both upper limbs, but without objective motor, sensory, or reflex abnormalities. Such syndromes often occur after seemingly minor injuries such as "fender-bender" car accidents. Some clinicians suspect psychosocial factors such as litigation for the persistence of pain in some patients with whiplash injuries. Studies have generally shown a close relationship between persistent pain and the severity of the initial injury, the intensity of pain in the early period after the injury, older age, and the presence of apparent cognitive dysfunction, which often seems to accompany whiplash injuries just as it does minor head injuries. Findings of cervical spondylosis on x-rays or magnetic resonance imaging (MRI) scans of the cervical spine are present in some patients without symptoms, but their presence also correlates with persistent pain after whiplash injuries. One study indicated a much lower incidence of persistent pain after cervical strain injuries in countries such as Lithuania, in which disability and litigation for such injuries are much less common than in the U.S. and Western Europe.

Low back pain

Low back pain is even more common than neck pain, literally one of the scourges of mankind, and next to headache the most common pain syndrome causing visits to physicians. Low back pain is the leading cause of work-related disability and workers' compensation claims. The mechanisms of pain, symptoms, and diagnosis by physical examination are similar to those of cervical spine problems, discussed above. As in neck pain, inflammation of the structures of the spine can cause local pain, or the pain can be referred into the territories of nerve roots, but spinal cord involvement is usually not seen, since the spinal cord ends at about L1 in most adults. As in the cervical spine, the pathological process may involve either degenerative changes in the bones of the spine or protrusions of disk material as a result of a direct injury. Also as in cervical spine disorders, the pain can be either spontaneous or the apparent result of a traumatic injury. In the lumbar spine, only the history of an injury separates the post-traumatic *lumbar strain* or *lumbar sprain* injury from an idiopathic low back pain syndrome.

The most common disk protrusions are at L4-5 and L5-S1, with L3-4 a distant third. L1-2 and L2-3 protrusions are very uncommon. The common symptoms and signs of disk protrusions at the various lumbar levels can be found in Table 2-2, Chap. 2. The presence of symptoms and signs in a nerve root distribution helps in diagnosis of these conditions. The diagnosis is best made by careful examination of muscle strength, reflexes, and sensory function, with special attention to the specific areas listed in the table. Increase in radicular symptoms by coughing, straining, or bending also increases diagnostic confidence in a lumbar radiculopathy. The straight leg raising test can also be used to bring on radicular symptoms. Finally, local bony tenderness to palpation of the spine is a clue to diagnosis of low back pain syndromes not due to the usual lumbar spondylosis/disk mechanism, but by infections or tumors affecting the lumbar spine.

Rarely, a large, midline disk or tumor will affect not just one exiting root, but several roots of the cauda equina. The *cauda equina syndrome* is a medical emergency, in that only prompt surgery can prevent long-term nerve root damage, with weakness and sensory loss in the legs and loss of bowel, bladder, and sexual function.

The diagnosis of lumbar radiculopathy parallels that of cervical radiculopathy. The MRI is a rapid, noninvasive test for imaging the lumbar spine, disks, and nerve root foramena. Increasingly, surgeons are basing decisions on whether or not to operate on MRI, as long as a straightforward, single disk protrusion is found. CT/myelography can be used for confirmation. The electromyogram can be used to document denervation in a nerve root distribution.

The management of lumbar spondylosis and radiculopathy also parallels that of cervical spondylosis and radiculopathy. A variety of conservative treatment strategies is widely employed, but the evidence for efficacy of most of them is very weak. Bed rest was formerly recommended for people with acute back strain or injury, but there is no evidence to support this. Likewise, transcutaneous nerve stimulators (TENS units), local injections, exercise and therapy techniques are performed with mainly anecdotal evidence of effectiveness. Surgery, in this case posterior lumbar laminectomy, generally improves radicular syndromes in patients with intractable pain and radicular numbness and weakness for the weeks to months after surgery, but long-term results differ little between medically and surgically managed patients.

Neuropathic (dysesthetic) pain

Pain is defined as an unpleasant sensory or emotional experience associated with actual or potential tissue damage. Neuropathic pain may be defined by pain that is caused by abnormal firing of a peripheral or central nerve fiber, rather than by a pathological process in an organ, muscle, or bony structure. In normal physiology, pain is induced by nociceptors, sensory axons in tissues, which project via dorsal root ganglion cells, then via thinly myelinated A delta and unmyelinated C fibers, traveling via the spinothalamic tracts to the thalamus. If pain exists to warn the organism of impending risk of injury, neuropathic pain has no such purpose, and the pain tends to worsen as it becomes chronic. Neuropathic pain involves activation of these pain pathways not because of a normal stimulation of a nociceptive neuron by peripheral tissue injury or disease, but because of pathology in the neural pathways themselves. Abnormal activation of glutamatergic nociceptors leads to overactivity of dorsal root ganglion neurons and increased central transmission of pain signals.

Neuropathic pain is often described as burning, itching, stabbing, or having a "pins and needles" quality. Such feelings are called *paresthesias* or *dysesthesias*. These terms have somewhat varying definitions, with paresthesias referring either to spontaneous sensations or altered but not painful sensations, and dysesthesias usually referring to a painful distortion of a true stimulus. Other terms used to describe neuropathic pain are *hyperalgesia*, in which a painful stimulus is transmitted in an exaggerated form, or *allodynia*, pain experience from an ordinarily nonpainful stimulus. Neuropathic pain may occur spontaneously, or it may follow sensory stimuli, with an unpleasant, painful after-effect of a normal sensation. In most cases, the threshold for feeling a stimulus at all is elevated, reflecting a degree of sensory loss. Once the stimulus is above the threshold, however, the sensation seems out of proportion to the stimulus, as if the patient is *hypersensitive* to pain.

Neuropathic pain is not specific to any one neurological diagnosis. Patients who have had strokes and suffer areas of sensory loss often develop neuropathic pain weeks or months after the stroke. The classic example is the *thalamic pain syndrome* of Dejerine and Roussy. These unfortunate patients, many with a small, thalamic lacune and no motor disability at all, have severe, burning pain for which they seek multiple treatments. Although thalamic pain is the classic example of a post-stroke pain syndrome, any stroke involving the spinothalamic pain pathways, whether in the brainstem, thalamus, white matter, or parietal cortex, can result in chronic, neuropathic pain. Similar, central neuropathic pain is seen in multiple sclerosis, traumatic brain or spinal cord injuries, and in tumors of the spine or brain.

Neuropathic pain may also follow peripheral nerve injuries. In the past, *causalgia* was defined as a pain syndrome related to severe damage to an identified peripheral nerve. The neuropathic pain in causalgia is often accompanied by autonomic changes such as swelling, cool temperature, skin discoloration, and ultimately atrophy of the soft tissues. Other patients develop similar changes without an identified nerve injury, after seemingly minor injuries to limbs, or after disuse of a limb, as when a cast is removed after a fracture. This pain syndrome was formerly referred to as *reflex sympathetic dystrophy* (RSD), on the theory that cross-talk between the afferent sensory nerve and efferent sympathetic nerve explains both the painful distortion of sensory inputs and the abnormal autonomic outputs. It is not clear, however, that all such pain is truly related to sympathetic overstimulation, or *sympathetically-mediated pain*. Current terminology refers to these peripheral pain syndromes as *Complex Regional Pain Syndrome* (CRPS), types I and II. CRPS I corresponds to causalgia, or pain in the distribution of an identifiable peripheral nerve injury, and CRPS II corresponds to pain in the absence of a single nerve injury, as in RSD.

One very specific focal neuropathic pain syndrome is post-herpetic neuralgia, or pain following Herpes zoster (*shingles*) rash. This is a typical burning, tingling neuropathic pain, more common in older patients who have developed Herpes zoster. The pain usually starts after the rash has been present, but occasionally, pain is a prodrome before the rash. Some evidence supports early treatment of the zoster rash with corticosteroids such as prednisone and antiviral agents such as acyclovir or valacyclovir (Valtrex), in order to prevent or minimize the development of post-herpetic neuralgia.

The treatment of neuropathic pain is one of the most problematic areas in neurology, perhaps in all of medicine. Many medications have been tried. As mentioned in the first section of this chapter, lancinating pains analogous to trigeminal neuralgia may respond to the antiepileptic drugs carbamazepine (Tegretol) and oxcarbazepine (Trileptal). Many other antiepileptic drugs have been evaluated in neuropathic pain, including gabapentin (Neurontin), pregabilin (Lyrica), topiramate (Topamax), valproic acid (Depakote), lamotrigine (Lamictal), and levatiracetam (Keppra). None of these drugs is approved by Food and Drug Administration (FDA) specifically for neuropathic pain, though gabapentin and pregabilin have proved effective in post-herpetic neuralgia and in painful diabetic neuropathy. Antidepressants such as amitriptyline and the newer drug duloxetine (Cymbalta) also appear to help neuropathic pain. The evidence for efficacy of duloxetine is mainly in diabetic neuropathy. For very focal pain, of which the best example is post-herpetic neuralgia, placement of a lidocaine (Lidoderm) patch may be helpful. Finally, narcotic analgesics are sometimes used chronically for neuropathic pain, usually in long-acting preparations.

As in the pain of cervical and lumbar radiculopathy, various nerve blocks and therapy techniques have been tried, with limited evidence of benefit. Surgical management is even more problematic. In the past, spinal cord tractotomy (of the spinothalamic tract) or of the dorsal column entry zone (DREZ procedure) were performed for pain below the level of the spinal procedure. More recently, dorsal column stimulators have been used more than ablative surgical procedures. Patients with very intractable pain can also be treated with the placement of an intrathecal morphine pump.

KEY REFERENCES

Ballantyne JC, Mao J. Opioid therapy for chronic pain. *N Engl J Med* 2003;349: 1943–1953.

Barker FG, Jannetta PJ, Bissonette DJ, et al. The long-term outcome of microvascular decompression for trigeminal neuralgia. *N Engl J Med* 1996;334:1077–1083.

Carragee EJ. Persistent low back pain. *N Engl J Med* 2005;352:1891–1898.

Carette S, Fehlings MG. Cervical radiculopathy. *New Engl J Med* 2005;353:392–399.

Chen H, Lamer TJ, Rho RH, et al. Contemporary management of neuropathic pain for the primary care physician. *Mayo Clin Proc* 2004;79:1533–1545.

Cheshire WP. Trigeminal neuralgia. A guide to drug choice. *CNS Drugs* 1997;7:98–110.

Cross SA. Pathophysiology of pain. *Mayo Clin Proc* 1994;69:375–383.

Curtis P, Spanos A, Reid A. Persistent symptoms after whiplash injuries. Implications for prognosis and management. *J Clin Rheumatology* 1995;1:149–156

Deyo RA, Weinstein JN. Low back pain. *N Engl J Med* 2001;344:363–370.

Deyo RA, Walsh NE, Martin DC, et al. A controlled trial of transcutaneous electrical nerve stimulation (TENS) and exercise for chronic low back pain. *N Engl J Med* 1990;322:1627–1634.

Eisenberg E, McNicol ED, Carr DB. Efficacy and safety of opioid agonists in the treatment of neuropathic pain of nonmalignant origin. Systematic review and meta-analysis of randomized controlled trials. *JAMA* 2005;293:3043–3052.

Gilron I, Bainey JM, Dongsheng T, et al. Morphine, gabapentin, or their combination for neuropathic pain. *N Engl J Med* 2005;352:1324–1334.

Green MW, Selman JE. The medical management of trigeminal neuralgia. *Headache* 1991;31:588–1592.

Hooshmand H, Hashmi M. Complex regional pain syndrome (Reflex sympathetic dystrophy syndrome): diagnosis and therapy—A review of 824 patients. *Pain Digest* 1999;9:1–24.

Houser OW, Onofrio BM, Miller GM, et al. Cervical disk prolapse. *Mayo Clin Proc* 1995;70:939–945.

Jahnke RW, Hart BL. Cervical stenosis, spondylosis, and herniated disc disease. *Rad Clinics NA* 1991;29:777–791.

Jensen MC, Brant-Zawadzki MN, Obuchowski N, et al. Magnetic resonance imaging of the lumbar spine in people without back pain. *N Engl J Med* 1994;331:69–73.

Kost RG, Straus SE. Postherpetic neuralgia—pathogenesis, treatment, and prevention. *N Engl J Med* 1996;335:32–42.

Lahad A, Malter AD, Berg AO. The effectiveness of four interventions for the prevention of low back pain. *JAMA* 1994;272:1286–1291.

Malanga GA, Nadler SF. Nonoperative treatment of low back pain. *Mayo Clin Proc* 1999;74:1135–1148.

Nardin RA, Patel MR, Gudas TF, et al. Electromyography and magnetic resonance imaging in the evaluation of radiculopathy. *Muscle Nerve* 1999;22:151–155.

Rho RH, Brewer RP, Lamer TJ, Wilson PR. Complex regional pain syndrome. *Mayo Clin Proc* 2002;77:174–180.

Schrader H, Obelieniene D, Bovim G, et al. Natural evolution of late whiplash syndrome outside the medicolegal context. *Lancet* 1996;4:1207–1211.

Smed A. Cognitive function and distress after common whiplash injury. *Acta Neurol Scand* 1997;95:73–80.

Taha JM, Tew JM. Comparison of surgical treatments for trigeminal neuralgia: reevaluation of radiofrequency rhizotomy. *Neurosurgery* 1996;38:865–871.

Vroomen PCAJ, De Krom CTFM, Wilmink JT, et al. Lack of effectiveness of bed rest for sciatica. *N Engl J Med* 1999;340:418–423.

Wahlig JB, McLaughlin MR, Subach BR, et al. Management of low back pain. *The Neurologist* 2000;6:326–337.

NUMBNESS AND PARESTHESIAS

INTRODUCTION

Numbness and paresthesias denote loss or disturbance of sensory function. In the clinical history, numbness means a loss of sensation, whereas paresthesias imply spontaneous, positive symptoms such as tingling, burning, or itching. As mentioned in Chap. 17, some authorities define *dysesthesias* as distorted responses to sensory stimuli, whereas paresthesias occur spontaneously. Sensory symptoms are subjective, part of the history; sensory signs are also largely subjective, since they require the patient to report the reduction or absence of feeling of a specific sensory stimulus, such as a sharp object, a light touch, or a vibrating tuning fork. Objective information can sometimes be drawn from the sensory examination, however; if a patient grimaces after the examiner jabs the leg with a sharp Q-tip, the patient clearly felt the stimulus. Accurate reporting of vibration or position also indicates intact sensation objectively, though incorrect reporting could result from a failure to feel the stimulus or a willful intent to mislead the examiner.

Sensory symptoms can result from lesions at multiple levels of the nervous system. Peripheral nerve lesions, in the form of a mononeuropathy (as in carpal tunnel syndrome) or a polyneuropathy, can cause both numbness and paresthesias. Central lesions of the spinal cord or brain can also cause both numbness and paresthesias.

CLINICAL PRESENTATION: SYMPTOMS AND SIGNS

The symptoms of sensory dysfunction involve either a feeling of numbness, indicating reduced or absent sensation, or a positive symptom such as tingling, pins and needles, feeling a constricting band around a part of the body, burning, or itching. These symptoms may occur in isolation, or in association with other symptoms. Patients often differ in their use of terms like *numbness* or *weakness*. It is important to pin the patient down and make sure that the complaint is truly of sensory loss or distortion. Injury to peripheral nerves clearly causes sensory symptoms, both numbness and paresthesias.

Within the spinal cord, spinothalamic lesions tend to cause just numbness, whereas posterior column lesions are more likely to be associated with symptoms of tightness, a constricting band, or feeling as if there is an extra wad of sock material inside one's shoe. In the brain, lesions of the white matter, thalamus, or sensory cortex may be associated with either sensory loss or paresthesias, or both. Lesions of the thalamus often cause sensory deficits of the entire contralateral side of the body, including splitting of the midline. Sometimes this midline splitting, along with an absence of motor deficits, may create a misimpression that the patient could have a functional, or psychogenic illness. Great care should always be taken before labeling a patient with a psychogenic diagnosis, and this applies also to the purely sensory findings in an early Guillain-Barré syndrome patient (see Chap. 33). Thalamic lesions are also especially likely to be associated with painful paresthesias and dysesthesias, often including not only tingling, but burning, pins and needles, and itching sensations. This syndrome, called *thalamic pain syndrome* or the *Dejerine-Roussy syndrome*, is often a major cause of suffering in patients who have experienced thalamic strokes.

A final deficit related to sensory loss is sensory ataxia. Patients with severe sensory loss, especially joint position sense, cannot feel where their limbs are, and they appear ataxic in walking and in performing "cerebellar" tests, such as finger-nose-finger and heel-knee-shin coordination. In the days of neurosyphilis, severe sensory deficits related to tabes dorsalis, or disease of the dorsal root ganglia, caused numb limbs with secondary injuries such as Charcot joints (damage to joints such as the knee from repeated trauma, not felt by the patient). In diabetic neuropathy, loss of sensation may be at least partially responsible for the poorly healing pressure sores and areas of skin ulceration that can lead to amputation of a limb. Severe sensory loss is also a feature of peripheral neuropathy in leprosy. Such profound sensory deficits are more often seen in peripheral nerve and root than central nervous system disease, but even in stroke patients, sensory loss in an affected limb can severely impair coordination and gait.

DIFFERENTIAL DIAGNOSIS

The first differential diagnosis is to make sure that the patient's complaint is sensory, and not motor. Familiar examples are Bell's palsy and Guillain-Barré syndrome (GBS). In both entities, the patient often complains first of tingling sensations. Bell's palsy patients may even say that the face on the affected side *feels numb*, or even "like novocaine", even though the examination shows only motor weakness, with normal sensory function. The exact explanation for these apparently sensory symptoms in lesions of a purely motor nerve is unclear. Heaviness of the sagging muscles may be part of the reason. In GBS, patients often complain of tingling of the toes and feet before any obvious weakness develops. As the numbness ascends, weakness supervenes. Once the limbs have become severely weak, sensory function may seem normal. In GBS, the peripheral neuropathy involves primarily motor nerves, but sensory nerves may also be affected to some degree.

Sensory dysfunction may differ among lesions at different levels of the nervous system. When a peripheral nerve is the source of the numbness, the sensory complaints should be very localized. In carpal tunnel syndrome, for example, the numbness should involve only the median nerve distribution of the hand and fingers, whereas ulnar nerve compression at the elbow affects only the ulnar distribution. A combination of history and careful sensory examination may be required to demonstrate the very focal nature of the sensory disturbance. If the lesion involves a mixed sensory and motor nerve, weakness and reflex loss in the distribution of the nerve can help to localize the lesion. Lesions of nerve roots should also affect very local areas in dermatomal distributions, again with motor and reflex changes in the distribution of the nerve root. In the spinal cord, the lesion is more likely to affect predominantly the spinothalamic or posterior column pathways, sometimes with involvement of the sensory nerve roots. Spinal cord localization is discussed in Chap. 2. In the brainstem, crossed sensory loss in the ipsilateral face and contralateral body can be a clue to localization. In the hemisphere, sensory loss often involves the face, arm, and leg on the contralateral side of the body.

LABORATORY AND RADIOLOGICAL INVESTIGATION

Laboratory investigation of the patient with a sensory deficit depends critically on the neurological localization and likely diagnosis. If the history and physical findings suggest a mononeuropathy, the diagnosis can be confirmed by electrodiagnostic testing with nerve conduction velocity/electromyography (NCV/EMG) (see Chap. 38). Electrodiagnostic testing can also delineate a peripheral neuropathy or nerve root syndrome. Blood and urine tests may be needed to define the cause of a neuropathy (see Chap. 33). Within the spinal cord and brain, imaging studies such as magnetic resonance imaging (MRI), myelography, and related tests may be indicated. Isolated sensory deficits can be seen in thalamic infarctions. I have seen one patient with a thalamic glioma whose only symptom was tingling and numbness on the contralateral side of the body.

TREATMENT

The treatment of a sensory disorder involves first the diagnosis, with treatment of the cause of the sensory loss or disturbance if that is possible. If it is not possible, treatment can be directed at symptomatic relief of uncomfortable paresthesias and neuropathic pain. This topic was discussed in Chap. 17 on focal pain. Drugs including the antidepressants amitriptyline and duloxetine (Cymbalta) and a variety of antiepileptic drugs can be prescribed to reduce neuropathic pain. If the pain is localized, as in post Herpetic neuralgia, a lidocaine (Lidoderm) patch may be helpful. Devices such as transcutaneous electric nerve stimulators (TENS) provide some relief, though clinical trials supporting their efficacy are scarce. Finally, spinal cord stimulators and neurosurgical ablation procedures can be performed in patients with very refractory, life-altering neuropathic pain.

COURSE AND PROGNOSIS

The course and progression of numbness and paresthesias varies according to the etiology. One important variable, however, is time. Sensory loss may improve as edema goes down after an acute insult. In patients with sensory loss related to strokes or trauma, initial numbness may give way over time to active paresthesias and neuropathic pain. In the thalamic pain syndrome after thalamic infarctions, the pain typically begins days, weeks, or even months after the initial infarction. Some patients have active paresthesias that make them fear that another stroke is occurring. Over a period of years, neuropathic pain tends to diminish, but the patient may just become accustomed to it.

KEY REFERENCES

Fishbain D. Evidence-based data on pain relief with antidepressants. *Ann Med* 2000;32:305–316.

Kost RG, Straus SE. Postherpetic neuralgia. *Arch Intern Med* 1997;157:1166–1167.

Mogyros I, Bostock H, Burke D. Mechanisms of paresthesias arising from healthy axons. *Muscle Nerve* 2000;23:310–320.

Pappagallo M. Newer antiepileptic drugs: possible uses in the treatment of neuropathic pain and migraine. *Clin Ther* 2003;25:2506–2538.

Waxman SG. The molecular pathophysiology of pain: abnormal expression of sodium channel genes and its contributions to hyperexcitability of primary sensory neurons. *Pain*. 1999;Aug(Suppl. 6):S133–S140. Review.

Waxman SG, Cummins TR, Dib-Hajj S, et al. Sodium channels, excitability of primary sensory neurons, and the molecular basis of pain. *Muscle Nerve* 1999;22:1177–1187.

TRANSIENT OR EPISODIC
FOCAL SYMPTOMS

INTRODUCTION

Transient or episodic focal neurological symptoms are common, and they may be the key to the diagnosis of a neurological condition. These symptoms are only rarely witnessed by the neurologist, so the information must be gleaned from a careful history. In Chap. 1 we said that localizing information for neurological diagnosis is largely obtained from the physical and neurological examinations, because the information is objective. Careful history taking, however, also provides important localizing information, and transient symptoms are a good example.

CLINICAL PRESENTATION: SYMPTOMS AND SIGNS

One of the most common causes of transient neurological symptomatology is transient ischemia to a part of the brain, ingrained in medical culture as a TIA, or transient ischemic attack. These symptoms are very important to recognize, as they are the "warning signs" of stroke. Common manifestations in the internal carotid artery territory are transient blindness in one eye, often with a sensation of a shade descending over the vision; transient difficulty in speaking or in understanding language; and transient numbness and/or weakness in the contralateral side of the body, such as arm and face, arm and leg, or face, arm, and leg. In the vertebrobasilar artery territory, TIAs can take the form of attacks of vertigo, often accompanied by other brainstem symptoms such as diplopia, dysarthria, dysphagia, facial or body paresthesias, weakness or incoordination.

TIAs are defined as transient symptoms lasting less than 24 hours and leaving no permanent, residual damage. In fact, most TIAs last a few minutes. In the era of magnetic resonance imaging (MRI) scanning, up to 40% of patients presenting with TIA symptoms are found to have small infarctions by diffusion weighted imaging (DWI). If such imaging is available, the attack would be reclassified as a stroke, rather than a TIA, according to current guidelines.

Transient ischemic attacks are considered to be medical emergencies, in that they warn of an impending stroke. In a study of over 1700 patients discharged from emergency departments in Northern California, fully 10.5% suffered a stroke within 3 months, half of them within 48 hours of the initial TIA. Other adverse outcomes such as myocardial infarction and death were also increased after TIA. The British Oxfordshire study found an even higher rate of stroke, 8–10% in the first 7 days following transient ischemic attacks. Predictors of increased risk of stroke included age over 60 years, presence of unilateral weakness or speech difficulty with the attack, duration over 10 minutes and especially >60 minutes, systolic blood pressure >140 mm Hg or diastolic blood pressure >90 mm Hg, and presence of diabetes. Increasingly, patients with TIA are being admitted to hospitals or stroke centers for observation and for testing including carotid imaging, echocardiography, fasting lipid panels, and other diagnostic tests for stroke (see Chap. 24), so that the appropriate preventive therapies can be undertaken before the patient is discharged.

DIFFERENTIAL DIAGNOSIS

The differential diagnosis of TIA involves other causes of transient symptoms or "spells". Migraine is a frequent source of confusion, since migraine can cause visual symptoms, though only rarely a monocular visual loss like the *transient monocular blindness* (also called *amaurosis fugax*, or transient blindness) cited above. In the aura of a migraine, sensory disturbances on one side are common, and occasionally even motor paralysis can develop. In general, migraines are characteristic from one attack to another, and they often feature a progression of symptoms over minutes, whereas TIA symptoms more often present simultaneously or march from one part of the body to another over seconds. In migraines, the aura is usually followed by a throbbing headache with nausea and photophobia, which would be much less frequent in stroke. Variants of migraine that can resemble stroke are hemiplegic and ophthalmoplegic migraine (see Chap. 30). Migraine usually begins at an earlier age than stroke, though exceptions occur. Occasionally, a migraine will be associated with an actual stroke (*migrainous infarction*). Criteria for migrainous infarction include the requirement that the spell begins with symptoms characteristic of the patient's usual migraines.

Another source of confusion with TIA and stroke is the epileptic seizure, sometimes followed by a postictal (Todd's) paralysis. Seizures are typically accompanied by active jerking, not usually a feature of strokes. Seizures, like migraines, often have a "march", but the epileptic march usually occurs over seconds, rather than over minutes. The postictal Todd's paralysis is usually brief, lasting minutes to hours, but occasionally the postictal period can last days, especially when associated with a structural lesion such as a brain tumor or infarction.

A last source of confusion with TIAs is the differential diagnosis of transient alterations of consciousness, such as light-headedness or syncope. These are discussed in Chap. 20.

LABORATORY AND RADIOLOGICAL INVESTIGATION

The laboratory investigation of a TIA patient is geared to exclude other diagnoses and also to look for a cause of the TIA, so that preventive treatment can be initiated before the patient experiences a stroke. MRI of the brain, usually with magnetic resonance angiography (MRA), is becoming a standard, in that it can detect small strokes in some patients with TIA, and it is also the most sensitive diagnostic tool for detecting structural brain lesions such as tumors and arteriovenous malformations. MRA of the head can detect intracranial artery stenoses, and the neck arteries can be imaged by MRA of the neck. Currently, a variety of imaging modalities is available for imaging of the cervical and cerebral vessels, including ultrasound (carotid Doppler and transcranial Doppler), computed tomographic (CT) angiography, MRA, and catheter angiography. Individual hospitals and stroke centers have protocols for which imaging technique to order, and there is no general consensus on which is best. Patients also undergo echocardiography to detect cardiac sources of embolism. If suspicion is strong, a transesophageal echocardiogram is much more sensitive than a standard, transthoracic echocardiogram. Heart monitoring, either by telemetry in the hospital, or an outpatient Holter monitor, is indicated to look for paroxysmal atrial fibrillation. Blood tests are also important, including a fasting lipid profile in all patients, and testing for hypercoagulable states or conditions associated with vasculitis when appropriate. Of the hypercoagulable states, anticardiolipin antibody is the most common entity associated with arterial disorders such as TIA and stroke.

TREATMENT

The treatment of a patient with TIA depends on the results of the diagnostic assessment. We recommend risk factor modification in all patients. This includes treatment of hypertension, β-hydroxy-β-methylglutaryl-coenzyme A (HMG-CoA) reductase inhibitor ("statin") therapy for elevated lipids (especially LDL >100), smoking cessation, and institution of a program of exercise and healthy diet. If a carotid stenosis is found, ipsilateral to the TIA symptoms, and the stenosis is greater than 70%, carotid endarterectomy is indicated. Currently, carotid angioplasty with stenting is gaining in popularity.

As of now, the only studies suggesting superiority of stenting over surgery are those supporting greater safety in patients considered to be at high risk for carotid endarterectomy, such as those with unstable angina, prior carotid surgery, prior neck irradiation, or a contralateral carotid artery occlusion. If the patient has atrial fibrillation or a related, definite cardiac source of embolus (prosthetic mitral or aortic valve, recent myocardial infarction (MI) with mural thrombus, ventricular aneurysm, or low output congestive heart failure with left ventricular ejection fraction <30%), anticoagulation with warfarin is indicated. For patients without such a cardiac source of embolus, antiplatelet therapy is recommended. The three current options for antiplatelet therapy are aspirin, aspirin plus extended release dipyridamole (Aggrenox), and clopidogrel (Plavix). Clinical trials suggest that both aspirin and extended release dipyridamole and clopidogrel are superior to aspirin in preventing stroke.

COURSE AND PROGNOSIS

As mentioned above, the occurrence of a transient ischemic attack presages a greatly increased risk of stroke, and prompt, preventive measures are essential. Aggressive management of patients with TIA can reduce the incidence of stroke and irreversible disability in this population.

KEY REFERENCES

Albers GW, Caplan LR, Easton JD, et al. Transient ischemic attack—proposal for a new definition. *New Engl J Med* 2002;347:1713–1716.

Albers GW, Amarenco P, Easton JD, et al. Antithrombotic and thrombolytic therapy for ischemic stroke: the Seventh ACCP Conference on Antithrombotic and Thrombolytic Therapy. *Chest* 2004;126 (Suppl.3):483S–512S.

Johnston SC, Gress DR, Browner WS, et al. Short-term prognosis after emergency department diagnosis of TIA. *JAMA* 2000;284:2901–2906.

Kirshner HS, Biller J, Callahan, AS III. Long-term therapy to prevent stroke. *J Am Board Fam Pract* 2005;18:528–540.

Levine SR. Hypercoagulable states and stroke: a selective review. *CNS Spectr* 2005;10: 567–578.

Rothwell PM, Giles MF, Flossmann E, et al. A simple score (ABCD) to identify individuals at high early risk of stroke after transient ischemic attack. *Lancet* 2005;366: 29–36.

North American Symptomatic Carotid Endarterectomy Trial Collaborators. Beneficial effect of carotid endarterectomy in symptomatic patients with high-grade carotid stenosis. *N Engl J Med* 1991;325:445–453.

Rosenberg RD, Aird WC. Vascular-bed-specific hemostasis and hypercoagulable states. *N Engl J Med* 1999;340:1555–1564.

The ESPRIT Study Group. Aspirin plus dipyridamole versus aspirin alone after cerebral ischaemia of arterial origin (ESPRIT): randomized controlled trial. Lancet 2006;367:1665–73.

The Stroke Prevention by Aggressive Reduction in Cholesterol Levels (SPARCL) Investigators. High-dose atorvastatin after Stroke or Transient Ischemic Attack. New Engl J Med 2006;355:549–559.

Yadav JS, Wholey MH, Kuntz RE, et al. Protected carotid-artery stenting versus endarterectomy in high-risk patients. *N Engl J Med* 2004;351:1493–1501.

Welch KMA, Levine SR. Migraine-related stroke in the context of the International Headache Society classification of head pain. *Arch Neurol* 1990;47:458–462.

TRANSIENT ALTERATION

OF CONSCIOUSNESS

INTRODUCTION

Much of neurology involves the diagnosis of "spells", in which there is alteration or loss of consciousness. The key to diagnosis is a careful history, as many patients will have a completely normal physical and neurological examination. As in transient ischemic attack (TIA) (Chap. 19), the history in this instance provides not only the temporal history, but also localizing information about the nervous system.

   Syncope, or transient loss of consciousness, is a very common symptom. It has been estimated that syncope accounts for as many as 3% of emergency department visits, 6% of hospitalizations, and nearly a third of young adults report a history of syncope. Many resources are committed to the diagnosis and treatment of syncope, but frequently the cause is obvious, based on a careful history.

CLINICAL PRESENTATION: SYMPTOMS AND SIGNS

Syncope is related to a transient global reduction in cerebral blood flow and most commonly results from decreased cardiac output, decreased blood volume, decreased peripheral resistance, or combinations of these factors. A cardiac origin, such as an arrhythmia, is more common in older individuals. Other cardiac causes of syncope include outflow obstruction in aortic stenosis, or in hypertrophic cardiomyopathy syndromes such as *asymmetric septal hypertrophy* or idiopathic hypertrophic septal hypertrophy. Carotid sinus hypersensitivity is another, rare cause of syncope. Orthostatic hypotension related to autonomic nervous system disorders or dehydration can cause syncope in the upright position, and taking the blood pressure lying, sitting, and standing can confirm this etiology.

In adolescents and young adults, syncope is most often neurally mediated; this type of syncope is variably referred to as vasovagal, reflex, or neurocardiogenic syncope. Syncopal episodes can be provoked by nociceptive stimuli, strong emotions, or rapid emptying of a distended bladder. In the case of an emotional stimulus or a severe anxiety state, hyperventilation, with vasoconstriction induced by hypocarbia, may be a contributing factor to syncope. Neurocardiogenic syncope is more likely to occur in the upright posture. There is commonly a prodrome of nausea, "cold sweats", light-headedness, and blurring or graying of vision, symptoms often referred to together as a "presyncopal feeling". An observer may witness pallor and limp posture. Recovery is usually very fast with syncope, without a "postictal state". Many syncopal episodes are associated with motor activity, predominantly brief myoclonic jerks, lasting a few seconds, and sometimes confused with tonic clonic activity associated with a seizure.

DIFFERENTIAL DIAGNOSIS

The most common differential diagnosis is between syncope and seizure. The aura of a syncopal episode is usually longer than that of a seizure, and the light-headedness is different from the peculiar odors, emotions, and psychic states that can precede a seizure (see Chap. 25). Patients who suffer syncope usually have enough warning to sit down, or at least to reach out an arm to break their fall. Patients with seizures often collapse so quickly that they may suffer broken limbs. As mentioned above, myoclonic jerks may accompany a syncopal episode, but prolonged, rhythmic jerking of the limbs on one or both sides would favor a seizure. Syncope usually ends quickly, with rapid resumption of normal mental status, whereas a seizure is usually followed by a postictal state of lethargy, headache, and confusion. Many patients go to sleep after a seizure. This differential diagnosis is usually easy when the spell is witnessed, but patients with epilepsy frequently do not remember the events surrounding a seizure, and this can lead to diagnostic confusion. If there is doubt, an electroencephalogram (EEG) may detect interictal electrical discharges, suggestive of epilepsy. The myoclonic activity associated with syncope is not accompanied by a cortical discharge on the EEG. The EEG shows progressive slowing leading to generalized attenuation, with rapid reversal during recovery, as opposed to the rhythmic discharges of an epileptic seizure.

Hyperventilation can produce dizziness, altered consciousness, and paresthesias, especially in the perioral area and in the fingertips. Hyperventilation can be performed in the clinic or during the EEG to reproduce symptoms.

Patients with pulmonary embolus may suddenly become hypoxic and lose consciousness, but most patients have associated shortness of breath and hypoxemia, as well as pleuritic chest pain, and often hemoptysis. None of these symptoms would be expected in association with a typical syncopal episode or epileptic seizure.

Migraine is usually not confused with syncope, since most migraine attacks do not involve loss of consciousness. Migraine attacks are frequently preceded by an aura, as discussed in Chap. 30, and migraine occasionally causes alteration of consciousness or a transient confusional state. The typical, throbbing headache and nausea usually make the diagnosis clear.

Transient ischemic attacks most often cause transient focal symptoms, such as numbness, visual loss, weakness, or inability to speak. Loss of consciousness is uncommon. Occasionally, a vertebrobasilar TIA will cause alteration or even loss of consciousness, usually preceded by brainstem symptoms such as vertigo, ataxia, dysarthria, dysphagia, diplopia, or unilateral weakness or sensory loss. This would be a rare differential diagnosis for syncope. One cause of vertebrobasilar symptoms is the subclavian steal syndrome, in which a subclavian artery stenosis causes the shunting of blood from the brain to the arm via retrograde blood flow down one vertebral artery. Rarely, exercise of the arm can precipitate vertigo or syncope in this condition. Measuring blood pressure in both arms provides a clue to reduced subclavian artery blood flow.

Transient global amnesia (TGA) is a TIA-like episode of transient memory loss. The patient is usually alert, knows his or her own identity, but cannot say why he or she is at the present location. Many patients ask repetitive questions about their location, what has happened, and why they are there. This symptom complex lasts less than 24 hours, by definition. The cause is not fully understood. The TGA syndrome occurs mostly in middle-aged and elderly people, raising the question of a true TIA, but the risk of stroke appears to be small. Some patients do have magnetic resonance imaging (MRI) abnormalities in the temporal lobe or hippocampal area, raising the question of ischemia in the memory structures of the brain, but many do not. The differential diagnosis of TGA involves seizure, migraine, drug effects, and others.

Another TIA-like syndrome is the *drop attack of the elderly* , a syndrome of sudden falling, without any presyncopal warning symptoms, and without self-described loss of consciousness or postictal state. Most patients with such drop attacks are elderly, and fractured hips and related injuries are not uncommon, making the syndrome a major diagnostic problem. Like TGA, drop attacks are of unknown cause. TIA in the vertebrobasilar distribution, simple syncope with amnesia for the loss of consciousness, cardiac arrhythmia, and epileptic seizure are within the differential diagnosis. A history from an eyewitness is often very helpful in coming to a correct diagnosis.

A few other, less common episodic syndromes complete the differential diagnosis of syncope. Hypoglycemia can cause light-headedness, a sense of hunger, and an alteration of consciousness which can lead to loss of consciousness if the patient does not ingest glucose. Diabetic patients often wear bracelets with medical information for this reason, and most keep glucose-containing snacks with them. Carcinoid syndrome, in which sero- tonin and its metabolites are released by tumors, may cause peculiar, transi- tory symptoms including light-headedness and flushing. Similar symptoms can be seen in systemic mastocytosis, related to release of histamine.

Sleep disorders do not enter into the differential diagnosis of syncope, except for events that occur during waking, such as the sudden sleep attacks and cataplexy, which are part of the narcolepsy syndrome. Sleep attacks are usually preceded by an overwhelming desire to sleep, which the patient may try to resist, and this history is obviously quite different from that of syncope. Cataplexy involves a sudden loss of muscle tone, often causing the patient to collapse to the floor. This may occur in response to a sudden emotion, such as laughing at a joke or hearing some sad or upset- ting news. Cataplexy does not involve loss of consciousness; the patient is fully awake during the event. Further discussion of sleep disorders is included in Chap. 21.

Of the differential diagnoses discussed, the typical, neurally-mediated or neurocardiogenic syncope is a benign condition. Attention should be paid to a search for a cardiac origin such as arrhythmia or cardiac outflow obstruction, which can be life-threatening, or for seizures, which are likely to recur unpredictably, and also put the patient at risk of harm.

LABORATORY TESTING

The laboratory testing for a patient with syncope follows from the differen- tial diagnosis discussed above. A careful physical examination is essential and should include provoking factors such as deliberate hyperventilation and sudden standing from a lying or sitting position with documentation of pulse and blood pressure changes. Comparing the blood pressure in the two arms can help in detection of vascular abnormalities such as the sub- clavian steal syndrome. A careful cardiac examination is also important. Twenty-four-hour Holter monitoring, or more prolonged *cardiac loop* recorders are used for detecting arrhythmias, and an echocardiogram can exclude an aortic stenosis or other outflow obstruction in the heart. EEG or EEG monitoring is used to detect seizures. A brain imaging study such as an MRI scan can exclude a lesion that would cause a seizure, though this is usually not needed in the more typical work-up for syncope. MRA can be done to exclude vertebrobasilar transient ischemic attacks. If pulmonary embolism is suspected, a blood oxygen saturation measurement, or a heli- cal CT scan of the chest or ventilation-perfusion isotope lung scan is indi- cated. Chemistry monitoring, glucose tolerance testing, screening of indolamines (for carcinoid syndrome) or histamine (for mastocytosis) can be done in selected cases. Finally, tilt table testing can be used to look for hypotension. Most of the time, detailed work-ups are not very fruitful, and the routine use of EEG or brain imaging in cases of simple syncope is probably not warranted.

COURSE AND PROGNOSIS, TREATMENT

Most syncope is benign. Single episodes in someone who has had a strong emotional trigger such as bad news or venopunture (vasovagal syncope) probably do not require any diagnostic testing or any treatment other than reassurance. The most important aspect of the management of syncope is the identification of the more serious causes such as cardiac arrhythmia, cardiac outflow obstruction, or pulmonary embolism, so that these conditions can be treated. The correct diagnosis of syncope also requires the examiner to exclude the mimicking conditions, such as epileptic seizure, TIA, hypoglycemia, and sleep disorder, which would require entirely different treatment measures.

KEY REFERENCES

Syncope

Chen LY, Gersh BJ, Hodge DO, et al. Prevalence and clinical outcomes of patients with multiple potential causes of syncope. *Mayo Clin Proc* 2003;78:414–420.

Grubb BP. Neurocardiogenic syncope. *New Engl J Med* 2005;352:1004–1010.

Kapoor WN. Syncope. *New Engl J Med* 2000;343:1856–1862.

Kapoor WN. Evaluation and management of the patient with syncope. *JAMA* 1992; 268:2553–2560.

Parry SW, Kenny RA. The management of vasovagal syncope. *Q J Med* 1999;92: 697–705.

Soteriades ES, Evans JC, Larson MG, et al. Incidence and prognosis of syncope. *New Engl J Med* 2002;347:878–885.

Other spells

Meissner I, Wiebers DO, Swanson JW,et al. The natural history of "drop attacks". *Neurology* 1986;36:1029–1034.

Palardy J, Havrankova J, Lepage R, et al. Blood glucose measurements during symptomatic episodes in patients with suspected postprandial hypoglycemia. *New Engl J Med* 1989:321:1421–1425.

Young WF, Maddox DE. Spells: in search of a cause. *Mayo Clin Proc* 1995;70:757–765.

SLEEP DISORDERS

Kim Hutchison, MD

INTRODUCTION

Sleep disorders represent a rapidly growing, multidisciplinary field of medicine. Many of the primary sleep disorders have their origin in the brain, and it is therefore important for the neurologist and medical student to understand the various presentations, diagnostic tests, and treatments of common sleep disorders.

Hypersomnia

The most common complaint evaluated in a sleep disorders clinic is excessive daytime sleepiness. The *Sleep in America* poll reported in 2002 that 22% of Americans are excessively sleepy 2 or more days per week. This common condition has a wide range of negative consequences. Excessive sleepiness results in a greater risk of automobile, industrial, and household accidents, poor school or work performance, and impaired interpersonal relationships. Excessive daytime sleepiness has become an important public health concern.

The most frequent cause of excessive sleepiness is inadequate sleep time. Increased waking demands often relegate sleep to a level of secondary importance. For those who are obtaining a sufficient amount of sleep (typically 7–8 hours per night in adults), excessive sleepiness may result from disrupted sleep continuity, caused by a comorbid sleep or medical disorder. Disorders of the circadian rhythm (e.g., time zone changes, jet lag, and shift work sleep disorder) and soporific medications can also produce excessive daytime sleepiness. Lastly, excessive sleepiness can result from pathology of the sleep-wake system of the central nervous system, as seen in persons with narcolepsy.

Narcolepsy

Narcolepsy is a chronic neurological disorder, in which the brain cannot regulate sleep-wake cycles normally. The hallmark of narcolepsy is excessive daytime sleepiness and sleep attacks, but narcolepsy is also commonly associated

with other rapid eye movement (REM) sleep phenomena, including cataplexy, hypnogogic hallucinations, and sleep paralysis. Cataplexy occurs in
approximately 70% of narcoleptics. Cataplexy is defined as a sudden, transient loss of muscle tone triggered by an intense emotional stimulus such as
laughter, fright, or anger. Cataplexy may be subtle, such as jaw sagging or
knee-buckling, or more dramatic, resulting in collapse and injury. The duration of the loss of muscle tone is typically seconds to a few minutes, and consciousness is always preserved. Other REM sleep abnormalities include
hypnagogic or hypnapompic hallucinations (vivid dream-like experiences
that occur during the transition between wakefulness and sleep) and sleep
paralysis (inability to move during sleep onset or upon awakening from
sleep, while the patient is awake). Other, commonly reported but less specific symptoms for the diagnosis of narcolepsy include automatic behaviors
(time lapses during daytime activities), short-term memory difficulty, and
depression.

Narcolepsy also disrupts nocturnal sleep. Ironically, narcoleptics may
complain of insomnia (difficulty falling asleep or staying asleep). Less common, but more dramatic, are sleep attacks. These are sudden, irresistible
urges to fall asleep, often at inappropriate times, such as during a meal or
conversation. The excessive sleepiness noted in narcolepsy is worse during
passive activities, and patients often report falling asleep during classes.
Brief naps typically offer a transient, "refreshed" feeling. Narcolepsy can
have significant negative effects on family and social situations, in addition
to interfering with performance at school or work.

The etiology of narcolepsy is still being investigated. Narcolepsy has
recently been associated with decreased levels of hypocretin, a neuropep-
tide found in the lateral hypothalamus, and with specific human leukocyte
antigen (HLA)-types (HLA–DQB1*0602). The HLA-type predilection suggests a possible genetic or autoimmune cause. Neuroimaging studies are
typically normal.

Narcolepsy is diagnosed by a combination of clinical symptoms and
polysomnographic studies. An overnight polysomnogram (PSG) is performed primarily to eliminate other causes of excessive daytime sleepiness.
Short sleep-onset and REM latencies may be observed. In the normal PSG,
the patient falls asleep in Stage 1, slow-wave sleep, and progresses through
Stages 2–4 before entering the first REM period. In narcolepsy, the patient
may enter REM sleep immediately from wakefulness. The overnight PSG is
followed by a daytime multiple sleep latency test (MSLT). This study consists of four–five nap opportunities lasting approximately 20 minutes each
and scheduled 2 hours apart. Two or more sleep-onset REM periods are
generally required for the diagnosis of narcolepsy. The mean sleep latency
(average time to fall asleep) is less than 8 minutes. Many of the symptoms
of narcolepsy can also occur in people who are sleep deprived; cataplexy,
however, is unique to narcolepsy.

Once the diagnosis of narcolepsy is established, the disease is not progressive but usually persists for life, though some of the symptoms may improve over time. Treatment is symptomatic and geared toward maintaining daytime alertness and alleviating REM phenomena. Central nervous system stimulants, such as modafinil (Provigil) or amphetamines, are the mainstay of treating daytime sleepiness. Tricyclic antidepressants and selective serotonin reuptake inhibitors (SSRIs) are the most effective for cataplexy and other REM phenomena. More recently, gamma-hydroxybutyrate (GHB) has been used in the treatment of cataplexy and for the consolidation of nocturnal REM sleep. Several behavioral treatments should also be utilized. These include scheduled daytime naps, particularly before attention-demanding tasks, keeping a regular sleep-wake schedule, and avoiding alcohol and large, carbohydrate-rich meals. Education and support services are essential to the long-term well-being of the patient with narcolepsy. Teachers, employers, and family members also need to be educated. Information for these support services is available through the Narcolepsy Network and the National Sleep Foundation.

Sleep-disordered breathing

Sleep-disordered breathing encompasses a spectrum of breathing abnormalities resulting from increased upper airway resistance. Obstructive sleep apnea (OSA), the most severe form of sleep-disordered breathing, is characterized by repetitive episodes of reduced (hypopneas) or total cessation (apneas) of airflow during sleep. These obstructions are most commonly the result of excessive relaxation of the upper airway dilating muscles. The reduced airflow leads to blood oxygen desaturation and arousal from sleep. The patient thus wakes up, consciously or unconsciously, frequently throughout the night. The cumulative effect of the hypoxemia and sleep fragmentation can result in excessive daytime sleepiness, as well as a number of cardiovascular and neurobehavioral effects. Obstructive sleep apnea has recently been found to be an independent risk factor for myocardial infarction and stroke.

The most common symptoms of obstructive sleep apnea include excessive daytime sleepiness, habitual snoring, and witnessed apneas during sleep. Less common symptoms include morning headaches, insomnia/restless sleep, nocturia, short-term memory loss, chronic fatigue, and erectile dysfunction. It is important to obtain information from a bed partner, as patients are often unaware of their nighttime symptoms. Predisposing factors include male gender, excessive weight, large neck circumference (greater than 43 cm.), narrow oropharynx (abnormal structure of the palate, uvula, or tongue), increasing age, alcohol usage, and family history. In children, enlarged tonsils are commonly associated with OSA.

An overnight polysomnogram (sleep study) is the best means to detect and quantify the apneic events associated with obstructive sleep apnea. The apnea-hypopnea index (AHI) is the number of apneas and/or hypopneas per hour of sleep. By consensus, OSA is defined by an AHI of 5 or greater, with evidence of daytime symptoms, or when the AHI is 15 or greater. Treatments include weight loss, nasal continuous positive airway pressure (CPAP), and dental devices that modify the position of the tongue or jaw. Upper airway and jaw surgical procedures may also be appropriate in selected patients, but these procedures are invasive and expensive.

Insomnia

Insomnia is a debilitating and often chronic condition that affects nearly one-third of the population at one time or another. Insomnia is characterized by difficulty initiating and/or maintaining sleep, resulting in sleep loss and decreased functioning during wakefulness. There are many different types of insomnia. Chronic, or psychophysiological, insomnia is the most common type evaluated in a sleep disorders clinic. Psychophysiological insomnia refers to a heightened level of arousal during attempted sleep, along with learned sleep-preventing associations. A cycle develops where, the more one tries to fall asleep, the more anxious one becomes, and the less able one is to fall asleep. Learned negative associations develop between the sleep environment and successful sleep. This results in an inability to relax the body and allow sleep onset. Individuals with insomnia tend to note decreased feelings of well-being during the day and complain of daytime fatigue, though typically they are unable to take naps.

Insomnia may also be a symptom of other conditions. Many medical and neurological disorders may give rise to acute or chronic insomnia. Pain, in particular, often results in sleep difficulties. Hormone changes, as seen in menopause and pregnancy, may disrupt sleep cycles. Other primary sleep disorders, such as obstructive sleep apnea and narcolepsy, may present with symptoms of insomnia. Mood and anxiety disorders frequently have associated sleep complaints. Lastly, medication use and substance use and abuse can interfere with natural sleep cycles. Alcohol is commonly used as a sleep aid, however individuals who use alcohol to induce sleep are more prone to fragmented and restless sleep later in the night. With prolonged use of alcohol, abstinence can cause rebound insomnia.

Initiation of appropriate insomnia treatment depends on identification of the underlying cause. Chronic insomnia is best treated by behavioral modification and improvement of sleep hygiene (see Table 21-1). Hypnotic medications may be beneficial for short periods, but most are not indicated for long-term use.

Parasomnias

Parasomnias are defined as unusual or undesirable behaviors during sleep. They often involve complex, seemingly purposeful behaviors enacted outside of conscious awareness. In most instances, there is no memory for the event the next morning. Parasomnias can occur during nonrapid eye movement (NREM) or rapid eye movement (REM) sleep.

Table 21-1 **Practicing Good Sleep Hygiene**

1. Develop a consistent bedtime routine
2. Go to bed and get out of bed at the same time 7 nights per week
3. Exercise and expose oneself to daylight every day (early in the day)
4. Limit alcohol, tobacco and caffeine, especially in the evenings
5. Avoid daytime naps
6. Go to bed only when sleepy and get out of bed if unable to sleep (read quietly)
7. Keep the bedroom cool and comfortable and hide your clock

NREM parasomnias, or disorders of arousal, include sleep walking, sleep terrors, and confusional arousals. These parasomnias are more common in children than in adults. REM parasomnias include REM-sleep behavior disorder (RBD) and nightmares. RBD is characterized by a loss of the normal motor paralysis that is part of REM sleep. This results in dream enactment, often with the sleeper defending against an attacker. These behaviors frequently result in injury to the patient or bed partner. RBD is associated with several neurological disorders, including Parkinson's disease, dementia with Lewy bodies, and multiple-system atrophy. Parasomnias do not typically cause insomnia or excessive sleepiness. They may be triggered by sleep deprivation, physical activity, emotional stress, alcohol, and medications. Treatment is required when the behaviors are potentially dangerous or cause significant disruption to family members. Low dose benzodiazepines or tricyclic antidepressant medications are usually effective in suppressing parasomnias.

Restless legs syndrome

The restless legs syndrome (RLS) is a common clinical syndrome characterized by uncomfortable sensations in the legs that are alleviated, at least in part, by movement. There are four diagnostic criteria (see Table 21-2). Other commonly associated features include sleep disturbance, especially difficulty initiating

Table 21-2 **Diagnostic Criteria for Restless Legs Syndrome**

1. Uncomfortable sensations in the limbs associated with an urge to move
2. Worsening of symptoms with rest or inactivity
3. Partial or total relief of symptoms with movement (such as walking or stretching)
4. Symptoms worse in the evening and/or at night

sleep, involuntary movements, and a family history of restless legs. The symptoms range in severity from mildly annoying to severe pain. Secondary restless legs syndrome occurs when there is a medical or neurologic condition associated with RLS. Such conditions include iron-deficiency anemia, uremia, Parkinson's disease, and pregnancy. Treatment is symptomatic and consists of dopaminergic agents such as pramipexole (Mirapex) and ropinirole (Requip), benzodiazepines, opiates, and avoidance of caffeine. In patients with decreased ferritin levels (below 50), oral iron replacement may significantly improve the symptoms. RLS overlaps with periodic limb movements in sleep (PLMS), a term used to describe frequent extension movements of the limbs while asleep.

Polysomnography

Polysomnography (PSG or "sleep study") is the recording, analysis, and interpretation of multiple, simultaneous physiologic parameters during sleep. PSG is an essential tool in the understanding of normal sleep and the diagnosis of sleep disorders. A PSG usually occurs overnight in a sleep laboratory and is performed by a trained technologist. Standard monitoring includes electroencephalography (EEG) to measure brain electrical activity, electro-oculography and electromyography (EMG) to measure eye and jaw muscle movements, electrocardiography (ECG) to measure heart rhythms, airflow and respiratory effort channels, oxygen saturation via pulse oximetry, limb EMG to measure leg movements, and sound and video recording. The recording is divided into epochs of 30 seconds and the predominant stage of sleep (NREM 1-4 or REM) is assigned. Each epoch is then analyzed for any neurophysiologic and/or respiratory abnormalities. Figure 21-1 shows an epoch from a PSG showing apnea during a REM sleep phase. A daytime multiple sleep latency test (MSLT) may follow an overnight PSG. This test is used to document the presence and severity of daytime sleepiness and the presence of REM sleep.

CASE HISTORY

A 64-year-old male with a 10-year history of Parkinson's disease presents with his wife, who is very concerned about some recent behaviors during her husband's sleep. She notes that several times over the past few months he seemed to be struggling during his sleep. He would yell and kick and even punched her once during the night. She reports that these behaviors are contrary to his character, and she is concerned that he has no memory of the events in the mornings. Once when she woke him after an episode, he reported dreaming that someone was attacking him. An overnight polysomnogram demonstrated increased muscle activity during REM sleep. The diagnosis of REM-sleep behavior disorder was made. He was treated with clonazepam 0.5 mg at bedtime, with complete resolution of the events.

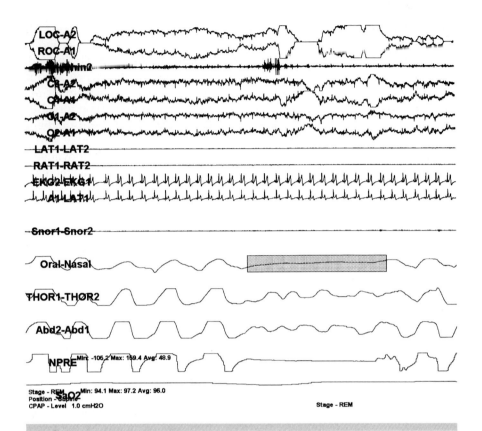

Figure 21-1 ***Epoch from PSG with apnea (during REM).*** Obstructive sleep apnea during a one-minute segment of rapid eye movement (REM) sleep. Event is shaded in the oral-nasal thermistor channel and represents a flattening of the signal lasting greater than 10 seconds, consistent with lack of airflow. A similar flattening is seen in the NPRE (nasal pressure tranducer) channel. The THOR and Abd (thoracic and abdominal) channels show that the patient has preservation of respiratory effort.

KEY REFERENCES

Aldrich MS. Narcolepsy. *N Engl J Med* 1990;323:389–394.

American Academy of Sleep Medicine. *International Classification of Sleep Disorder s.* 2nd ed. *Diagnostic and Coding Manual.* Westchester, IL: American Academy of Sleep Medicine; 2005.

Earley CJ. Restless legs syndrome. *N Engl J Med* 2003;348:2103–2109.

Flemons WW. Obstructive sleep apnea. *N Engl J Med* 2002;347:498–504.

Guilleminault C (2005). Narcolepsy: diagnosis and management. In: Kryger MH, Roth T, Dement WC, eds. *Principles and Practice of Sleep Medicine.* 4th ed. Philadelphia, PA: Elsevier Saunders 2005;780–790.

Krahn LE, Black JL, Silber MH. Narcolepsy: new understanding of irresistible sleep. *Mayo Clin Proc* 2001;76:185–194.

Mahowald MW. Parasomnias. *Med Clin North Am* 2004;88(3):669–678.

Olsen EJ, Moore WR, Morgenthaler TI, et al. Obstructive sleep apnea–hypopnea syndrome. *Mayo Clin Proc* 2003;78(12):1545–1552.

Overeem S, Mignot E, van Dijk JG, et al. Narcolepsy: clinical features, new pathophysiologic insights, and future perspectives. *J Clin Neurophysiol* 2001;18:78–105.

Overeem S, Scammell TE, Lammers GJ. Hypocretin/orexin and sleep: implications for the pathophysiology and diagnosis of narcolepsy. *Curr Opin Neurol* 2002;15:739–745.

Shamsuzzaman ASM, Gersh BJ, Somers V. Obstructive sleep apnea. Implications for cardiac and vascular disease. *JAMA* 2003;290:1906–1914.

Siegel JM. Narcolepsy. *Sci Am* 2000;282:58–63.

Silber MH, Ehrenberg BL, Allen RP, et al. An algorithm for the management of restless legs syndrome. *Mayo Clin Proc* 2004;79:916–922.

Yaggi HK, Concato J, Kernan WN, et al. Obstructive sleep apnea as a risk factor for stroke and death. *N Engl J Med* 2005;353:2034–2041.

DEVELOPMENTAL
DISORDERS

Gerald M. Fenichel, MD
and Howard S. Kirshner, MD

INTRODUCTION

Developmental disorders are somewhat different from other neurological disturbances, in that the brain disorders, whether focal or diffuse, affect the nervous system before it fully forms and organizes. These disorders are generally in the purview of a developmental pediatrician or pediatric neurologist, but medical students should have knowledge of at least the major developmental disorders. This chapter is introductory in nature. More complete discussion of the genetic and metabolic diseases associated with developmental delay can be found in textbooks of pediatric neurology.

Cerebral palsy

Cerebral palsy (CP) is a motor impairment present from birth or shortly thereafter, caused by a nonprogressive brain disturbance (a static encephalopathy). The encephalopathy may be of prenatal or perinatal origin. Possible motor disturbances include spasticity, hypotonia, ataxia, and dyskinesia. The clinical features are the basis for diagnosis, but determining the etiology often requires a brain imaging study. The incidence of CP is 2 per 1000 children, and low birth weight/preterm infants account for more than half of the cases.

The categorization of CP is by the pattern of motor disturbance. *Hemiplegic CP* refers to weakness of the limbs on one side of the body. The usual causes are perinatal stroke or cerebral malformation. *Diplegia* is weakness of all limbs with the legs affected more than the arms. Diplegia is the most common pattern in children born prematurely. The prevalence is 60 per 1000 among children weighing less than 1,000 g at birth. In *spastic quadriplegia*, all four limbs are equally weak and spastic. This pattern is most common with intrauterine disorders (malformations, infections, and hypoxic ischemic encephalopathy at term). *Ataxic CP* refers to a disorder in which incoordination or ataxia on one or both sides of the body is the principal neurological disorder. *Dyskinetic CP* refers to children who have a movement disorder, usually associated with spastic quadriplegia. Dyskinesia is never present at birth but develops during infancy or early childhood. Dyskinetic CP was common in children with kernicterus, a now preventable condition secondary to bilirubin encephalopathy. Dyskinesia in the absence of spasticity suggests an underlying inborn error of metabolism, or one of a large number of inherited metabolic diseases of the nervous system.

ETIOLOGY OF CEREBRAL PALSY

Modern brain imaging techniques, computerized tomography (CT), and especially magnetic resonance imaging (MRI), clarify the etiology in almost all cases of CP. Genetic disorders are the most common cause of *ataxic CP* syndromes. Brain malformations are an important cause of CP in term infants, while periventricular leukomalacia (PVL) is the most common cause of CP in preterm infants. Periventricular leukomalacia is usually the consequence of hypoxic-ischemic encephalopathy in infants born prematurely.

TREATMENT

Prevention is a more important strategy than treatment for cerebral palsy. The most cost-effective strategies are the prevention of prematurity, the avoidance of maternal high-risk behavior during pregnancy (alcohol, drugs, and exposure to infection), the delivery of high-risk pregnancies in regional perinatal centers, and the availability of neonatal intensive care units.

Treatment of affected infants is symptomatic. The main goals of rehabilitative treatment are to improve motor function and to modify the environment to improve mobility. Factors that shorten life expectancy are immobility, profound retardation, and feeding difficulty. Seizures often accompany CP and require medication (see Chap. 25).

Mental retardation

The traditional definition of mental retardation (MR) is an intelligence quotient (IQ) less than 70. A more useful definition, however, is one that combines IQ and functional ability. The American Association of Mental Retardation links degree of severity to the degree of community support required to achieve optimal independence. Mild retardation (IQ 55–70) means intermittent support; moderate retardation (IQ 45–55) indicates limited support; severe retardation (IQ 25–50) indicates extensive support; and profound retardation (IQ below 25) indicates pervasive support.

Mild MR represents three-quarters of the total. These individuals tend to come from socially disadvantaged backgrounds and often have a family history of borderline IQ or mild retardation. Individuals with severe retardation are more likely to have a definable biological cause. X-linked inheritance is responsible for more than 150 known mental retardation syndromes. Fragile X syndrome is the most common X-linked disorder among children with moderate and mild MR. Several other gene loci are associated with mental retardation. In addition, mental retardation can result from many inborn errors of metabolism, infections, and toxic exposures. Epilepsy is the most common comorbid condition.

Treatment is supportive. Those with mild MR require a special educational setting, which may focus on vocational training. Those with severe and profound impairments often require institutional placement.

Autistic spectrum disorders

The initial definition of *infantile autism* was a single syndrome with onset during infancy. The characteristic features included a triad of impaired sociability, impaired verbal and nonverbal communication skills, and restricted activities and interests. Other, commonly observed features include stereotyped behaviors, rigid adherence to routines, and failure to empathize or share activities with others. A spectrum of developmental disorders with a range of disabilities comprises the autistic spectrum disorders (ASD). The broader category, *pervasive developmental disorders*, applies to children who do not meet the full criteria for autism (above). Most people with ASD are functionally retarded, but some have normal or even superior IQ, often in isolated areas of mental function (*idiot savant*). One of the bases of the disorder is thought to be a disturbed *theory of mind*, meaning the inability of autistic children to understand what other people are thinking, and thereby lacking empathy for them. The most common specific cause of autism appears to be maternally inherited duplications of chromosome 15q11–13, accounting for 1–3% of cases. Autistic behavior is associated with other genetic disorders, including other chromosomal abnormalities, the Fragile X syndrome, Rett syndrome, Williams syndrome, and tuberous sclerosis, among many others. It is also associated with inborn errors of metabolism such as phenylketonuria, mucopolysaccharidoses, and peroxisomal disorders, and with infections such as rubella, herpes, and cytomegalovirus.

Asperger disorder represents the high-functioning end of the spectrum. Table 22-1 shows the criteria for the diagnosis of Asperger disorder. A 90% concordance in monozygotic twins suggests a genetic etiology.

Among children with ASD, 40% show improvement during adolescence and one third deteriorate. The neurological examination is generally normal. The onset of seizures or mood disorders usually underlies the deterioration. Approximately two-thirds of adults with autism show poor social adjustment and one-half require institutional care.

The treatment of autism spectrum disorders is challenging. Much of the management is behavioral. Preschool children with ASD should receive special education in a therapeutic nursery or in a home-based behavioral

Table 22-1 **Asperger's Disorder: Diagnostic Criteria**

A. Qualitative impairment in social interaction, manifested by ≥2 of:
   1. Impairment in use of nonverbal behaviors to regulate social interaction
   2. Failure to develop peer relationships
   3. Lack of spontaneous sharing of enjoyments and interests
   4. Lack of social or emotional reciprocity
B. Restricted repetitive and stereotyped behavior, interests, and activities, manifested by ≥1 of:
   1. Preoccupations
   2. Inflexible adherence to routines
   3. Stereotyped, repetitive motor mannerisms
   4. Persistent preoccupation with parts of objects
C. The abnormal behaviors cause significantly impaired functioning
D. No clinically significant language delay
E. No clinically significant cognitive deficit
F. Criteria not met for another pervasive developmental disorder or schizophrenia

Source: *Diagnostic and Statistical Manual of Mental Disorders*. 4th ed. Washington, DC: American Psychiatric Association; 1994.

modification program. Drug treatment may help some symptoms of the disorder, though there is no specific treatment for autism itself. Attention deficit hyperactivity disorder (ADHD)-like behavior can be managed with stimulants; obsessive compulsive behavior with clomipramine (Anafranil), selective serotonin reuptake inhibitors, or atypical antipsychotic drugs; aggressive behaviors with mood stabilizers such as carbamazepine (Tegretol) or beta blockers; tics with neuroleptic drugs such as haloperidol; and psychosis with neuroleptic or atypical antipsychotic drugs.

Learning disabilities

Approximately 10% of school-aged children have learning disabilities (LD) that affect one or more cognitive skills. LDs may involve one or more specific skills; reading (dyslexia), motor function (dysgraphia and dyspraxia), and attention deficit disorder with or without hyperactivity (ADD or ADHD). ADD is also one element of the Tourette triad of tics and obsessive-compulsive disorder.

DYSLEXIA

Dyslexia affects 10% of school-aged children and often has a genetic basis. The definition of developmental dyslexia is an unexpected difficulty in learning to read. A major neurological abnormality is an exclusionary criterion for the diagnosis of dyslexia. The diagnosis requires normal intelligence and exposure to a social and educational environment conducive to learning to read. Although dyslexia is a permanent condition, children identified at an early age and provided remediation are able to read functionally, though rarely for pleasure.

ATTENTION DEFICIT HYPERACTIVITY DISORDER

Attention deficit disorder, formerly called the "hyperactive child" syndrome, can occur with or without hyperactivity. The prevalence of ADHD in school-aged children varies with class size but may be as high as 20%. Complete recovery is not the rule; ADHD persists in 60–70% of adults diagnosed with ADHD in childhood and is an under-recognized cause of cognitive difficulty and work-related stress in adults. ADHD is more common in males than females. Affected females have less hyperactivity. The main features of ADHD are inappropriate inattention, impulsivity, distractibility, and hyperactivity for chronological and mental age. Physical examination is generally normal. Neuropsychological testing reveals normal IQ but low scores on subtests that demand attention or rapid processing.

Most ADHD has a genetic basis. Ten percent of ADHD children probably have the Tourette gene (see Chap. 5). Tics often become manifest when treating the child with drugs that increase attention span. Stimulant use indicated for ADHD, however, is not contraindicated. Atomoxetine (Strattera), a nonstimulant medication used to treat ADHD, does not increase tic frequency.

The treatment of attention deficit disorder involves stimulant drugs and counseling. Stimulants such as methylphenidate (Ritalin, Concerta) and dexamphetamine (Dexedrine, Adderal) are available in long-acting forms, administered once daily. A weaker stimulant is pemoline (Cylert), little used currently because of liver toxicity. Much current controversy surrounds the very common prescribing of stimulants to school-age children who may have mild ADHD. Atomoxetine (Strattera), a reuptake inhibitor of norepinephrine, is not primarily a stimulant and is non-habit-forming. This drug appears to have some efficacy in ADHD.

KEY REFERENCES

General

Diagnostic and Statistical Manual of Mental Disorders. 4th ed. Washington, DC: American Psychiatric Association; 1994.

Fenichel GM. *Clinical Pediatric Neurology. A Signs and Symptoms Approach.* 5th ed. Philadelphia, PA: Elsevier Saunders; 2005.

Pastores GM, Kolodny EH. Inborn errors of metabolism of the nervous system. In: Bradley WG, Daroff RB, Fenichel GM, Jankovic J, eds. *Neurology in Clinical Practice.* Chap. 68. Philadelphia, PA: Elsevier; 2004:1811–1832.

Cerebral palsy

Bax M, Goldstein M, Rosenbaum P, et al. Proposed definition and classification of cerebral palsy, April 2005. *Dev Med Child Neurol* 2005;47:571–576.

Ferriero DM. Neonatal brain injury. *N Engl J Med* 2004;351:1985–1995.

Goldstein M. The treatment of cerebral palsy: what we know, what we don't know. *J Pediatr* 2004;145:S42–S46.

Koman LA, Smith BP, Shilt JS. Cerebral palsy. *Lancet* 2004;363:1619–1631.

Nelson KB. Can we prevent cerebral palsy? *N Engl J Med* 2003;349:1765–1769.

Nelson KB, Grether JK. Causes of cerebral palsy. *Curr Opin Pediatr* 1999;11:487–491.

Petersen MC, Palmer FB. Advances in prevention and treatment of cerebral palsy. *Met Retard Dev Disabil Res Rev* 2001;7:30–37.

Phelan JP, Martin GI, Korst LM. Birth asphyxia and cerebral palsy. *Clin Perinatol* 2005;32:61–76.

Shapiro SM. Definition of the clinical spectrum of kernicterus and bilirubin-induced neurologic dysfunction. *J Perinatol* 2005;25:54–59.

Wasiak J, Hoare B, Wallen M. Botulinum toxin A as an adjunct to treatment in the management of the upper limb in children with spastic cerebral palsy. *Cochrane Database Sys Rev* 2004;3:CD003469.

Mental retardation, genetic syndromes

Baker E, Hinton L, Callen DF, et al. Study of 250 children with idiopathic mental retardation reveals nine cryptic and diverse subtelomeric chromosomal anomalies. *Am J Med Genet* 2002;107:285–293.

Daily DK, Ardinger HH, Holmes GE. Identification and evaluation of mental retardation. *Am Fam Physician* 2000;61:1059–1067.

Geneclinics http://www.geneclinics.org/profiles/ataxias/details.html

Online Mendelian Inheritance in Man

http://www.ncbi/nlm.nih.gov/Omim/

Shevell M, Ashwal S, Donley D, et al. Practice parameter: evaluation of the child with global developmental delay. *Neurology* 2003;60:367–380.

Visootsak J, Warren ST, Anido A, et al. Fragile X syndrome: an update and review for the primary pediatrician. *Clin Pediatr* 2005;44:371–381.

Learning disabilities, dyslexia

Alexander AW, Slinger-Constant AM. Current status of treatments for dyslexia: critical review. *J Child Neurol* 2004;19:744–758.

Demonet JF, Taylor MJ, Chaix Y. Developmental dyslexia. *Lancet* 2004;363:1451–1460.

Hall N. Developmental language disorders. *Semin Pediat Neurol* 1997;4:77–85.

Price CJ, Mechelli A. Reading and reading disturbance. *Curr Opin Neurobiol* 2005;15:231–238.

Rumsey JM. The biology of developmental dyslexia. *JAMA* 1992;268:912–915.

Shaywitz SE. Dyslexia. *N Engl J Med* 1998;338:307–312.

Attention deficit hyperactivity disorder

Barton J. Atomoxetine: a new pharmacotherapeutic approach in the management of attention deficit hyperactivity disorder. *Arch Dis Child* 2005;90(Suppl.1):i26–i29.

Biederman J, Faraone SV. Attention deficit hyperactivity disorder. *Lancet* 2005;366: 237–248.

Brown RT, Amler RW, Freeman WS, et al. Treatment of attention deficit hyperactivity disorder: overview of the evidence. *Pediatrics* 2005;115:e749–e757.

Elia J, Ambrosini PJ, Rapoport JL. Treatment of attention deficit hyperactivity disorder. *N Engl J Med* 1999;340:780–788.

Rappley MD. Attention deficit hyperactivity disorder. *N Engl J Med* 2005;352:165–173.

Steer CR. Managing attention deficit hyperactivity disorder: unmet needs and future directions. *Arch Dis Child* 2005;90(Suppl.1):i19–i25.

Wilens TE, Faraone SV, Biederman J. Attention deficit hyperactivity disorder in adults. *JAMA* 2004;292:619–623.

Wolraich ML, Wibbelsman CJ, Brown TE, et al. Attention deficit hyperactivity disorder among adolescents: a review of the diagnosis, treatment, and clinical implications. *Pediatrics* 2005;115:1734–1746.

Zametkin AJ, Ernst M. Problems in the management of attention deficit hyperactivity disorder. *N Engl J Med* 1999;340:40–46.

Autism and autism spectrum disorders

Chakrabarti S, Fombonne E. Pervasive developmental disorders in preschool children. *JAMA* 2001;285:3093–3099.

Chez MG, Memon S, Hung PC. Neurologic treatment strategies in autism: an overview of medical intervention strategies. *Semin Pediatr Neurol* 2004;11:229–235.

Cohen D, Pichard N, Tordjman S, et al. Specific genetic disorders and autism: clinical contribution towards their identification. *J Autism Dev Disord* 2005;35:103–116.

Deuel RK. Autism: a cognitive developmental riddle. *Pediatr Neurol* 2002;26:349–357.

Francis K. Autism interventions: a critical update. *Dev Med Child Neurol* 2005;47: 493–499.

Muhle R, Trentacoste SV, Rapin I. The genetics of autism. *Pediatrics* 2004;113:e472–e486.

Palermo MT, Curatolo P. Pharmacologic treatment of autism. *J Child Neurol* 2004;19: 155–164.

Prater CD, Zylstra RG. Autism: a medical primer. *Am Fam Physician* 2002;66: 1667–1674.

Rapin I, Dunn M. Update on the language disorders of individuals on the autistic spectrum. *Brain Dev* 2003;25:166–172.

Shastry BS. Molecular genetics of autism spectrum disorders. *J Hum Genet* 2003;48: 495–501.

Shea V. Autism. A perspective on the research literature related to early intensive behavioral intervention (Lovaas) for young children with autism. *Autism* 2004;8:349–367.

Tuchman R. Autism. *Neurol Clin* 2003;21:915–932.

APPROACHES
TO SPECIFIC
NEUROLOGICAL
DISEASES

NEUROLOGICAL

EMERGENCIES

COMA AND INCREASED INTRACRANIAL PRESSURE

The examination of the comatose patient, which was presented in Chap. 1, is absolutely critical to the emergency management of neurological patients. The clinician must be able to evaluate a patient with decreased responsiveness promptly and create a rapid anatomic and etiologic differential diagnosis, as concomitant steps are being taken to minimize or reverse further injury. Confirmatory laboratory tests are then obtained quickly. The examination indicates whether the comatose patient has symptoms and signs that indicate: (1) metabolic brain dysfunction, or (2) anatomic brain dysfunction. Metabolic insults are identified by the typical absence of localizing signs, suggesting that the process is diffuse (for example, drugs intoxications, hepatic encephalopathy, hypoxia, hypoglycemia), affecting the cerebral hemispheres. Anatomic lesions usually cause localizing signs that point to a hemisphere lesion, with or without secondary herniation and compression of the brain stem, or a primary brainstem lesion. Examples include traumatic brain injury, stroke, and cerebral hemorrhage. If a mass lesion with secondary herniation is present, emergency surgery may be needed, but medical measures are always needed to stabilize the patient. Much of the initial management involves treatment of increased intracranial pressure (increased ICP).

Increased intracranial pressure denotes the presence of an elevated spinal fluid pressure within the head. Increased ICP can be caused by many mechanisms, including localized, space-occupying lesions such as brain tumor, brain abscess, or stroke, intracerebral, or extracerebral hemorrhages; hydrocephalus, either of the obstructive or communicating type; venous sinus thrombosis, or blockage in the venous drainage of the brain; benign intracranial hypertension, a syndrome of unknown cause possibly related to decreased egress of cerebrospinal fluid (CSF); or even metabolic disorders such as diffuse hypoxic encephalopathy with edema. The symptoms of increased intracranial pressure include whatever symptoms the localized mass lesion may cause, plus headache; drowsiness, leading to obtundation, stupor, or coma; nausea; and vomiting. Signs of increased intracranial pressure include arterial hypertension, bradycardia, sometimes hyperreflexia, sometimes signs related to the focal lesion (and also signs secondary to a cerebral herniation syndrome), and sometimes optic disc edema (*papilledema*). Papilledema, however, can be a delayed sign, such that the neurologist should never rely on its presence or absence.

The pathophysiology of increased intracranial pressure is based upon the simple fact that the brain rests in a closed, noncompliant space, containing only the three compartments of brain, spinal fluid, and blood within blood vessels. If a mass lesion increases pressure, this will compress adjacent structures and lead to midline shift, herniation of the brain tissue of the frontal lobe under the falx, of the temporal lobe under the tentorium, or of the cerebellar tonsils downward through the foramen magnum. These herniation syndromes are associated with distinctive patterns of evolution of clinical symptoms and signs, as discussed in Chap. 1. In addition, increased intracranial pressure may compromise blood flow to the brain, worsening tissue ischemia. Cerebral perfusion pressure (CPP) is the difference between mean arterial blood pressure and intracranial pressure. In most cases, the CPP should be maintained above 60–70 torr. If CPP drops below about 40 torr, global hypoxia and coma rapidly ensue.

Diagnostic testing of the patient with increased ICP includes rapid brain imaging, usually with computed tomography (CT) scanning, since it is faster than magnetic resonance imaging (MRI). Lumbar puncture can be performed to measure the CSF pressure, but this can increase the risk of herniation in the presence of a mass lesion. CT scanning should always be carried out first, unless the patient has no focal signs and bacterial meningitis is suspected. Even then, most experts now recommend broad spectrum antibiotic coverage first, then a CT scan, and then a lumbar puncture.

Emergency management

If the patient has a space occupying lesion, the definitive treatment is neurosurgery to remove the mass. The patient must be stabilized with medical therapies, however, before it is safe to take the patient to the operating room. This includes, as in any emergency patient, the "ABC's" of airway, breathing, and circulation. The physician must ensure that the patient has a stable airway and respirations, as well as stable and adequate vital signs, and venous access for treatments.

Emergency management of increased ICP includes immediate tracheal intubation and mechanical ventilation. Hyperventilation to PCO_2 levels of approximately 30 torr will induce vasoconstriction and reduce the intravascular blood volume, thus reducing ICP, but care must be taken to avoid hypoperfusion of brain tissue. In general, hyperventilation is an emergency measure, used for only brief periods until more definitive therapy can be initiated. After such brief treatment, maintenance of the PCO_2 in a more normal range of 40 ± 5 torr is safest.

Osmotic agents such as mannitol can also be given to "pull" fluid from the brain tissue into the intravascular space, and then out in the venous drainage. Mannitol is usually given in bolus doses, at a dose of approximately 0.25 g/kg every 4–6 hours. Many critical care specialists give an initial bolus dose of as much as 100 g, and then smaller doses of 25–50 mg every 6 hours. Care must be taken not to dehydrate the patient to the point of vasoconstriction and shock. During mannitol therapy, serum osmolarity should be measured as often as every 6 hours, and osmolarities in the range of 300–320 mOsm are the target. Like hyperventilation, osmotic therapy is a time-limited treatment, since the brain seems able to generate "idiogenic osmoles", and the effect declines over the first few days. Some critical care specialists use hypertonic saline (3–23.4%) rather than or in addition to mannitol.

Corticosteroids such as dexamethasone can help to reduce intracranial pressure, if there is evidence of edema around a mass lesion, often referred to as *vasogenic* or blood-brain barrier breakdown edema, the type of edema usually found around a mass lesion such as a tumor or abscess. The usual dose is a 10 mg loading dose, followed by 4–6 mg every 6 hours. This treatment may take several hours to work, even in patients with edema related to breakdown of the blood-brain barrier. Corticosteroids are not effective in patients with *cytotoxic* or intracellular edema, such as is seen in acute stroke and hypoxic encephalopathy, and they increase the risk of secondary complications such as infection and gastrointestinal bleeding. For this reason, corticosteroids are not recommended for increased intracranial pressure secondary to stroke or cardiac arrest.

Barbiturates and anesthetic agents such as propofol (Diprivan) can also help to reduce intracranial pressure, largely by reducing the metabolism of brain cells. Of course, the patient must be intubated before these agents can be used safely.

Close management of increased ICP requires hour to hour knowledge of the ICP level, which can be accomplished by an ICP monitor such as a subdural pressure bolt or an extraventricular drain (EVD). The bolt has less risk of infection and hemorrhage, but the EVD permits drainage of CSF, thereby lowering pressure. This maneuver is especially helpful in cases of hydrocephalus, as in an obstructive lesion, or in the setting of subarachnoid hemorrhage or meningitis. More permanent drainage of CSF can be accomplished by placement of a ventriculo-peritoneal shunt.

ENCEPHALOPATHY/DELIRIUM

A discussion of the causes and evaluation of delirium is found in Chap. 13. Delirium represents a global brain dysfunction, sometimes a harbinger of impending coma. When delirium has an abrupt onset, rapid diagnosis of the treatable factor or factors is essential in avoiding any permanent complications.

The first issue, as in any emergency patient, is to insure that the patient has a stable airway, stable breathing and oxygenation, and stable heart rate and blood pressure. Hypoxia or hypotension can cause delirium, as can severely elevated blood pressure (hypertensive encephalopathy). The second issue in acute delirium is the identification of an etiology. Blood sampling for complete blood count (CBC), electrolytes, blood urea nitrogen (BUN) and creatinine, glucose, calcium, magnesium, and liver function tests can reveal the cause of delirium secondary to hypo- or hypernatremia, hypo- or hyperglycemia, hypo- or hypercalcemia, renal or hepatic failure. Thyroid tests are also warranted for impending myxedema coma, cortisol level for Cushing's disease, and B_{12} level for pernicious anemia. Wernicke's encephalopathy is a medical emergency that is difficult to diagnose and easy to treat. It can present as sudden coma, or with ataxia, extraocular movement abnormalities, and confusion. It is seen in malnourished individuals, including alcoholics. Prompt treatment with intravenous thiamine can prevent long-term memory loss.

The patient's medications should be carefully screened for agents that cause encephalopathy, as well as the possibility of withdrawal from alcohol or drugs such as benzodiazepines, or of accidental or deliberate overdose of medications. A brain imaging test, CT or MRI scan, is necessary to look for focal brain lesions, subdural hematoma, hydrocephalus, and other structural abnormalities. If the patient is febrile or has a stiff neck, lumbar puncture is needed to look for meningitis, encephalitis, or subarachnoid hemorrhage; as mentioned earlier, a CT scan should virtually always be performed before lumbar puncture, unless the suspected diagnosis is bacterial meningitis and a CT scan is not available quickly. Finally, electroencephalography is needed to exclude seizures or status epilepticus (see below).

Emergency treatment

Once the patient is stabilized in terms of airway, breathing, and circulation, the blood samples are drawn, and the patient is given intravenous thiamine 100 mg to prevent or treat Wernicke's encephalopathy, an ampule of D50W, and 0.4 mg of naloxone (Narcan) diluted in 9 mL of NS, given in 1–2 ml IV boluses, to reverse any narcotic analgesic overdose. If an oral drug overdose is suspected, gastric lavage via a large tube should be carried out, usually after the patient is intubated to avoid aspiration. These measures should be almost automatic in any patient with a severely altered level of consciousness. Further management must await the definition of the causative factors, through the diagnostic tests summarized above.

SUBARACHNOID HEMORRHAGE

Subarachnoid hemorrhage (SAH) denotes bleeding into the spaces around the brain, beneath both the arachnoid and the dura. The most common cause, in over 90% of cases, is a ruptured intracranial aneurysm, though

SAH can also be caused by trauma, arteriovenous malformations, or coagu-lopathies. In a small percent of cases, no cause is found.

The symptoms of SAH usually involve headache and stiff neck. The key to diagnosis is the very sudden onset of headache, and most patients with SAH describe the headache as the worst they have ever experienced. Another key to diagnosis is that many patients who present with SAH give a history of one or several previous sudden headaches, interpreted as "sen-tinel headaches" indicating "warning leaks" from an aneurysm. Failure to recognize such an acute headache as a serious problem is a frequent source of lawsuits in patients who go on to have serious subarachnoid hemorrhage with the next episode. The level of illness in patients with SAH varies greatly from one patient to the next. The Hunt and Hess scale was devised to prog-nosticate based on the patient's initial status (Table 23-1). Most patients with ruptured aneurysms have subarachnoid hemorrhage only, but in some cases the bleed causes focal signs either because of the aneurysm itself (aneurysms of the posterior cerebral artery (PCA) or internal carotid artery at the poste-rior communicating artery junction often cause a III nerve palsy) or because of associated intraparenchymal hemorrhage (anterior communicating artery aneurysms may bleed into the frontal lobe, middle cerebral artery (MCA) aneurysms may bleed into the temporal lobe).

The diagnosis of SAH is usually accomplished by CT scan, without con-trast, showing blood in the subarachnoid space. Occasionally, with small bleeds, CT will be negative, so lumbar puncture must be performed in patients who present with typical symptoms of SAH but have a negative CT scan. Xanthochromia develops in the CSF about 4–6 hours after SAH. The aneurysm will be seen on CT only if it is large or calcified, but sometimes the location of the aneurysm can be surmised by the presence of hemorrhage in a focal area, such as the sylvian fissure on only one side for an MCA aneurysm, or intraparenchymal hemorrhage in the frontal region (anterior communicating artery) or temporal lobe (MCA). Magnetic resonance (MR) angiography or CT angiography may confirm the presence of an aneurysm, but catheter angiography is the gold standard for aneurysm diagnosis. Many neurosurgeons insist on cerebral angiography because they feel that it

Table 23-1 **Hunt and Hess Scale**

Grade	Criteria
I	Asymptomatic or mild headache, nuchal rigidity
II	Moderate to severe headache, nuchal rigidity, cranial nerve deficit
III	Drowsiness, confusion, lethargy
IV	Stupor, moderate or severe hemiparesis
V	Coma, decerebrate posturing

is essential to see the precise anatomic relationships of the aneurysm and also to exclude the presence of other, smaller aneurysms (approximately 20% of patients with SAH have more than one aneurysm).

Ruptured aneurysms can lead to multiple medical complications. First, the aneurysm can rebleed, usually a devastating event. This may occur within the first 24 hours, but the peak time for rebleeding is several days later, when the thrombus over the ruptured portion of the aneurysm dissolves. The incidence of rebleeding then gradually declines over several weeks, but even after the acute period there is a risk of 2–3% per year of a recurrent subarachnoid hemorrhage. Second, arteries can go into *vasospasm*, resulting in ischemic strokes. This complication appears to correlate with the presence of localized collections of subarachnoid blood, causing a localized arteritis. Third, the blood in the subarachnoid space can lead to obstruction of the spinal fluid pathways, producing dilated ventricles or hydrocephalus. Occasional patients have seizures, hyponatremia, and other complications. In about a third of the patients a cerebral salt-wasting syndrome will develop, which is treated with salt replacement and not by fluid restriction (as in the syndrome of inappropriate secretion of antidiuretic hormone [SIADH]). Overall morbidity and mortality of SAH is in the range of 40–50%.

Emergency treatment

The first key to treatment of the patient with SAH is proper diagnosis, since, as mentioned above, many patients are not diagnosed at the time of the initial "sentinel headache". Once the diagnosis is made, the patient should be admitted emergently to an intensive care unit, hydrated with intravenous normal saline and kept normovolemic, and gently sedated if the patient is anxious, placed on stool softeners to prevent straining at stool. Some experts recommend antiepileptic drugs such as phenytoin (Dilantin) or valproic acid (Depakote, Depacon) to prevent seizures. In our neurological intensive care unit, empiric antiepileptic therapy is ordered for 1 week and then rapidly tapered off, unless there is a cerebral hematoma. If the patient is Grade I or II, prompt identification of the aneurysm and definitive treatment by surgical clipping or endovascular coiling (see below) is indicated. If surgery is delayed, prevention of ischemia related to vasospasm becomes an important issue. The patient is hydrated, with blood pressure (BP) maintained at normal or even mildly elevated levels. The calcium channel blocker, nimodipine, is given at a dose of 60 mg every 4 hours for 21 days to prevent ischemia. Vasospasm can be detected noninvasively by transcranial Doppler ultrasound, with serial measurement of the velocities of blood flow within the major intracranial arteries. Occasionally, endovascular procedures such as infusion of papaverine or angioplasty can be carried out to dilate vasospastic arteries. For patients with hydrocephalus, placement of an external ventricular drain (EVD) is critical, and sometimes a permanent ventriculoperitoneal shunt becomes necessary.

The ultimate plan is to treat the aneurysm definitively. This can be accomplished by a neurosurgeon via craniotomy and clipping of the aneurysm or by an interventional neuroradiologist via placement of endovascular coils to thrombose the aneurysm. Some aneurysms have a thick neck and are not amenable to coiling, others are difficult to approach surgically and more appropriate for coiling than clipping. For aneurysms amenable to either procedure, an international study found that coiling is safer than clipping, but there appears to be a higher risk of incomplete obliteration of the aneurysm.

One last topic under cerebral aneurysms is the management of patients who are found to have asymptomatic, unruptured aneurysms. An international study showed that unruptured aneurysms of the anterior circulation less than 7 mm in diameter have a low enough risk of bleeding that surgery is probably not warranted. Some neurosurgeons dispute this finding, based on cases of small aneurysms presenting with subarachnoid hemorrhage. Management of the patient with an incidentally discovered, unruptured aneurysm remains controversial.

MENINGITIS, ENCEPHALITIS

Meningitis is an inflammation involving the meninges, or coverings of the brain, whereas encephalitis refers to an infection of the brain substance itself. One of the most critical of all neurological emergencies is acute bacterial meningitis. The symptoms include headache, fever, stiff neck, confusion or delirium, and occasionally seizures. In recent series, usually at least two of the four symptoms of headache, fever, stiff neck, and altered mental status are present in the vast majority of patients with meningitis. Conditions that increase the risk of bacterial meningitis include immunodeficiency states, alcoholism, cancer and chemotherapy, recent head injury or neurosurgery, and parameningeal infections such as sinusitis. Spinal fluid testing usually shows a pleocytosis with predominantly polymorphonuclear cells, low glucose, and high protein. Gram stains of the spinal fluid can be done to identify the specific organism. The most common organisms in the past were pneumococcus (streptococcus pneumoniae), meningococcus, and Hemophilus influenzae, but in recent series staphylococcal species have become more prevalent.

Acute bacterial meningitis is usually a fulminating illness, in which patients become rapidly ill. Coma at presentation, focal symptoms and signs (excluding cranial nerve palsies), and specific organisms, such as pneumococcal illness, predict a poor outcome or death. Meningitis was almost uniformly fatal before the introduction of antibiotics, but current mortality rates are under 25%. Antibiotic therapy for bacterial meningitis is a changing subject, depending on what organisms are prevalent in a community, and based on the latest information about antibiotic resistance. The most common organisms are still streptococcus pneumoniae, or *pneumococcal meningitis*, meningococcus, or meningococcal meningitis, and Hemophilus influenzae, or *H flu meningitis*. Less common forms include staphylococcal meningitis, gram negative meningitis, listeria, and spirochetal meningitis. Cerebrospinal fluid (CSF) usually shows elevated counts of polymorphonuclear leukocytes, low glucose, and elevated protein. Currently, ceftriaxone and vancomycin are often started empirically, with further decisions based on the culture and sensitivity results and response to treatment.

Other infectious agents can cause meningitis. Tuberculous meningitis may present somewhat more subacutely, usually in chronically ill individuals. Again, headache, confusion, stiff neck, and seizures are frequent symptoms and signs. Fever is less reliably present in tuberculous as compared to bacterial infection. CSF formulas are likely to show more mononuclear cells, low CSF glucose, and high CSF protein. Fungal meningitis, such as cryptococcal meningitis, can be even more chronic than tuberculosis (TB) meningitis. Patients occasionally present with chronic headaches or confusion, without any fever or stiff neck. Diagnostic lumbar puncture is essential to diagnose these very treatable conditions. In the era of human immunodeficiency virus (HIV) infection, cryptococcal meningitis has become more common.

Viral or *aseptic meningitis*, in comparison to bacterial meningitis, is a benign syndrome of headache, fever, and stiff neck, usually without any focal neurological symptoms or signs or seizures. Viral meningitis often occurs in epidemics. The virus is often not known except by antibody titers in the acute and convalescent periods; a 4-fold rise in antibody titer indicates that the infection was probably caused by that virus.

Encephalitis is usually a viral syndrome of lethargy, confusion, and often seizures and fever. Many viruses can cause encephalitis. The arboviruses, such as St. Louis, California, Eastern, and Western Equine encephalitis, are epidemic illnesses with headache, obtundation, and fever. Another epidemic viral encephalitis, which has become common in the United States over the past few years, is West Nile Virus encephalitis. This illness is a typical encephalitis, but the virus also has a predilection for the spinal cord, and back pain, and paraparesis are often associated findings. The diagnosis is made by serological testing. No specific treatment other than supportive care is available.

Herpes simplex encephalitis (HSE) occurs year-round in nonepidemic occurrence. HSE has a predilection for the orbital frontal and temporal lobes. Patients typically present with headache, fever, confusion, and often aphasia, and seizures. Diagnosis can be made by a genetic polymerase chain reaction (PCR) test on CSF; in previous years, brain biopsy was often required. Electroencephalography (EEG) often shows focal, temporal lobe epileptiform discharges, and CT and MRI scans may show structural abnormalities in the orbital frontal, and temporal lobes. CSF shows elevated mononuclear cells, usually normal glucose and mildly elevated protein. HSE is important to diagnose because it is treatable, with antiviral agents such as acyclovir.

If the disease is not treated early, severe tissue damage, with death or permanent neurogical deficits, is likely.

Emergency management

Diagnosis of bacterial meningitis is a medical emergency. A frequent debate in meningitis therapy has been whether to recommend a CT scan before lumbar puncture, to avoid herniation from downward displacement of an intracranial mass. Patients with such mass lesions usually have focal neurological symptoms or signs and a depressed level of consciousness; without these factors, lumbar puncture is probably safe. Most experts, however, still recommend a pre-lumbar puncture CT scan, and antibiotic therapy should therefore be started before the CT scan, since delay in initiation of antibiotic treatment increases the risk of death and other complications of meningitis.

The specific antibiotics used in acute meningitis vary with the organism and with the latest information about antibiotic resistance. In the United States, so many pneumococcal infections have become resistant to penicillin that standard recommendations for bacterial meningitis now include a combination of a third generation cephalosporin such as ceftriaxone and vancomycin. If listeria is suspected, a combination of ampicillin and a cephalosporin is standard treatment.

The use of corticosteroids in acute bacterial meningitis to reduce inflammation and secondary cranial complications such as deafness has been supported by several studies. Such treatment should be begun early, before or concurrent with initiation of antibiotics if possible, and the duration of treatment can probably be limited to 4 days, at a dose of approximately 0.15 mg/kg q 6 hours.

STATUS EPILEPTICUS

Status epilepticus (SE) is a medical emergency, currently defined as recurrent epileptic seizures without an intervening return of consciousness, or seizure activity lasting more than 5 minutes. Both experimental and clinical evidence indicates that prolonged seizure activity can damage the brain, and the longer into status epilepticus that treatment is initiated, the harder it will be to bring the seizures under control.

Status epilepticus is divided into generalized convulsive SE and nonconvulsive SE. Generalized convulsive SE begins with physical convulsions, or tonic-clonic activity, bilaterally, and always associated with loss of consciousness once the bilateral jerking has begun. If the status epilepticus is prolonged, the motor activity may diminish into *subtle nonconvulsive SE*, in which the motor phenomena may be limited to nystagmoid jerking of the eyes, lip smacking, or automatic behaviors such as picking with the fingers. The other types of nonconvulsive status epilepticus do not begin with convulsive activity; these are divided into partial complex status epilepticus, absence status epilepticus, focal status epilepticus (or *epilepsia partialis continua*, or myoclonic status epilepticus. These syndromes are closely related to the epileptic syndromes discussed in Chap. 25, diagnosed both by clinical symptomatology and electroencephalographic (EEG) changes.

Emergency management

As in any medical emergency, the patient must first be stabilized, in terms of airway, breathing, and circulation. Hypoxia or hypotension can greatly accentuate the degree of neuronal damage caused by status epilepticus, and these must be treated aggressively. Hyperthermia is also thought to have adverse effects, and use of acetaminophen or body cooling techniques is an important part of the management of SE. When the patient with status epilepticus is first seen, intravenous glucose and thiamine should be administered, as blood is drawn for electrolytes, glucose, calcium, magnesium, complete blood count, drug levels (if patient known to take antiepileptic medications), and toxicology.

   Pharmacological therapy for status epilepticus generally occurs in a series of steps. A suggested protocol for the management of status epilepticus is shown in Table 23-2. Usually the initial treatment is an intravenous benzodiazepine, of which the most popular agent is lorazepam (Ativan, 0.1 mg/kg). Benzodiazepines act at the $GABA_A$ receptor, hyperpolarizing the resting

Table 23-2 **Management of Acute Status Epilepticus**

Step 1
Airway, breathing, circulation
Give thiamine 100 mg IV and glucose 1 ampoule D50W
Send blood for electrolytes, BUN, glucose, calcium, magnesium
Step 2
Administer lorazepam 2 mg/min, maximum dose 6 mg
Step 3
Administer phentytoin 20 mg/kg by slow IV infusion (<50 mg/min)
Or
Fosphenytoin 20 mg/kg dilantin equivalents (<150 mg/min)
Step 4 (for refractory status epilepticus only)
Propofol, loading intravenous dose of 3–5 mg/kg, followed by an infusion of 1–15 mg/kg/hour
Or
Pentobarbital, loading intravenous dose of 5–15 mg/kg over 1 hour, then maintained at 0.5–10 mg/kg/hour

membrane potential of neurons and inhibiting neural transmission. Lorazepam is preferred over the older agent diazepam (Valium) because of its longer duration of antiepileptic action. Intubation may be necessary to ensure adequate ventilation. If intravenous access is a problem, as in out-of-hospital treatment of status epilepticus, rectal diazepam (Diastat) is a treatment option.

After the initial benzodiazepine treatment, a longer-acting antiepileptic agent is usually the next step in management. Phenytoin (Dilantin) is still the most widely used agent for generalized, tonic-clonic status epilepticus. Phenytoin reduces repetitive firing of neurons through its effect on voltage-activated sodium channels in neurons. Intravenous phenytoin must be given at an infusion rate slower than 50 mg/minute, meaning that the average 1000 mg loading dose takes a minimum of 20 minutes to infuse. In fact, larger patients need larger doses, in the range of 20 mg/kg. Adverse effects include local necrosis if this very alkaline solution infiltrates into the subcutaneous tissues, hypotension, cardiac arrhythmias, and allergic reactions. The newer prodrug, fosphenytoin (Cerebyx) can be given at a faster rate, up to 150 mg of phenytoin equivalents/minute, and this agent appears to have a lower risk of local tissue damage, or systemic hypotension, or cardiac arrhythmias. The only disadvantage is that this drug is considerably more expensive than phenytoin.

An alternative to phenytoin or fosphenytoin is Phenobarbital, an older drug that, like benzodiazepines, increases $GABA_A$ mediated neuronal inhibition. This drug has lost favor in recent years because of its sedative, respiratory depressant, and hypotensive effects. Patients should always be tracheally intubated before administration of a full, loading dose of Phenobarbital.

Valproic acid (Depacon) is another antiepileptic drug which has only recently become available in an intravenous form. This drug has a number of antiepileptic mechanisms, including effects on sodium channels, calcium channels, and GABA metabolism. It can be given with loading doses of 15–20 mg/kg, but the efficacy of this drug in SE has not been confirmed in large, randomized clinical trials, and it is not approved by Food and Drug Administration (FDA) for this indication.

When status epilepticus is refractory to a benzodiazepine and phenytoin or fosphenytoin, the next step involves tracheal intubation, mechanical ventilation, and use of an anesthetic agent such as propofol (Diprivan) or pentobarbital. These agents must be administered in an intensive care unit (ICU) or critical care setting. Propofol is a very short-acting anesthetic agent that likely suppresses seizures by a $GABA_A$ mechanism similar to that of barbiturates and benzodiazepines. It is popular because the drug effects wear off quickly when the drug is discontinued. It can be given in a loading dose of 3–5 mg/kg, followed by an infusion of 1–15 mg/kg/hour. The drug can produce hypotension, metabolic acidosis, and occasionally idiosyncratic acute renal failure. Pentobarbital is a barbiturate, given by loading dose of 5–15 mg/kg over one hour, maintained at 0.5–10 mg/kg/hour. Pentobarbital, taken to *barbiturate coma* level, is very effective in suppressing even refractory seizure activity. Both propofol and pentobarbital are usually maintained for 24 hours at an anesthetic level, or one associated with a *burst-suppression* pattern on the EEG, then weaned off. Occasionally, seizure activity will resume. The other problem with pentobarbital is the extensive drug storage in fatty tissue, ensuring a very slow recovery from the sedative effects of the drug. Skeletal muscle paralytic agents should be avoided, since they mask clinical seizures, even when the brain continues discharging. Continuous EEG monitoring should be considered for patients in SE.

ACUTE STROKE AND CEREBRAL HEMORRHAGE

The acute treatment of stroke differs between cerebral hemorrhage and infarction. As will be discussed in Chap. 24 on stroke, hemorrhages can occur into four potential spaces: extradural, intradural, subarachnoid, and intracerebral. The first two are mostly related to traumatic brain injury, whereas subarachnoid and intracerebral hemorrhage usually occur spontaneously. The management of extradural hematoma is a medical emergency, usually treated by neurosurgical evacuation of the hematoma as quickly as possible. Subdural hematomas also usually require surgery, though small ones can sometimes be treated conservatively, without surgery.

Intracerebral hemorrhage (ICH) is usually related to hypertension, with a small vessel presumably rupturing from the direct effect of sustained, elevated blood pressures on a thin-walled, small cerebral artery. Other causes of ICH include vasculopathies such as amyloid angiopathy in elderly patients, arteriovenous malformations or aneurysms, bleeding into cerebral tumors, trauma, or coagulopathies such as warfarin therapy. Hypertensive intracerebral hemorrhages usually occur deep in the brain, roughly half in the lateral basal ganglia area, 10% each in the thalamus, brainstem (usually pons), and cerebellar regions, with the other 20% mainly in lobar locations. Surgery has had limited application in intracerebral hemorrhage. Cerebellar hemorrhages greater than 3 cm in diameter, especially if enlarging, represent the clearest indication for evacuation of a hematoma. Occasionally, an enlarging lobar hemorrhage is surgically decompressed, especially when cerebral herniation and death are imminent. The more common, deep, basal ganglia hemorrhages have not been shown to have improved outcome with surgery as compared to medical therapy, though there are advocates for "minimally invasive" surgery aimed at draining the hemorrhage. A recent, international surgical trial for ICH (ISTICH) did not show a clear advantage of surgical versus medical therapy for intracerebral hemorrhages, though patients with bleeds within 1 cm of the cortical surface appeared to do better with surgery. Some neurosurgeons place a thrombolytic agent such as tissue plasminogen activator (tPA) into the hematoma to facilitate its drainage.

Medical therapy of ICH includes blood pressure management. In the early hours after a hemorrhage the blood pressure is almost invariably high, and antihypertensive treatment may reduce the growth of the hematoma, which takes place in about 40% of cases. Later, when intracranial pressure is elevated, care must be taken to keep the blood pressure high enough to perfuse the brain. Cerebral perfusion pressure (CPP, mean arterial pressure-ICP) should be maintained above 70 mm Hg. The other key medical management of ICH is reduction of increased intracranial pressure. As discussed earlier in this chapter, hyperventilation, osmotic agents, and external ventricular drains serve to reduce ICP, but the first two have very temporary effects. Despite these measures, some patients die of herniation after an acute bleed. The most recent addition to the armamentarium in the treatment of ICH is concentrated recombinant Factor VII (Novo 7), shown in a preliminary study to reduce growth of an intracerebral hemorrhage when introduced within the first four hours after a bleed. This product is being tested currently.

Treatment of acute ischemic stroke includes many of the same initial measures as just described under treatment of intracerebral hemorrhage. The patient must be stabilized like any other emergency patient, with attention to airway, breathing, and circulation, placement of IV access. We avoid hypotonic solutions such as D5W, which can increase brain edema; we recommend normal saline solutions. Oral feeding of food or liquids is delayed until the patient's ability to swallow can be assessed. Attempts at acute treatment of stroke include those geared to break up a clot and restore circulation to the brain (*thrombolytic* or *reperfusion* therapies), and those geared to protect the brain against ischemia, so-called *neuroprotective* therapies. To date, no neuroprotective drug has been proved effective in acute stroke, despite many clinical trials of agents which had appeared beneficial in animal models of stroke. Several clinical trials of neuroprotective agents are currently in progress.

With regard to thrombolytic therapy, only one agent has received approval by the FDA, intravenous tPA. This drug must be given within 3 hours of the first symptoms of a stroke. Table 23-3 is a simplified list of the indications and contraindications for use of IV tPA. Proper use of the drug requires a hospital to have a stroke team physician on call 24 hours per day, 7 days per week, a CT scanner that can be activated within 20 minutes, a physician able to read the scan immediately, and ability to obtain at least three laboratory blood tests within 45 minutes: platelet count, prothrombin time/international normalized ratio (PT/INR), and glucose. The hospital should be able to have the tPA running via an IV ("door-to-needle time") within 60 minutes of the patient's arrival. This treatment has been shown to improve chances of a nearly complete recovery by about 12% (absolute percentage benefit), or 30% (relatively increased chance of normal recovery); stated another way, the odds ratio of a good outcome is 1.7:1 with the use of tPA versus placebo treatment. In the National Institute of

Table 23-3 **Guidelines for Use of tPA**

Inclusions:
  Acute stroke
  <3 hours post-onset
  NIHSS 4–21
Exclusions:
  Rapidly improving deficit, mild deficit (NIHSS <4) or severe deficit (NIHSS >22)
  History of stroke, head injury within 3 months, surgery within 14 days
  History of intracerebral hemorrhage, or suspected subarachnoid hemorrhage
  Systolic BP >185 mm Hg, diastolic BP >110 mm Hg
  History of GI/GU hemorrhage within 21 days, arterial puncture at a
  noncompressible site within 7 days, use of heparin, seizure at onset
  Laboratory: INR >1.5, platelets <100,000, glucose <50 or >400

Source: Practice Advisory: thrombolcytic therapy for acute ischemic stroke. *Neurology* 1996;47:835–839.

Neurological Disorders and Stroke (NINDS) trial, there was a 6% risk of intracerebral hemorrhage, but deaths were not more likely in the treated group. This treatment has revolutionized the field of stroke, and a national program is currently underway for certification of hospitals as stroke centers. To date, however, only 2–3% of stroke patients nationally are receiving this treatment.

Other, more experimental treatments of acute stroke are under development. Ultrasound waves, using a transcranial Doppler probe directed at the clot, may improve the chances of clot lysis. Intra-arterial thrombolytic agents, placed via an arterial catheter, may have greater efficacy in restoring circulation, but these treatments are not currently FDA approved. Recently, the FDA approved a clot retrieval device, the MERCI clot retriever, for use in snaring and removing intracranial clots. This device was successful in reopening cerebral vessels in about 50% of cases, but the mortality in the treated group was quite high. Clinical trials to determine whether a clinical outcome benefit can be proved are underway.

There is some evidence that the early use of aspirin in ischemic stroke is beneficial. The use of aspirin and anticoagulants for secondary stroke prevention is discussed in Chap. 24.

SPINAL CORD OR CAUDA EQUINA SYNDROMES

Acute spinal cord syndromes include traumatic injuries; compression by a tumor, hematoma, spinal arteriovenous malformation, abscess, or disc; and intrinsic spinal cord syndromes such as acute transverse myelitis and spinal cord infarction. The annual incidence of spinal cord injury in the United States is 5–6 cases/100,000 population/year, with over 3,500 deaths and 5,000 patients left with permanent paralysis. The first key to management is prompt diagnosis, based on clinical suspicion, the findings of segmental motor and sensory deficits, especially with a "sensory level". Some of the common presentations of spinal cord syndromes were presented in Chap. 2.

One cause of acute paraparesis of which physicians should be aware is an abdominal aortic aneurysm with dissection or frank rupture. In the process, aortic branches supplying the spinal cord can be affected. The spinal cord syndrome resulting from ischemia is the *anterior spinal artery syndrome*, with paralysis below the level, but sparing of posterior column sensory function. Attention should be directed to diagnosing the problem by abdominal ultrasound or CT scanning, to permit treatment of the aneurysm before full rupture. Less commonly, aortic dissections can cause acute spinal cord syndromes at thoracic or even cervical levels, or an aortic dissection can affect the great vessels, including the carotid or vertebral arteries, and lead to a stroke syndrome. Pain radiating from the chest to the back is often a harbinger of an acute dissection of the aorta.

Emergency management

The first issue, as in any emergency, is to stabilize the patient and arrive at the correct diagnosis. In the case of spinal cord injury, stabilization means not only ensuring airway, breathing, and circulation, but also using a spine board, neck collar, or other measures to prevent motion of an unstable spine. Formerly, emergency myelography was often needed for diagnosis, but currently MR or CT imaging of the spine has made noninvasive spinal cord diagnosis easier and more practical. The first treatment issue is the identification of patients who can benefit from surgery. Spinal cord compression from an extradural disc or mass is the most favorable indicator for surgery. Corticosteroids are often used for acute antiedema and anti-inflammatory effects. The standard protocol for corticosteroid administration within 8 hours of an acute spinal cord injury is intravenous methylprednisolone, 30 mg/kg as a bolus, followed by 5.4 mg/kg hourly for 24–48 hours.

TRAUMATIC BRAIN INJURY

Traumatic brain injury (TBI) is one of the most common afflictions of mankind. Annually in the United States, over two million people suffer head injuries, of whom an estimated 500,000 require hospitalization, 70,000–90,000 have permanent, severe disabilities, and up to 50,000 die. Head injury is also the leading cause of death in persons under the age of 24 years. Traumatic brain injuries are more common than breast cancer, AIDS, and multiple sclerosis.

TBIs are traditionally divided into severe, moderate, and mild, based on the Glasgow Coma Scale (GCS) (Teasdale and Jennett 1974; Table 23-4). Severe head injuries are those with initial Glasgow Coma Scale scores of 3–8, moderate head injuries are those with scores of 9–12, and mild head injuries are those with GCS scores of 13–15. The severe and moderate injuries are all treated in the hospital, whereas patients with minor head injuries frequently present to a physician days or weeks after the initial injury.

The brain is suspended in spinal fluid, covered by a thick, dural membrane, and encased by a hard yet pliable skull, all of which render the brain relatively resistant to trauma. When the head is struck on one side, however, the brain may move to the opposite direction and strike the inside of the skull, causing a *contrecoup* injury. The hard surfaces of the inner skull base, particularly the jagged bony contours of the frontal and temporal areas, can contuse and injure the brain. Hemorrhages occur into the epidural, subdural, or subarachnoid spaces, or into the brain parenchyma. In addition to hemorrhage, there are shear injuries of the brain tissue, sometimes referred to as *diffuse axonal injury*. The combination of focal and diffuse injury is at the heart of the presentation of patients with traumatic brain injury. Axonal injury and edema in the hemispheres or brainstem cause initial stupor or coma. The closed skull that protects the brain against acute injury becomes a problem in restricting room for the brain when edema develops. Hypotension or hypoxia after the initial trauma can also increase the degree of brain injury. Subarachnoid

Table 23-4 **The Glasgow Coma Scale**

Best motor response	Obeys commands	6
	Localizes	5
	Withdraws	4
	Flexion response (decorticate)	3
	Extensor response (decerebrate)	2
	No response	1
Best verbal response	Oriented, conversational	5
	Disoriented but conversational	4
	Inappropriate words	3
	Incomprehensible sounds	2
	No response	1
Eye opening	Spontaneous	4
	To verbal stimuli	3
	To pain	2
	Never	1

Source: Teasdale G, Jennett B. Assessment of coma and impaired consciousness: a practical scale. *Lancet* 1974;2:81–84.

bleeding may obstruct the cerebrospinal fluid pathways and lead to hydro-cephalus. Scars from brain injury also lead to post-traumatic epilepsy.

Initial management of the patient with severe traumatic brain injury involves the use of CT scanning to look for hematomas or edematous contusions. Neurosurgical intervention can be lifesaving if an epidural or subdural hematoma threatens brain herniation. Occasionally, a lobar intracerebral hematoma can be successfully evacuated. Decompressive craniectomy (removal of portions of the skull to allow room for the brain to expand) can be used to allow room for otherwise fatal brain swelling. An external ventricular drain EVD (see above) can be placed to reduce the cerebrospinal fluid volume. Medical management is similar to that discussed above for intracerebral hemorrhage. We treat brain edema with brief periods of hyperventilation and osmotic agents such as mannitol or hypertonic saline. Many patients undergo intracranial pressure monitoring, in order to optimize the use of other medical managements. The management of acute traumatic brain injuries has become much more aggressive in recent years, with improved outcomes in major trauma centers.

Patients who survive major head injuries are often left with profound neurobehavioral impairments. Frontal lobe signs such as excessive passivity, or alternatively a disinhibited or agitated state, are prominent. Some patients also have focal signs of brain injury, such as hemiparesis, hemianopsia, and aphasia or neglect resembling stroke deficits. Patients with severe closed head injuries had 36% mortality in a series of 1030 patients, ranging from 76% for patients with a GCS score of 3 to 18% for those with GCS scores of 6–8. Most patients who survive such injuries need intensive rehabilitation and are left with significant neurobehavioral deficits.

Another challenge in the management of patients with TBI is the treatment of mild head injury or concussion. Concussion refers to a traumatic brain injury with either loss of consciousness or a feeling of being "stunned" or "seeing stars", often associated with an aftermath of headaches, irritability, dizziness, and difficulty with memory and concentration. The *post-concussive syndrome* is the subject of much litigation in the United States. About 15% of minor head injury patients have persistent disability at 1 year following injury. According to a review article by Alexander (1995), predictors for the persistent post-concussive syndrome include: (1) ongoing litigation, (2) low socioeconomic status, (3) history of prior head injuries, (4) persistent headache, (5) other significant injuries, (6) female gender, and (7) prior history of psychological disorders.

Athletes who suffer concussions also pose important treatment issues. As many as 300,000 concussions occur each year in sports and recreation. Repeated minor head injuries in college athletes result in deficits of attention, memory, and planning. Cases of second concussions occurring before complete recovery from the first (*second impact syndrome*) have occasionally led to malignant brain swelling and even death. High-school and college athletes who have sustained a concussion should be counseled before being permitted to return to competitive sports; the American Academy of Neurology issued a practice guideline in 1997, supporting these restrictions. Even minor concussions should keep an athlete out of competition for at least a week, or until the symptoms have completely resolved. If the athlete has a definite loss of consciousness, and if a CT or MRI scan is abnormal, the guidelines suggest keeping the athlete out of competition for the season, and possibly for life.

ACUTE RESPIRATORY DISTRESS SECONDARY TO NEUROMUSCULAR DISEASE

Any neurological disorder associated with weakness on both sides of the body can result in respiratory insufficiency. In clinical practice, among the most common syndromes are acute inflammatory demyelinating polyradiculoneuropathy (AIDP or Guillain-Barre syndrome), myasthenia gravis, botulism, and occasionally a critical care polyneuropathy or myopathy. Neuromuscular disorders are discussed in Chaps. 33–35.

The key to emergency management is to detect the incipient respiratory failure before it becomes critical. An important point is that oxygen saturation tends to remain relatively normal, as CO_2 rises, until ventilation is on the point of collapse. For this reason, monitoring of oxygen saturations alone is not sufficient to predict impending respiratory failure. Patients with neurological weakness should be monitored by serial pulmonary function tests (especially vital capacity and negative inspiratory force), as well as arterial blood gases. When vital capacity falls below 30–50% of normal, or below an absolute limit of one liter, elective tracheal intubation should be planned. Other clinical signs that predict need for tracheal intubation are loss of muscle strength in the neck muscles such that the patient cannot lift the head up from the bed, or bilateral facial paralysis. Patients with neuromuscular weakness sufficient to threaten respiration should always be managed in an intensive care setting.

TEMPORAL ARTERITIS

Temporal arteritis is a giant cell inflammatory arteritis, occurring in medium-sized arteries of the brain and extracranial circulation. The disease is common in elderly people, rare before age 50. Most patients present with headaches, but many patients also have the diffuse muscle aches, malaise, and low grade fever of polymyalgia rheumatica, as well as pain on chewing (*jaw claudication*). The most feared complication of temporal arteritis is the sudden loss of vision in one eye, rarely both eyes. Occasionally, strokes or seizures may ensue. The diagnosis is aided by an elevated erythrocyte sedimentation rate (ESR). C-reactive protein (CRP) levels have also proved helpful in diagnosing this condition. The diagnosis is confirmed by biopsy of the superficial temporal artery, usually in its preauricular portion.

Treatment of temporal arteritis involves corticosteroids, usually in the form of oral prednisone, beginning with 60–100 mg daily dose. The biopsy is still helpful even after a week of corticosteroid therapy; if the disease is suspected, treatment should not be delayed until after the biopsy is performed. Corticosteroid therapy can prevent the development of blindness in an unaffected eye or a stroke. The course of steroid therapy is usually at least several months, and the ESR or CRP can be used to monitor therapy. Occasionally, other immunosuppressive agents are used to "spare" the amount of steroid required, but there has been limited clinical trial evidence to guide such treatment.

KEY REFERENCES

General

Bleck TP, Klawans HL. Neurologic emergencies. *Med Clin North Am* 1986;70: 1167–1184.

Diringer, MN, Zazulia, AR. Osmotic therapy. *Neurocrit Care*. 2004;1:219–233.

Grant IS, Andrews PJ. ABC of intensive care. Neurological support. *BMJ* 1999;319: 110–113.

Subarachnoid hemorrhage

Brisman JL, Song JK, Newell DW. Cerebral aneurysms. *New Engl J Med* 2006;355: 928–939.

Edlow JA, Caplan LR. Avoiding pitfalls in the diagnosis of subarachnoid hemorrhage. *N Engl J Med* 2000;342:29–36.

International Study of Unruptured Intracranial Aneurysms Investigators. Unruptured intracranial aneurysms: natural history, clinical outcome, and risks of surgical and endovascular treatment. *Lancet* 2003;362:103–110.

International Subarachnoid Aneurysm Trial (ISAT) Collaborative Group. International subarachnoid aneurysm trial (ISAT) of neurosurgical clipping versus endovascular coiling in 2143 patients with ruptured intracranial aneurysms: a randomized trial. *Lancet* 2002;360:1267–1274.

Leblanc R. The minor leak preceding subarachnoid hemorrhage. *J Neurosurg* 1987;66: 35–39.

Meyer FB, Morita A, Puumala MR, et al. Medical and surgical management of intracranial aneurysms. *Mayo Clin Proc* 1995;70:153–172.

Mitchell P, Gholkar A, Vindlacheruvu RR, et al. Unruptured intracranial aneurysms: benign curiosity or ticking bomb? *Lancet Neurol* 2004;3:85–92.

Roy D, Milot G, Raymond J. Endovascular treatment of unruptured aneurysms. *Stroke* 2001;32:1998–2004.

Schievink WI. Intracranial aneurysms. *New Engl J Med* 1997;336:28–40.

Weaver JP, Fisher M. Subarachnoid hemorrhage: an update of pathogenesis, diagnosis and management. *J Neurol Sci* 1994;125:119–131.

Wijdicks FFM, Kallmeo DF, Manno EM, et al. Subarachnoid hemorrhage: neurointensive care and aneurysm repair. *Mayo Clin Proc* 2005;80:550–559.

Cerebral hemorrhage

Hankey GJ, Hon C. Surgery for primary intracerebral hemorrhage: is it safe and effective? A systemic review of case series and randomized trials. *Stroke* 1997;28: 2126–2132.

Manno EM, Atkinson JLD, Fulgham JR, et al. Emerging medical and surgical management strategies in the evaluation and treatment of intracerebral hemorrhage. *Mayo Clin Proc* 2005;80:420–433.

Mayer SA, Brun NC, Begtrup K, et al. Recombinant activated factor VII for acute intracerebral hemorrhage. *N Engl J Med* 2005;352:777–785.

Mendelow AD, Gregson BA, Fernandes HM, et al. Early surgery versus initial conservative treatment in patients with spontaneous intracerebral hematomas in the International Surgical Trial in Intracerebral Hemorrhage (ISTICH): a randomized trial. *Lancet* 2005;365:387–397.

Qureshi AI, Tuhrim S, Broderick JP, et al. Spontaneous intracerebral hemorrhage. *N Engl J Med* 2001;344:1450–1460.

Acute ischemic stroke

Alexandrov AV, Molina CA, Grotta JC, et al. Ultrasound-enhanced systemic thrombolysis for acute ischemic stroke. *N Engl J Med* 2004;351:2170–2178.

Brott T, Bogousslavsky J. Treatment of acute ischemic stroke. *N Engl J Med* 2000;343: 710–722.

Furlan A, Higashida R, Wechsler L, et al. Intra-arterial prourokinase for acute ischemic stroke. The PROACT II study: a randomized controlled trial. *JAMA* 2003;282:2003–2011.

The NINDS rt-PA Stroke Study Group. Tissue plasminogen activator for acute ischemic stroke. *N Engl J Med* 1995;333:1581–1587.

Practice advisory: thrombolytic therapy for acute ischemic stroke-summary statement Report of the Quality Standards Subcommittee of The American Academy of Neurology. *Neurology* 1996;47:835–839.

Smith WS, Sung G, Starkman S, et al. Safety and efficacy of mechanical embolectomy in acute ischemic stroke. Results of the MERCI trial. *Stroke* 2005;36: 1432–1440.

Meningitis and encephalitis

De Gans J, Van de Beek D. Dexamethasone in adults with bacterial meningitis. *N Engl J Med* 2002;347:1549–1556.

Durand ML, Calderwood SB, Weber DJ, et al. Acute bacterial meningitis in adults. A review of 493 episodes. *N Engl J Med* 1993;328:21–28.

Hasbun R, Abrahams J, Jekel J, et al. Computed tomography of the head before lumbar puncture in adults with suspected meningitis. *N Engl J Med* 2001;345: 1727–1733.

McIntyre PB, Berkey CS, King SM, et al. Dexamethasone as adjunctive therapy in bacterial meningitis. *JAMA* 1997;278:925–931.

Quagliarello V, Scheld WM. Bacterial meningitis: pathogenesis, pathophysiology, and progress. *N Engl J Med* 1992;327:864–872.

Rosenstein NE, Perkins BA, Stephens DS, et al. Meningococcal disease. *N Engl J Med* 2001;344:1378–1388.

Swartz MN. Bacterial meningitis– a view of the past 90 years. *N Engl J Med* 2004;351:1826–1828.

Van de Beek D, de Gans J, Spanjaard L, et al. Clinical features and prognostic factors in adults with bacterial meningitis. *New Engl J Med* 2004;351:1849–1859.

Status Epilepticus

Alldredge BK, Gelb AM, Isaacs SM, et al. A comparison of lorazepam, diazepam, and placebo for the treatment of out-of-hospital status epilepticus. *N Engl J Med* 2001;345:631–637.

Limdi NA, Shimpi AV, Faught E, et al. Efficacy of rapid IV administration of valproic acid for status epilepticus. *Neurology* 2005;64:353–355.

Lowenstein DH, Alldredge BK. Status epilepticus. *N Engl J Med* 1998;338:970–976.

Manno EM. New management strategies in the treatment of status epilepticus. *Mayo Clin Proc* 2003;78:508–518.

Rossetti AO, Reichhart MD, Schaller MD, et al. Propofol treatment of refractory status epilepticus: a study of 31 episodes. *Epilepsia* 2004;45:757–763.

Treiman DM, Meyers PD, Walton NY, et al. A comparison of four treatments for generalized convulsive status epilepticus. *N Engl J Med* 1998;339:792–798.

Working Group on Status Epilepticus. Treatment of convulsive status epilepticus. Recommendations of the Epilepsy Foundation of America's Working Group on Status Epilepticus. *JAMA* 1993;270:854–859.

Spinal cord syndromes

Bracken MR, Shepard MJ, Collins WF, et al. A randomized controlled trial of methylprednisolone or naloxone treatment in treatment of acute spinal cord injury. *N Engl J Med* 1990;322:1405–1411.

Cheshire WP, Santos CC, Massey EW, et al. Spinal cord infarction: etiology and outcome. *Neurology* 1996;47:321–330.

Geisler, FH, Coleman WP, Benzel, et al. Spinal cord injury. *Lancet* 2002;359(9304):417–425.

Schiff D. Spinal cord compression. *Neurol Clin* 2003;21:67–86.

Walters BC, Hadley MN. Development of evidence-based guidelines for the management of acute spine and spinal cord injuries. *Clin Neurosurg* 2003;50:239–248.

Traumatic brain injury

Alexander MP. Mild traumatic brain injury: pathophysiology, natural history, and clinical management. *Neurology* 1995;45:1253–1260.

Ghajar J. Traumatic brain injury. *Lancet* 2000;356:923–929.

Macciocchi SN, Barth JT, Alves W, et al. Neuropsychological functioning and recovery after mild head injury in college athletes. *Neurosurgery* 1996;39:510–514.

Marshall LF, Gautille T, Klauber MR, et al. The outcome of severe closed head injury. *J Neurosurg* 1991;75:S28–S36.

Matser EJT, Kessels AG, Lezak MD, et al. Neuropsychological impairment in amateur soccer players. *JAMA* 1999;282:971–973.

Report of the Quality Standards Subcommittee, American Academy of Neurology. Practice parameter: the management of concussion in sports (summary statement). *Neurology* 1997;48:581–585 (http://aan.com/professionals/practice/guideline/index.cfm).

Stein SC, Ross SE. Moderate head injury: a guide to initial management. *J Neurosurg* 1992;77:562–564.

Thurman D, Guerrero J. Trends in hospitalization associated with traumatic brain injury. *JAMA* 1999;282:954–957.

White RJ, Likavec MJ. The diagnosis and initial management of head injury. *N Engl J Med* 1992;327:1507–1511.

Williams DH, Levin HS, Eisenberg HM. Mild head injury classification. *Neurosurgery* 1990;27:422–428.

Temporal arteritis

Caselli RJ, Hunder GG. Giant cell (temporal) arteritis. *Neurol Clin* 1997;15:893–902.

Smetana GW, Shmerling RH. Does this patient have temporal arteritis? *JAMA* 2002;287:92–101.

Younge BR, Cook BE Jr, Bartley GB, et al. Initiation of glucocorticoid therapy: before or after temporal artery biopsy? *Mayo Clin Proc* 2004;79:483–491.

STROKE

INTRODUCTION

Stroke is the most common "serious" neurological disease, the third leading cause of death in the United States, and the most common cause of neurological disability in adults. Over 700,000 strokes occur in the United States, more than one each minute. Many additional, small strokes, perhaps as many as 11 million per year in the United States, may be asymptomatic, but the accumulated effects can lead to vascular dementia and chronic mental deterioration.

A stroke is a focal abnormality of brain function, caused by either an obstruction in blood flow from occlusion of an artery (ischemic stroke) or hemorrhage from a ruptured blood vessel (hemorrhagic stroke). About 80–85% of strokes are ischemic, 15–20% hemorrhagic. The management of the stroke patient begins with diagnosis, based on symptoms and signs. Stroke must be understood in terms of the risk factors to develop the condition, the premonitory symptoms beginning before the stroke, and the mode of evolution of the stroke itself. Treatment includes acute stroke management, rehabilitation after the stroke, and secondary prevention efforts.

CLINICAL PRESENTATION: SYMPTOMS AND SIGNS

In general, stroke symptoms reflect dysfunction of focal areas of the brain, affected by either ischemia or hemorrhage. This presentation of a focal deficit in an awake patient, especially a patient of older age or with known risk factors, is instantly recognizable as a stroke to most people, including non-medically-trained family members.

As discussed in Chap. 19, transient ischemic attacks (TIAs) involve temporary focal ischemia, resolving completely within minutes or hours. TIAs are the "warning signs of stroke." Carotid distribution TIAs include transient obscuration of the vision of one eye (*transient monocular blindness* or *amaurosis fugax*), or symptoms of hemisphere ischemia, including slurred speech or language difficulty and weakness or numbness of the contralateral side of the body. TIAs in the vertebrobasilar artery distribution include dizziness, diplopia, slurred speech, numbness or weakness on one or both sides of the body, ataxia, or decreased level of consciousness.

The American Heart Association also lists "sudden, severe headache" as a warning sign of stroke. A sudden, severe headache, especially the worst headache of one's life, should be of concern for a subarachnoid hemorrhage (SAH), usually caused by rupture of a cerebral aneurysm (see Chap. 23). Stiff neck makes the diagnosis of SAH even more likely. While most headaches do not reflect SAH, this diagnosis is a medical emergency, one that physicians do not want to miss.

The symptoms of stroke are, in general, the same as those of TIAs. Patients presenting to an emergency department 1–2 hours after the onset of ischemic symptoms are very likely to have a stroke, since most TIAs begin to resolve within minutes.

In the case of a hemorrhage, the location of the hemorrhage is of obvious importance in determining the stroke syndrome. As discussed in Chap. 23, intracranial hemorrhage (ICH) can occur into one of four separate spaces: the extradural, subdural, subarachnoid, and intracerebral spaces. Extradural hemorrhage usually occurs after head trauma in a young patient, with most commonly a skull fracture that tears a dural artery such as the middle meningeal artery. This is a rapidly progressive, acute syndrome that requires emergency neurosurgical evacuation. Sometimes a "lucid interval" occurs between the head injury and the development of symptoms, as the blood accumulates. Progression can then be rapid, and prompt diagnosis and neurosurgical consultation is critical. Subdural hemorrhage (SDH) also occurs most often after trauma, but SDH may be either acute or chronic. The subacute or chronic SDH may develop very gradually, sometimes without a clear history of trauma or one of trivial trauma. Chronic SDHs are more common in elderly patients, in whom brain atrophy leaves a space between the brain and the skull, traversed by fragile veins. Drowsiness and subtle neurological symptoms and signs are the hallmark of SDH, and the physician must have a high index of suspicion to send patients for diagnostic computed tomography (CT) or magnetic resonance imaging (MRI) scans. SAH most commonly results from a ruptured aneurysm. Headache and stiff neck are the most common symptoms of SAH, though a variety of other syndromes can occur.

The fourth type of hemorrhage, ICH, occurs directly into the substance of the brain and mimics the localized syndromes of ischemic stroke. The most common cause of ICH, hypertension, tends to produce bleeds deep in the brain, in the putamen and basal ganglia most commonly, followed by the thalamus, brainstem, and cerebellum. Cerebellar hemorrhage is the most amenable to neurosurgical treatment (see below) and is therefore especially crucial to diagnose early. This hemorrhage syndrome often causes seemingly nonspecific symptoms such as dizziness, nausea, vomiting, and headache. The key to diagnosis is early gait ataxia. Patients who are dizzy from vestibular function can usually walk, but patients with cerebellar hemorrhage usually cannot. CT scan will then be diagnostic. Hemorrhages in the pons tend to cause bilateral hemiparesis, and often coma. The prognosis is poor, unless the hemorrhage is small. Hemorrhages into the basal ganglia usually cause hemiparesis. Occasionally, hemorrhages in the caudate or thalamus break into the ventricular system and cause symptoms of increased intracranial pressure (increased ICP), without obvious focal symptoms and signs. Hemorrhages into the cortical-subcortical areas of the brain, termed *lobar hemorrhages*, may occur with hypertension but are more characteristic of bleeds related to coagulopathies (e.g., warfarin therapy) or structural changes in small arteries that occur with aging (*amyloid angiopathy*). Figure 24-1 is a CT image of an intracerebral hemorrhage into the right basal ganglia.

Ischemic stroke, the result of an obstruction of blood flow to the brain, can have several mechanisms. The most common ones are: (1) large vessel, atherothrombotic strokes; (2) small vessel or *lacunar* thrombotic strokes; (3) cardioembolic strokes; (4) strokes caused by a variety of clinically definite, but less common mechanisms; and (5) cryptogenic strokes, or those for which a precise mechanism or cause is not discovered.

A brief review of vascular anatomy is necessary for the understanding of clinical stroke. Figures 24-2, 24-3 and 24-4 depict the normal circulatory anatomy. The two internal carotid arteries (ICAs) supply most of the blood flow to the cerebral hemispheres. The carotid artery distribution is often referred to as the *anterior circulation*, whereas the vertebrobasilar distribution is referred to

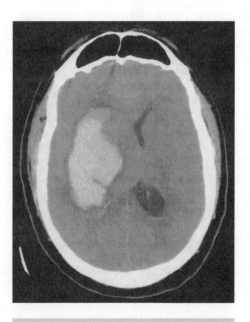

Figure 24-1 **CT from a patient with an acute R basal ganglia intracerebral hemorrhage.**

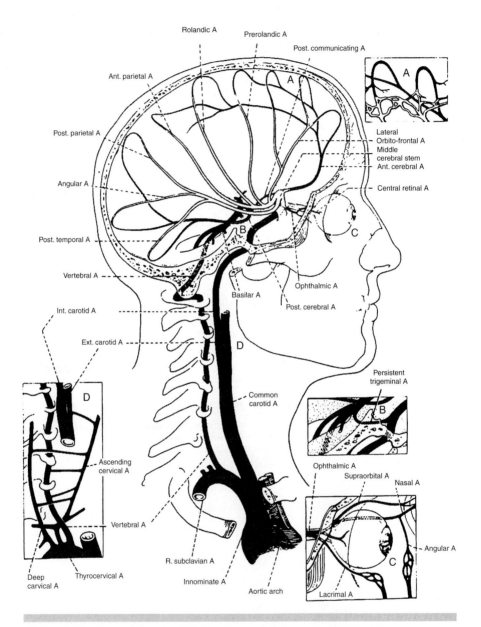

Figure 24-2 **Arrangement of the major arteries on the right side of the neck and head, including the L internal carotid artery and major branches, and the vertebral artery.** (From Victor, Ropper Adams and Victor's Principles of Neurology, Fig. 34-1, P. 826.)

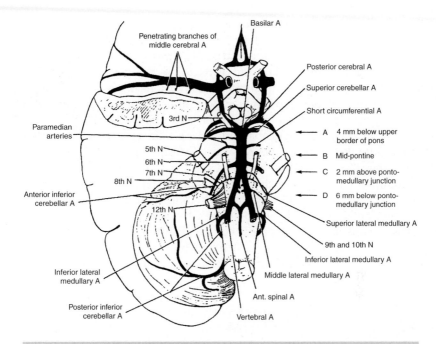

Figure 24-3 **Diagram of the brainstem showing the principal vessels of the vertebrobasilar system.** (From Victor, Ropper, Fig. 34-2, P. 827)

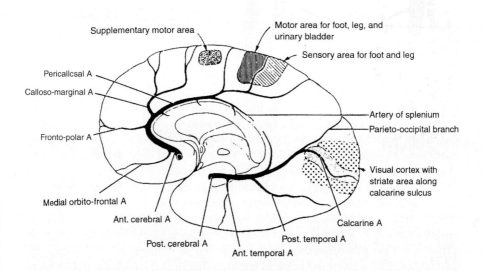

Figure 24-4 **Diagram of the medial aspect of the cerebral hemisphere, showing the anterior cerebral and posterior cerebral arteries.** (From Victor, Ropper, Fig. 24-3, P. 833)

as the *posterior circulation*. The bifurcation of the common carotid artery into the ICA and external carotid artery (ECA) is a frequent site of lipid plaque accumulation in atherosclerosis, and disease at this location is often the cause of large vessel, thrombotic TIA and stroke. Less commonly, stenosis of the ICA develops higher up, in the intracranial portions of the ICA. Intracranial large vessel disease develops in advanced atherosclerosis, in patients with chronic risk factors such as hypertension and diabetes mellitus, and more commonly in African Americans and Asians than in Caucasians. The ICA bifurcates into the anterior cerebral artery (ACA) and middle cerebral artery (MCA). Since the MCA takes more of a straight course from the ICA, emboli more commonly travel there, though occasionally emboli involve the ACA or posterior cerebral artery (PCA) territories. In general, disease of the MCA is more commonly caused by emboli than by local atherosclerotic disease, whereas disease of the ACA is more equally distributed between embolic and local disease. MCA territory strokes are much more common than ACA territory strokes. The ICA also gives rise to a posterior communicating artery, joining the carotid circulation with the PCA, which arises from the basilar artery of the posterior circulation. Occasionally, the posterior communicating artery supplies most of the blood to the PCA on one or both sides, a normal variant sometimes referred to as a *fetal circulation*.

The vascular territories of the ACA, MCA, and PCA are depicted in Fig. 24-5. Each has a superficial (cortical) and deep component. The precise correlation between the area of damage in a stroke and the clinical syndrome constitutes much of clinical neurology, which is why one preeminent neurologist (Dr. C. Miller Fisher) famously declared that "we learn neurology stroke by stroke." The MCA bifurcates into an upper division of branches and a lower division; the upper division of the left MCA supplies the motor speech area (Broca's area), the motor strip in the precentral gyrus (face and arm areas), and the sensory strip in the postcentral gyrus, leading to the common syndrome of Broca's aphasia and right hemiparesis in left MCA stroke. If only single branches are involved, more restricted deficits, such as Broca's aphasia with only right facial weakness, may occur. Involvement of the inferior division branches causes a fluent, Wernicke's aphasia, sometimes accompanied by a right upper quadrant visual field defect if the optic radiations are involved. Involvement of both upper and lower divisions of the left MCA, as in an embolus that lodges in the left MCA stem, produces global aphasia and right hemiplegia, a severe and disabling stroke syndrome. In the case of the right MCA, visuospatial deficits and neglect behavior are commonly associated. Involvement of deep branches of the MCA on either side also produces weakness of the leg as well as the arm, since the descending fibers from the cortical leg area descend through the MCA territory and into the internal capsule, also largely supplied by deep branches of the MCA. Small vessel, lacunar infarctions in the territory of the deep, lenticulostriate branches of the MCA produce localized infarctions of the posterior

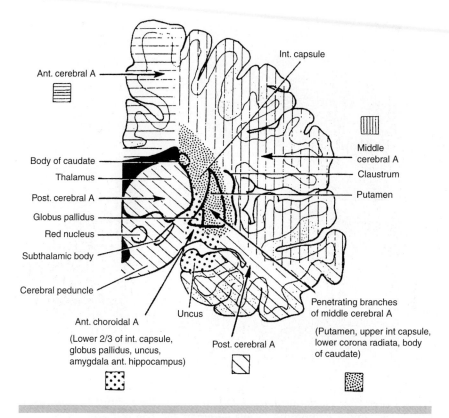

Figure 24-5 **Diagram of the left cerebral hemisphere, coronal section, showing the territories of the major cerebral vessels.** (From Victor, Ropper, Fig. 34-4, P. 832)

limb of the internal capsule, resulting in the stroke syndrome of pure motor hemiparesis, without sensory signs, cortical behavioral or cognitive deficits, or visual field abnormalities. Larger infarctions in the lenticulostriate territory produce more complex syndromes including combined motor and sensory deficits, dysarthria, and even cognitive deficits. Other small infarctions in the basal ganglia, sparing the internal capsule, may be relatively "silent," noted on brain imaging studies of patients without a clinical history of stroke.

Figure 24-6 shows an MR image with the new technology of "perfusion-weighted imaging" (PWI). The red (dark gray in the figure), core area of the infarction is colored red, indicating that perfusion is below limits of tissue viability. The surrounding, green area (light gray in the figure) represents tissue that is ischemic but not totally damaged. This area might be salvageable after reperfusion techniques such as thrombolytic therapy or deployment of

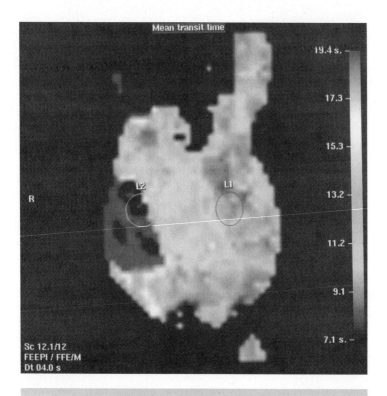

Figure 24-6 **MRI perfusion image from a patient about 4 hours after initial symptoms of left hemiparesis. The red area (dark gray) reflects severe ischemia likely to be associated with infarction, the green area (light gray) is a "penumbra" of ischemia that has not resulted in irreversible damage.** See color figure on the back cover.

an embolism extraction device (see Chapter 23). Figure 24.7 shows diffusion-weighted imaging showing infarcted tissue from an embolus to the left MCA. Figure 24-8 shows the MCA occlusion by MRA of the circle of Willis.

Strokes in the ACA territory cause a contralateral hemiparesis that is characteristically more severe in the leg than in the arm, and in the shoulder more than in the hand. In fact, many patients with ACA territory strokes have an involuntary grasp reflex in the affected hand. Behavioral disturbances are also characteristics of ACA territory strokes, including abulia or akinectic mutism and nonfluent speech (syndrome of transcortical motor aphasia in left ACA territory stroke, see Chapter 15).

Strokes in the PCA territory generally cause the most obvious symptoms in the contralateral visual field, often with a relatively isolated

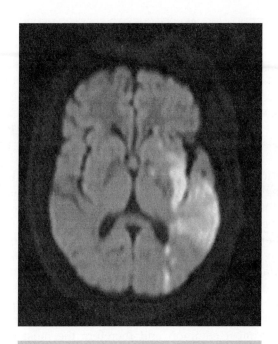

Figure 24-7 **MR diffusion image showing an infarction in the territory of the left middle cerebral artery.**

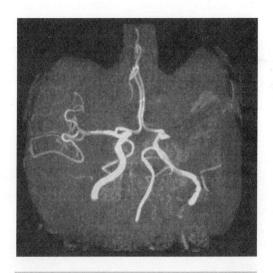

Figure 24-8 **MRA of the circle of Willis in the same patient as Figure 24.7, showing non-filling or occlusion of the left middle cerebral artery. This was an embolic stroke, with right hemiparesis and aphasia.**

homonymous hemianopsia. In left PCA territory strokes, alexia, or inability to read may be an associated symptom, together with color naming deficits and short-term memory loss (see Chapter 15). Usually, motor and sensory signs are absent, though occasional patients with PCA territory strokes develop motor or sensory deficits because of atypical arterial territories, including parts of the brainstem, thalamus, or posterior limb of internal capsule.

The posterior circulation of the brain is made up of the two vertebral arteries, arising from the subclavian artery on each side, merging within the skull to form the single, unpaired basilar artery. The vertebral arteries can be affected by atherosclerosis in their proximal portions, at the origin from the subclavian artery, or distally. The vertebral arteries are also a site of dissection, usually in more distal portions. The vertebral artery has one important branch intracranially, the posterior inferior cerebellar artery (PICA). The PICA supplies the lateral medulla and inferior, lateral, posterior portion of the cerebellum. The stroke syndrome that results from occlusion of either the vertebral artery or the PICA is the lateral medullary syndrome of Wallenberg, the most common and therefore the most important of the named brainstem stroke syndromes. The symptoms and signs of the Wallenberg syndrome are listed in Table 24-1. The "crossed sensory loss" of the ipsilateral face and contralateral body is one of the hallmarks of the syndrome, along with ipsilateral Horner syndrome (ptosis and miosis), ipsilateral palate paralysis and dysphagia, ipsilateral ataxia, and ipsilateral *lateral pulsion* (a tendency to lean toward the side of the stroke when sitting or standing).

At the level of the pontomedullary junction, the two vertebral arteries join to form the basilar artery. The basilar artery has two long, circumferential branches, the anterior inferior cerebellar artery (AICA) and the superior cerebellar artery (SCA). The AICA syndrome often involves ipsilateral

Table 24-1 **Symptoms and Signs of the Lateral Medullary Syndrome of Wallenberg**

Ipsilateral signs	Contralateral signs
Numbness of face	Numbness of arm, leg, body
Horner's syndrome	
Vertigo, nausea, hiccoughs	
Ataxia, lateral pulsion	
Dysphagia, palate paralysis	

VII (facial palsy) and VIII (deafness) cranial nerve abnormalities, ipsilateral ataxia, and contralateral motor and sensory deficits. The AICA syndrome has many variations, many with traditional eponyms. The SCA syndrome involves ipsilateral ataxia and contralateral sensory loss; other, variably associated symptoms include dysarthria, nausea and vomiting, ipsilateral tremor, palatal myoclonus, and partial deafness. The basilar artery also gives rise to many, small penetrating branches that supply portions of the brainstem. The stroke syndromes of the brainstem are quite variable, and I recommend that the student spend time on brainstem anatomy to make sense of these syndromes, rather than memorize the many eponymic syndromes.

DIFFERENTIAL DIAGNOSIS

Differential diagnosis must take place both at the stage of TIA and at the stage of stroke. TIA is an ominous symptom; as discussed in Chap. 19, TIA should be recognized as a medical emergency, and prompt diagnostic testing should be done to find the cause of the event and permit initiation of the proper preventive treatment. The differential diagnosis of TIA includes other causes of transient symptoms or "spells", including migraine, seizures, and other transient alterations of consciousness.

In the case of stroke, the presentation of a focal deficit in an awake patient, with appropriate risk factors, is so characteristic of stroke that, most of the time, the diagnosis is made by the family, by emergency medical technologists, and by emergency department triage nurses, even before the patient has seen a physician. Occasionally, however, other brain pathologies mimic stroke. Migraine can cause confusion with stroke as well as TIA, though most typically the focal symptoms occur during the aura, and these then improve as the severe headache ensues. *Complicated* migraine can include stroke symptoms, and sometimes a true infarction (see Chap. 30). Other focal brain pathologies such as tumors, abscesses, or inflammatory disorders such as multiple sclerosis occasionally present in an acute fashion. SDH in elderly patients is also frequently mistaken for stroke. A clear history of abrupt onset of symptoms usually favors stroke; the less clear the history, as in the patient "found down" at home, the more likely another diagnosis will emerge. About 15% of initial stroke diagnoses made by emergency medical technicians turn out to be incorrect.

A number of rapid screening tools for the diagnosis of stroke have been developed. One of the easiest to remember is the "Think FAST" paradigm developed at the University of Cincinnati. The "F" stands for facial weakness, the "A" for arm drift or weakness, the "S" for slurred speech or inability to speak or understand language, and the "T" for time, emphasizing the emergent nature of stroke treatment.

LABORATORY AND RADIOLOGICAL INVESTIGATION

The first aspect of stroke diagnosis, after clinical diagnosis, is a brain imaging study. The CT scan has traditionally served as the primary diagnostic test. CT has the capability to detect hemorrhage early and to delineate the location and extent of an ischemic lesion, but it may take 2–3 days before a cerebral infarction becomes clearly visible on CT. Occasionally, CT can image the thrombus in an occluded middle cerebral artery (*hyperacute MCA sign*), and an experienced interpreter can detect subtle, early signs of ischemia in stroke. In general, however, CT is less sensitive for the detection of early infarct changes than MRI. Recent additions to the CT armamentarium include CT angiography, imaging the cerebral and neck vessels with contrast infusion, and CT perfusion studies, mapping areas of cerebral blood flow after contrast infusion, such that areas of extremely low blood flow can be assumed to be associated with irreversible infarction. MRI scanning, by contrast, can delineate areas of ischemia very early in ischemic stroke (within minutes to an hour) via the diffusion weighted imaging (DWI) modality. If a timed contrast infusion is added, a perfusion weighted image (PWI) can identify areas of ischemia that have not yet become infarcted. The "mismatch" between the DWI and PWI lesion can indicate *tissue at risk* that can potentially be salvaged if the circulation can be restored. Figure 24-4 shows a perfusion MRI showing areas of profound ischemia, surrounded by a penumbra of ischemic but not infarcted tissue. There has been some concern about the ability of MRI to delineate intracerebral hemorrhage, but imaging with a T2* or gradient echo sequence shows both acute and chronic blood products as a black signal. Many centers now skip the CT scan entirely and go directly to MR imaging. Magnetic resonance (MR) angiography, or MRA, can also image the vessels, much like computed tomographic angiography (CTA), but the technology is such that MRA images can be "reconstructed" more readily into angiogram-like three-dimensional images, available for viewing shortly after the test is completed. CTA, on the other hand, can be performed more rapidly, though it has the disadvantages of requiring an iodinated contrast agent and more laborious reconstruction techniques. In the United States, stroke centers vary in their use of the CT/CTA and MRI/MRA technologies, and both techniques are becoming more accurate.

Other brain imaging techniques such as single photon emission computed tomography (SPECT) and positron emission tomography (PET) scanning are used in stroke, more as investigational procedures. The SPECT scan, with and without a vasodilator such as acetazolamide, can show whether brain perfusion is compromised by a vasodilator, suggesting decreased *cerebrovascular reserve*. New MRI techniques such as MR spectroscopy can also detect biochemical changes associated with ischemia.

Two other techniques permit visualization of cerebral vessels. Doppler ultrasound technology permits both real-time ultrasound imaging of the carotid bifurcations and Doppler signal analysis of blood flow. This rela- tively inexpensive, noninvasive vascular imaging technology detects steno- sis in the carotid vessels almost as accurately as MRA and CTA, though the imaging of the vertebral arteries is difficult. Transcranial Doppler (TCD) can insonate the major intracranial arteries. Finally, the traditional catheter arte- riogram is the "gold standard" of vascular diagnosis, since iodinated con- trast can be injected directly into the neck and cerebral vessels and imaged by standard X-ray technology. Arteriography is superior for detecting very small lesions such as aneurysms or changes in small arteries such as is seen in cerebral vasculitis, but it has the disadvantages of being invasive, with complications possible both from injury to vessels (dissection, breaking off of thrombus or plaque material that can embolize up to the brain) and from effects of the iodinated contrast agent.

Another area of diagnostic testing in patients with TIA or stroke is investigation of the heart, looking for a source of embolism to the brain. Electrocardiography (ECG) and heart rhythm monitoring are useful in stroke patients, since arrhythmias such as atrial fibrillation can occur inter- mittently, yet pose a serious risk of embolic stroke. Echocardiography images the heart, looking for thrombus within the left atrium or ventricle, poor contractility of the ventricle, valvular pathology, or an abnormal shunt between the right and left sides of the heart. Atrial septal defects or the more common patent foramen ovale occur in as many as 25% of the population. These shunts provide a conduit whereby clots from the venous circulation can cross from the right to left side of the heart and then embolize to the brain (*paradoxical embolization*). The echocardiogram is augmented by injec- tion of agitated saline, and the bubbles can be visualized crossing from the right to left atrium. Transesophageal echocardiography (TEE), in which the ultrasound probe is placed in the esophagus, directly behind the heart, has permitted more accurate diagnosis of cardiac conditions. Studies have shown that the TEE is more sensitive and more cost-effective than the stan- dard echocardiogram instroke patients, despite its increased discomfort and higher cost. Transcranial Doppler can also be combined with intravenous injection of agitated saline, and microemboli to the brain can then be detected.

Another important area of clinical testing in stroke patients involves blood tests. A complete blood count (CBC) is always indicated in stroke patients. Rarely, thrombocytosis or increased red blood cell counts can be a cause of stroke, as can severe anemia. Elevated platelet counts (thrombocytosis) can lead to clotting in cerebral vessels, whereas thrombocytopenia can lead to bleeding. Tests of clotting such as the prothrombin time (PT) and partial thromboplastin time (PTT) can detect clotting defects that lead to cerebral hemorrhage. A host of blood tests have been developed to detect increased clotting tendency, or *hypercoagulable states*. The *lupus anticoagulant* or *anticar- diolipin antibody* can be associated with arterial clotting and stroke syndromes.

Most of the other tests for hypercoagulability are more related to venous thrombosis and pulmonary embolism; these include protein C and S, antithrombin III, factor V Leiden, prothrombin gene mutation, and others. Elevated homocysteine levels are also associated with a higher risk of stroke. Finally, blood tests for endocrine (especially diabetes mellitus), metabolic, and organ function can be important in stroke. Plasma lipids are important to gauge risk of both myocardial infarction (MI) and stroke; fasting total cholesterol, high density lipoprotein (HDL), low density lipoprotein (LDL), and triglycerides should be tested in virtually all stroke patients. C-reactive protein (CRP) is as predictive of MI as is LDL cholesterol, and preliminary evidence also links this marker to stroke.

TREATMENT

The treatment of stroke is divided into acute interventions and chronic, preventive therapies. Acute management of aneurysmal SAH and ICH is discussed in Chap. 23. Treatment of acute ischemic stroke includes thrombolytic therapy or embolus extraction, and measures to reduce intracranial pressure, as discussed in Chap. 23. Aspirin has been found to have a small benefit as acute stroke treatment. Anticoagulation, either with intravenous, unfractionated heparin or low molecular weight heparin or heparinoids, has not been proved beneficial as acute stroke treatment. Some stroke experts recommend acute anticoagulation for patients with an acute stroke and evidence of an ipsilateral carotid bruit or carotid stenosis by ultrasound, carotid or vertebral artery dissection, and in those with atrial fibrillation or another, active source of embolism. These indications for acute anticoagulation have not been confirmed by evidence-based clinical trials, and some authorities do not recommend acute anticoagulation under any circumstances. Even when unfractionated heparin is used, bolus doses are generally avoided, because of fear of converting an infarction into a hemorrhage.

Once the stroke patient is stable, the treatment emphasis changes to avoidance of complications, provision of rehabilitative therapies, and measures to prevent future stroke recurrence. Speech/language pathologists check patients' ability to swallow before allowing the patient to take an oral diet or fluids. Prevention of deep vein thrombophlebitis (DVT) is an important aspect of stroke treatment, whether by sequential compression devices (SCDs), or subcutaneous heparin or enoxaparin. Studies have shown that enoxaparin 40 mg subcutaneously once daily is as effective as subcutaneous unfractionated heparin at 5000 units three times daily. Physical and occupational therapists prevent joint contractures and begin active exercises to help stroke patients regain function.

Secondary stroke prevention includes, first, the measures also effective in preventing first strokes, including smoking cessation, control of blood pressure (BP), healthy diet, medications to correct hyperlipidemia, and antiplatelet therapy; aspirin has been proved effective in preventing MI in healthy men, and stroke in women. In secondary stroke prevention, we avoid overtreating BP in the acute setting, when parts of the brain may depend critically on perfusion, but initiation of a BP regimen is a good strategy prior to discharge. Angiotensin converting enzyme inhibitors (ACE inhibitors) have been shown to have a primary stroke preventive effect in high-risk middle-aged and elderly patients, and also to prevent second strokes in stroke survivors. ACE receptor blockers also appear effective in preventing stroke. Likewise, stroke patients should all be tested for lipid levels. The recent Heart Protection Study and SPARCL study support the use of β-hydroxy-β-methylglutaryl-coenzyme A (HMG CoA) reductase inhibitors (*statins*) for all stroke patients. Patients should be screened for internal carotid artery stenosis, and surgery should be planned for patients with >70% stenosis of the carotid artery ipsilateral to the stroke, usually after a period of recovery. Echocardiography is carried out to look for a cardiac source of embolus. For patients with a definite cardiac source, anticoagulation is indicated with warfarin. Over the past few years, indications for anticoagulation in secondary stroke prevention have narrowed, mainly to patients with cardiac sources of embolism such as atrial fibrillation, carotid or vertebral artery dissections, cerebral venous sinus thrombosis, and documented hypercoagulable states. Management of patients with lower-risk sources of embolus, such as patent foramen ovale, is controversial. Patients with combined patent foramen ovale (PFO) and atrial septal aneurysm may be at increased risk of recurrent stroke, and some experts advocate anticoagulation for such patients. PFO closure devices are also being tested in patients with PFO who have sustained a stroke.

For all other noncardioembolic stroke patients, antiplatelet agents are used to prevent recurrent stroke. In the Warfarin Aspirin Recurrent Stroke Study, warfarin was not superior to aspirin, 325 mg daily, in preventing second strokes. Aspirin, combination aspirin and extended release dipyridamole, and clopidogrel are all recommended for secondary stroke prevention. The evidence indicates that both aspirin-extended release dipyridamole and clopidogrel are more effective than aspirin. Aspirin-dipyridamole has a robust effect in secondary stroke prevention (23% relative benefit over aspirin in the European Stroke Prevention 2 study, and similar benefit in the more recent ESPRIT trial). Clopidogrel had only about 9% relative benefit over aspirin in the clopidogrel versus aspirin in patients at risk of ischemic events (CAPRIE) study, but clopidogrel has more evidence of benefit than aspirin-dipyridamole in patients with coronary artery and peripheral vascular disease. The MATCH and CHARISMA trials have not supported the combination of aspirin and clopidogrel in stroke patients.

COURSE AND PROGNOSIS

As mentioned at the beginning of the chapter, stroke is the most serious of common neurological problems. Overall, about 10% of strokes are fatal, and most of the survivors have some level of disability. As many as one-third of stroke patients become demented in the year following an acute stroke. Many studies have shown that rehabilitative therapies improve outcome and should be initiated very early, to avoid complications such as aspiration pneumonia, DVT, and contractures of joints, as well as to optimize functional recovery. The risk of recurrent stroke is greatest over the first few years, and studies have shown that a stroke survivor's greatest risk over the next 2–3 years is another stroke. Long-term studies, however, have shown that the ultimate cause of death in the stroke patient is often cardiac, so prevention of both stroke and vascular disease in general is paramount.

KEY REFERENCES

Albers GW, Amarenco P, Easton JD, et al. Antithrombotic and thrombolytic therapy for ischemic stroke: the Seventh ACCP conference on antithrombotic and thrombolytic therapy. *Chest* 2004;126 (Suppl. 3):483S–512S.

Antithrombotic Trialists' Collaboration. Collaborative meta-analysis of randomised trials of antiplatelet therapy for prevention of death, myocardial infarction, and stroke in high risk patients. *BMJ* 2002;324:71–86.

Bhatt DL, Fox KAA, Hacke W, et al. Clopidogrel and aspirin versus aspirin alone for the prevention of atherothrombotic events. N Engl J Med 2006;354:1706–1717.

Brott T, Bogousslavsky J. Treatment of acute ischemic stroke. *N Engl J Med* 2000;343:710–722.

Caplan LR. Treatment of patients with stroke. *Arch Neurol* 2002;59:703–707.

CAPRIE Steering Committee. A randomised, blinded, trial of clopidogrel versus aspirin in patients at risk of ischaemic events (CAPRIE). *Lancet* 1996;348:1329–1339.

Chimowitz M, Lynn M, Howlett-Smith H, et al. Warfarin-Aspirin Symptomatic Intracranial Disease (WASID) trial: final results. *Stroke* 2004;35:235.

Diener HC, Cunha L, Forbes C, et al. European Stroke Prevention Study. 2. Dipyramidole and acetylsalicylic acid in the secondary prevention of stroke. *J Neurol Sci* 1996;143:1–13.

Diener HC, Bogousslavsky J, Brass LM, et al. Aspirin and clopidogrel compared with clopidogrel alone after recent ischemic stroke or transient ischemic attack in high-risk patients (MATCH): randomised, double-blind, placebo-controlled trial. *Lancet* 2004;364:331–337.

EAFT (European Atrial Fibrillation Trial) Study Group. Secondary prevention in non-rheumatic atrial fibrillation after transient ischemic attack of minor stroke. *Lancet* 1993;342:1255–1262.

Executive Committee for the Asymptomatic Carotid Atherosclerosis Study. Endarterectomy for asymptomatic carotid artery stenosis. *JAMA* 1995;273: 1421–1428.

Goldstein LB, Adams R, Becker K, et al. Primary prevention of ischemic stroke. A statement for healthcare professionals from the stroke council of the American Heart Association. *Circulation* 2001;103:163–182.

Goldstein LB, Simel DL. Is this patient having a stroke? *JAMA* 2005;293:2391–2402.

Grant EG, Benson CB, Monoeta GL, et al. Carotid artery stenosis: gray-scale and Doppler US diagnosis—Society of Radiologists in Ultrasound Consensus Conference. *Radiology* 2003;229:340–346.

Hanley D, Gorelick PB, Elliot WJ, et al. Determining the appropriateness of selected surgical and medical management options in recurrent stroke prevention: a guideline for primary care physicians from the National Stroke Association Work Group on Recurrent Stroke Prevention. *J Stroke Cerebrovasc Dis* 2004;13: 196–207.

Heart Protection Study Collaborative Group. Effects of cholesterol-lowering with simvastatin on stroke and other major vascular events in 20,536 people with cerebrovascular disease or other high-risk conditions. *Lancet* 2004;363:757–767.

Heart Protection Study Collaborative Group. MRC/BHF Heart protection study of cholesterol lowering with simvastatin in 20536 high-risk individuals: a randomised placebo-controlled trial. *Lancet* 2002;360:7–22.

Johnston SC, Gress DR, Browner WS, et al. Short-term prognosis after emergency department diagnosis of TIA. *JAMA* 2000;284:2901–2906.

Kidwell CS, Chalela JA, Saver JL, et al. Comparison of MRI and CT for detection of acute intracerebral hemorrhage. *JAMA* 2004;292:1823–1830.

Kirshner HS. Stroke mimicry: four cases eligible for tissue plasminogen activator. *Neurologist* 2000;6:220–223.

Kirshner HS. Medical prevention of stroke. *South Med J* 2003;96:354–358.

Kirshner HS, Biller J, Callahan AS III. Long-term therapy to prevent stroke. *J Am Board of Fam Pract* 2005;18:528–540.

Kizer JR, Devereux RB. Patent foramen ovale in young adults with unexplained stroke. *N Engl J Med* 2005;353:2361–2372.

Mas J-L, Arquizan, Lamy C, et al. Recurrent cerebrovascular events associated with patent foramen ovale, atrial septal aneurysm, or both. *N Engl J Med* 2001;345: 1740–1746.

Mayberg MR, Wilson SE, Yatsu F, et al. Carotid endarterectomy and prevention of cerebral ischemia in symptomatic carotid stenosis. Veterans Affairs Cooperative Studies Program 309 Trialist Group. *JAMA* 1991;266:3289–3294.

Mendelow AD, Gregson BA, Fernandes HM, et al. Early surgery versus initial conservative treatment in patients with spontaneous intracerebral hematomas in the International Surgical Trial in Intracerebral Hemorrhage (STICH): a randomized trial. *Lancet* 2005;365:387–397.

Mohr JP, Thompson JLP, Lazar RM, et al. A comparison of warfarin and aspirin for the prevention of recurrent ischemic stroke. *N Engl J Med* 2001;345:1444–1451.

North American Symptomatic Carotid Endarterectomy Trial Collaborators. Beneficial effect of carotid endarterectomy in symptomatic patients with high-grade carotid stenosis. *N Engl J Med* 1991;325:445 453.

Provenzale JM, Sorensen AG. Diffusion-weighted MR imaging in acute stroke. Theoretic considerations and clinical applications. *AJR* 1999;173:1459–1467.

Publications Committee for the Trial of ORG 10172 in Acute Stroke Treatment (TOAST) Investigators. Low molecular weight heparinoid ORG 10172 (danaparoid), and outcome after acute ischemic stroke. A randomized controlled trial. *JAMA* 1998;279: 1265–1272.

Pulsinelli W. Pathophysiology of acute ischemic stroke. *Lancet* 1992;339:533–537.

Qureshi AI, Tuhrim S, Broderick JP, et al. Spontaneous intracerebral hemorrhage. *N Engl J Med* 2001;344:1450–1460.

Report of the Quality Standards Subcommittee of the American Academy of Neurology. Practice advisory: thrombolytic therapy for acute ischemic stroke—summary statement. *Neurology* 1996;47:835–839.

Ridker PM, Cook NR, Lee I-M, et al. A randomized trial of low-dose aspirin in the primary prevention of cardiovascular disease in women. *N Engl J Med* 2005;352: 1293–1304.

Rosenberg C, Popelka GM. Post-stroke rehabilitation. A review of guidelines for patient management. *Geriatrics* 2000;55:75–81.

Sacco RL, Adams R, Albers G, et al. Guidelines for prevention of stroke in patients with ischemic stroke or transient ischemic attack: a statement for healthcare professionals from the American Heart Association/American Stroke Association Council on Stroke. Co-sponsored by the Council on Cardiovascular Radiology and Intervention. The American Academy of Neurology affirms the value of this guideline. *Stroke.* 2006;37:577–617.

Savitz SI, Caplan LR. Vertebrobasilar disease. *N Engl J Med* 2005;352:2618–2626.

Strauss S, Majumdar SR, McAlister FA. New evidence for stroke prevention. *JAMA* 2002;288:1388–1395.

The ESPRIT Study Group. Aspirin plus dipyridamole versus aspirin alone after cerebral ischaemia of arterial origin (ESPRIT): randomized controlled trial. Lancet 2006;367:1665–73.

The Stroke Prevention by Aggressive Reduction in Cholesterol Levels (SPARCL) Investigators. High-dose atorvastatin after Stroke or Transient Ischemic Attack. New Engl J Med 2006;355:549–559.

Warlow C, Sudlow C, Dennis M, et al. Stroke. *Lancet* 2003;362:1211–1224.

Wijdicks EFM. Management of massive hemispheric cerebral infarct; is there a ray of hope? *Mayo Clin Proc* 2000;75:945–952.

Yadav JS, Wholey MH, Kuntz RE. Protected carotid-artery stenting versus endarterectomy in high-risk patients. *N Engl J Med* 2004;351:1493–1501.

CHAPTER 25

SEIZURE DISORDERS

Bassel Abou-Khalil, MD
and Howard S. Kirshner, MD

INTRODUCTION

Epileptic seizures are among the most frightening acute manifestations seen in clinical medicine. Seizures are defined as episodes of symptoms and signs of excessive and/or hypersynchronous discharge of neurons. Epilepsy is defined as a recurrent tendency to have epileptic seizures. The diagnosis of epilepsy requires more than one spontaneous, unprovoked epileptic seizure. Recurrent seizures secondary to a recurrent metabolic disturbance such as hyponatremia do not indicate epilepsy.

Epilepsy is a very common condition. Each year in the United States, approximately 150,000 people receive a new diagnosis of epilepsy, and as many as 2 million people have epilepsy. The prevalence approaches 3% of the population, sometime in life. Idiopathic epilepsy is most common in the first two decades of life, but the incidence rises again later in life, largely related to acquired brain lesions that cause *symptomatic* or *secondary* epilepsy.

CLINICAL PRESENTATION: SYMPTOMS AND SIGNS

The clinical manifestations of epileptic seizures are variable, depending on which areas of the brain are involved in the *ictal* discharge, from seizure onset to termination. A classification of seizures is important to facilitate clinical diagnosis and communication, to assess prognosis, and to evaluate whether specific drugs are the most appropriate therapy. Dating back to the 1981 classification proposed by the International League Against Epilepsy (ILAE), seizures are classified first into partial or generalized seizures (see Table 25-1). Seizures are termed partial if there is either clinical or electroencephalogram (EEG) evidence indicating onset in a focal area of one hemisphere, whereas generalized seizures appear to begin simultaneously in both

Table 25-1 **Proposal for Revised Clinical and Electroencephalographic Classification of Epileptic Seizures**

I. Partial (focal, local) seizures
   A. Simple partial seizures
   B. Complex partial seizures
      1. with impairment of consciousness at onset
      2. simple partial onset followed by impairment of consciousness
   C. Partial seizures evolving to generalized tonic-clonic convulsions (GTC)
      1. Simple evolving to GTC
      2. Complex evolving to GTC (including those with simple partial onset)
II. Generalized seizures (convulsive or nonconvulsive)
   A. 1. Absence seizures
      2. Atypical absence
   B. Myoclonic seizures
   C. Clonic seizures
   D. Tonic seizures
   E. Tonic-clonic seizures
   F. Atonic seizures
III. Unclassified Epileptic Seizures

Source: The commission on classification and terminology of the International League Against Epilepsy. *Epilepsia* 1981;22:489–501.

hemispheres. Partial seizures are divided into three categories: (a) simple partial (not affecting consciousness); (b) complex partial seizures (involving alteration of consciousness); and (c) partial seizures evolving into secondarily generalized tonic, clonic (GTC) convulsions, which could begin as either simple partial or complex partial seizures. A simple partial seizure may involve jerking of a muscle in one hand or arm or may be purely subjective, with tingling in one body part; visual, auditory, or olfactory hallucinations; autonomic changes such as peculiar epigastric sensations or goosebumps; or a psychic feeling of familiarity or strangeness. A complex partial seizure may start with clouding of consciousness from the onset, or may be heralded by a subjective experience such as a feeling of familiarity or a peculiar smell. We call these phenomena the *aura* of a seizure, but electrographically they are actually part of the seizure. The seizure might then spread bilaterally, in which case we see clouding of consciousness and associated automatisms such as picking at objects or lip-smacking, or into the motor cortex, in which case there might be frank tonic clonic activity. The seizure may become secondarily generalized into a generalized tonic clonic seizure. Whether or not the patient loses consciousness, a *postictal* state of lethargy and confusion often follows the ictus.

Generalized seizures are divided into six types: (a) absence, (b) myoclonic, (c) clonic, (d) tonic, (e) tonic-clonic, and (f) atonic seizures. Generalized absence seizures are characterized by brief loss of awareness or responsiveness and arrest of activity. Absence seizures may be associated with minor motor components such as automatisms, blinking, slight twitching, decreased tone, or increased tone. Generalized tonic-clonic seizures are characterized by loss of consciousness at onset, with a sudden tonic muscular contraction, sometimes a movement of air through a closed glottis, producing a "cry," as well as cyanosis. After the tonic phase, the seizure then evolves into generalized clonic or rhythmic jerking activity, sometimes accompanied by grunting. The clonic activity is initially fast, and the frequency of the jerks decreases before the seizure stops. Generalized tonic-clonic seizures are often accompanied by tongue biting and urinary incontinence. Generalized myoclonic seizures are brief, sudden contractions that may be generalized or confined to a group of muscles, or even a single muscle. They can be single and isolated or repetitive in a cluster. Consciousness is usually preserved. Some forms of myoclonus are not epileptic. Myoclonic seizures usually have a concomitant discharge on the EEG. Generalized clonic seizures are characterized by repetitive clonic jerks, without an initial tonic component. Generalized tonic seizures manifest with a muscular contraction that may vary in duration, severity, and the parts of the body involved. The muscular contractions are more sustained than those of myoclonic seizures. If the contraction is prolonged, the seizure may resemble the tonic phase of a tonic-clonic seizure. Generalized atonic seizures are characterized by a sudden decrease in muscle tone, which is variable in severity and extent, so that there may simply be a slight head drop, or an abrupt fall to the ground.

The diagnosis of the specific seizure type is not always straightforward. A commonly encountered clinical differential diagnosis is that between complex partial seizures and generalized absence seizures. Absence seizures have no aura, have a sudden onset, short duration (generally less than 15 seconds), sudden termination, and no postictal confusion. They also tend to occur frequently, several times a day. Complex partial seizures may or may not have an aura, but they typically last more than 30 seconds. Postictal confusion or tiredness occurs commonly. The seizure frequency varies but is most commonly several times a month.

The classification of seizures just discussed applies only to individual seizures. There are also classifications of epileptic syndromes. Within these syndromes, a patient might have more than one seizure type. An epileptic syndrome is characterized by a cluster of characteristics, including types of seizures, age at onset, family history, response to drugs, and prognosis. The ILAE classification of 1989 (Table 25-2) is still the most widely used. The epilepsies are subdivided into two broad categories: partial and generalized. Most patients will have either partial or generalized seizure types, but a

Table 25-2 **Proposal for Revised Classification of Epilepsies and Epileptic Syndromes**

I. Localization-related (focal, local, partial) epilepsies and syndromes
    A. Idiopathic (with age-related onset)
    B. Symptomatic
    C. Cryptogenic
II. Generalized epilepsies and syndromes
    A. Idiopathic (with age-related onset)
    B. Cryptogenic or symptomatic
    C. Symptomatic
III. Epilepsies and syndromes undetermined whether focal or generalized
    A. With both generalized and focal seizures
    B. Without unequivocal generalized or focal features
IV. Special syndromes
    Situation-related seizures (Gelegenheitsanfälle)

Source: Commission on classification and terminology of the International League Against Epilepsy. Epilepsia 1989;30:389–399.

third category exists for those with both partial- and generalized-onset types. In each category there are three subcategories: idiopathic, symptomatic, and cryptogenic epilepsies. Idiopathic epilepsies are pure epilepsies, with no manifestations other than seizures, and with no known cause. They are usually genetically determined. Symptomatic epilepsies are acquired epileptic syndromes where the insult is known, such as traumatic brain injury (TBI), congenital brain malformation, tumor, or stroke. Cryptogenic epilepsies are those in which an acquired etiology is suspected, but the cause is not clear. The most recent ILAE classification scheme suggested replacing the term *cryptogenic* with *probably symptomatic*.

Idiopathic epileptic syndromes are the best defined and the most homogeneous. The partial symptomatic and cryptogenic epilepsies are further classified based on the anatomical location of the epileptogenic focus where the seizure discharge originates. The most common localization is temporal lobe, followed by frontal, then occipital and parietal. Temporal lobe epilepsies are subdivided into amygdalo-hippocampal or medial temporal epilepsies, the most common, versus lateral temporal varieties. Frontal lobe epilepsies are subdivided into those originating in the supplementary motor, cingulate, anterior frontopolar, orbitofrontal, dorsolateral, opercular, and motor cortex regions.

The ILAE Task Force on Classification and Terminology recently proposed a new diagnostic scheme, divided into five parts, or Axes, organized to facilitate a logical clinical approach to the diagnosis and treatment of

Table 25-3 **The ILAE Task Force on Classification and Terminology (2001)**

Axis 1: Ictal phenomenology (from the Glossary of Descriptive Ictal Terminology, can be used to describe ictal events with any degree of detail needed).

Axis 2: Seizure type (from the List of Epileptic Seizures. Localization within the brain and precipitating stimuli for reflex seizures should be specified when appropriate).

Axis 3: Syndrome (from the List of Epilepsy Syndromes, with the understanding that a syndromic diagnosis may not always be possible).

Axis 4: Etiology (from a Classification of Diseases Frequently Associated with Epileptic Seizures or Epilepsy Syndromes when possible, genetic defects, or specific pathologic substrates).

Axis 5: Impairment (this optional, but often useful, additional diagnostic parameter can be derived from an impairment classification adapted from the World Health Organisation International Classification of Impairment, Disability and Handicap–2 (WHO ICIDH–2).

patients with epilepsy. These axes are shown in Table 25-3. In this classification, axis 2 reflects the classifications for epileptic seizure type, and axis 3 the epilepsy syndrome; in addition, the scheme proposes axis 4 for "epileptic disease," to designate a pathologic condition with a single specific, well-defined etiology, such as a specific mutation. The next classification will include a few new seizure types, particularly generalized negative myoclonus, focal negative myoclonus, focal inhibitory motor seizures, and gelastic laughing seizures, and several new epileptic syndromes (see below).

An example of a partial idiopathic epileptic syndrome is the syndrome of *benign partial epilepsy with centrotemporal spikes* of childhood. This disorder has a genetic predisposition and a male predominance, suggesting a sex-linked inheritance pattern. The typical age of onset is 3–13 years, most commonly age 9–10. The seizures involve brief, motor manifestations, often involving the face on one side. Sensory symptoms are also seen frequently, and the seizures may secondarily generalize. The EEG shows high voltage, centrotemporal spikes, often coming out more in sleep, and often shifting between the two sides. The prognosis is excellent, typically with excellent control of seizures on medication. Most patients outgrow the epilepsy and remain seizure free off medication by age 15–16.

A common example of a generalized idiopathic epileptic syndrome is *juvenile myoclonic epilepsy* (JME). This disorder begins most commonly between 12 and 18 years, equally in the two genders. The principal seizure type is a myoclonic seizure, mainly involving the shoulders and arms, usually with no alteration of consciousness. Generalized tonic-clonic seizures also occur in a majority of patients, usually beginning with a series of clonic jerks. Myoclonic jerks typically precede the development of generalized tonic-clonic seizures by an average of 3 years. A few patients also have generalized absence seizures. All seizures tend to occur in the morning on awakening. Lack of sleep or premature awakening are precipitating factors. In some cases, flickering light or high musical notes may provoke seizures. The EEG typically shows 4–6 Hz generalized spike-and-wave discharges both during the myoclonic jerks and interictally. The prognosis is quite good; approximately 90% of patients achieve complete control of seizures with valproate (Depakote) as a single drug, but most patients have a life-long risk of seizures, and life-long antiepileptic treatment is usually necessary.

The international classification of epilepsies and epileptic syndromes has some limitations. The classification does not take into consideration patients who have both a genetic predisposition to epilepsy and acquired brain insults. Second, the classification breaks down in the continuum between symptomatic partial and symptomatic generalized epilepsy, which may include epilepsies with two, three, or multiple foci. Third, a number of new idiopathic, genetically determined epileptic syndromes, characterized in recent years, are not included in the current classification. Among the new localization-related epilepsy syndromes are benign familial infantile convulsions, autosomal dominant nocturnal frontal lobe epilepsy, benign familial temporal lobe epilepsy, familial partial epilepsy with variable foci, partial epilepsy with auditory features, and rolandic epilepsy with speech dyspraxia. One of the new generalized epilepsies is generalized epilepsy with febrile seizures plus (GEFS+), a genetically determined idiopathic generalized epileptic syndrome. Several of the idiopathic epileptic syndromes are now recognized to represent channelopathies, with mutations affecting the potassium, sodium, and calcium channels. In addition, some families with generalized epileptic syndromes have been found to have γ-aminobutyric acid$_A$ (GABA$_A$) receptor mutations.

DIFFERENTIAL DIAGNOSIS

The most important diagnostic tool is the seizure history, obtained from the patient and from observers who have witnessed typical attacks. The localizing information in epilepsy diagnosis is thus often obtained from the history, in contrast to other neurological disorders such as stroke, in which the most important localizing information usually comes from the neurological examination. In the description of clinical seizures, evidence for focal seizure onset should be sought, for example the presence of an aura, initial focal sensory symptoms, or motor signs. In addition, the type of aura and the first signs in partial seizures can help localize the seizure onset in the brain. The past history, including prenatal, birth, and early development, and family history may provide insight into the etiology. The neurological examination may occasionally provide focal findings, which would favor partial epilepsy. Generalized absence seizures are often easily precipitated by hyperventilation, which can be carried out as a part of the physical examination.

The diagnosis of epilepsy is typically based on the occurrence of transient, stereotyped seizure phenomena. The differential diagnosis is with other transitory neurological events. A listing of the differential diagnosis of seizures is presented in Table 25-4.

Simple syncope is a common confounding symptom, related to a transient global reduction in cerebral blood flow. Syncope most commonly results from decreased cardiac output, decreased blood volume, decreased peripheral resistance, or combinations of these factors. A cardiac origin, such as an arrhythmia, is more of a concern in older individuals, whereas in adolescents and young adults, syncope is most often neurally mediated (see Chap. 20). Neurally mediated syncope usually features a prodrome of nausea, light-headedness, and dimming of vision. An observer may witness pallor and limp posture. This prodrome is usually longer than the aura preceding an epileptic seizure. Recovery is usually much faster with syncope, without a *postictal state*. Up to 90% of syncope is associated with motor activity, predominantly brief multifocal myoclonus that lasts a few seconds. This is to be distinguished from epileptic tonic-clonic activity, which is longer in duration and synchronous on the two sides, and syncope is usually not associated with tongue-biting or incontinence. In syncope, the patient usually

Table 25-4 **Differential Diagnosis of Epileptic Seizures**

Physiologic disturbances
  Systemic
    Syncope (loss of consciousness due to decreased cerebral perfusion)
    Hyperventilation
    Hypoglycemia and other toxic/metabolic disturbances
  Neurologic
    Migraine
    Transient cerebral ischemia
    Transient global amnesia
    Movement disorders
    Sleep disorders (narcolepsy/ night terrors)
Psychogenic disturbances
  Psychogenic seizures (pseudoseizures)
  Episodic dyscontrol (with impulsively violent behavior)
  Dissociative states

has enough warning to sit down or at least break the fall, whereas patients with epileptic seizures may collapse suddenly, without any warning. If there is doubt, an EEG can be helpful.

Related causes of light-headedness or syncope involve hyperventilation and pulmonary embolism. These are discussed in Chap. 20.

Migraine can be preceded by positive visual or somatosensory symptoms, vertigo, or confusion, and occasionally patients experience "migraine equivalents" without headache. However, migraine symptoms tend to have a more gradual onset and a longer duration than those of seizures. Migraine occasionally causes alteration of consciousness, and even confusion, but the characteristic headache and nausea usually make the diagnosis clear. Both migraines and occipital lobe seizures may be preceded by an aura of visual hallucinations, but migraines usually develop into headache, nausea, and vomiting, whereas in seizures the spell is more likely to develop into motor manifestations such as jerking, or loss of consciousness. The "march" of symptoms from leg to arm to face, or vice versa is typically over seconds in a seizure, as opposed to minutes in migraine.

Transient ischemic attacks (TIAs) are usually characterized by negative symptoms and signs, such as numbness, visual loss, or weakness, whereas seizures most often produce positive phenomena, such as paresthesias, hallucinations, or involuntary motor activity. TIAs usually have no associated alteration of consciousness, with the exception of occasional vertebrobasilar TIAs. TIAs do not typically cause bladder incontinence, tongue-biting, or a postictal state. TIA episodes are often less stereotyped than seizures. Variants of TIA are transient global amnesia, a transient amnestic state that may mimic a temporal lobe seizure, and *drop attacks of the elderly*, a syndrome of sudden falling without self-described loss of consciousness or postictal state. For both transient global amnesia and drop attacks the cause is unknown in most cases, but seizure is always in the differential diagnosis.

Less common episodic syndromes complete the metabolic category in the differential diagnosis of epileptic seizures. Hypoglycemia can cause light-headedness, a sense of hunger, and an alteration of consciousness which can lead to syncope if the patient does not ingest glucose. Carcinoid syndrome, in which serotonin and its metabolites are released by tumors, may cause peculiar, transitory symptoms including light-headedness and flushing. Similar symptoms can be seen in systemic mastocytosis, related to release of histamine.

Movement disorders such as hemiballismus, dystonia, and myoclonus can occasionally be confused with seizures, especially when they are episodic or paroxysmal. These movement disorders do not affect consciousness and lack features associated with seizures, such as an aura, a postictal state, or ictal tongue-biting or incontinence. They also tend to disappear in sleep, whereas seizures may occur during sleep. A normal EEG during the manifestation can help to eliminate epilepsy from the differential diagnosis.

Simple partial seizures with motor manifestations, however, may also lack scalp EEG changes, because the cortical area involved does not reach the critical 6 cm^2 necessary for changes to appear on the scalp EEG.

A few sleep disorders such as parasomnias and rapid eye movement (REM) behavior disorder occasionally masquerade as seizures. Parasomnias such as sleep walking, sleep talking, or night terrors arise from deep, slow wave sleep, whereas seizures more often arise in light sleep. REM behavior disorder arises from an abnormal REM sleep in which inhibition of motor activity is impaired. Narcolepsy includes sleep attacks, cataplexy, or loss of tone with emotion or startle, visual hallucinations upon falling asleep or waking up, and sleep paralysis, an inability to move upon waking. These sleep manifestations occur in close association with sleep, whereas seizures often occur during waking; an exception is partial complex seizures, which often come on during light sleep. In these disorders, too, EEG or sleep studies with EEG leads can be helpful in diagnosis. Further discussion of sleep disorders can be found in Chap. 21.

Single seizures also raise a differential diagnosis of different seizure types. Most common is the distinction between complex partial and generalized absence seizures. Absence spells have no aura, sudden onset, duration less than 15 seconds, sudden termination, and no postictal state. They occur frequently, several times per day. Complex partial seizures often have an aura, last more than 30 seconds, and often have a postictal confusional-lethargic period. They occur less frequently than absence seizures.

A last issue concerns the diagnosis of nonepileptic seizures, often called *psychogenic seizures*, *pseudoseizures*, or *pseudoepileptic seizures*. These represent the most common condition in the differential diagnosis of epileptic seizures. Psychogenic seizures are episodes of alteration in movement, in responsiveness, or in sensory or cognitive experience, which resemble epileptic seizures but are purely emotional in nature and lack a concomitant cerebral electrical discharge. They occur most commonly through unconscious *conversion reactions*, but infrequently through voluntary malingering. Patients are commonly referred after they fail treatment for epilepsy. Psychogenic seizures may account for 20–30% of patients referred for intractable seizures. Psychogenic seizures are more common in young people, with a relative female predominance. The clinical manifestations of psychogenic seizures are extremely variable. There may or may not be a reported aura. The onset is often gradual, always in waking, even when the patient appears asleep. Psychogenic seizures often include motor manifestations, but collapse or altered responsiveness may be the only manifestations. Many clinical features have been used to diagnose psychogenic attacks and to distinguish them from epileptic seizures. Features that support a diagnosis of psychogenic seizures include out of phase upper and lower extremity movements, side-to-side head movement, and forward pelvic thrusting. Other clinical features suggestive of psychogenic seizures include a gradual onset, *preictal* behavioral changes, "pseudo-sleep" before seizure onset, discontinuous seizure activity, prolonged duration (*pseudostatus epilepticus* is common), gradual cessation, absence of postictal state, high seizure frequency, excessive variability in ictal manifestations, nonphysiologic progression, eye closure during unresponsiveness, eye fluttering, resistance to eye opening, vocalizations consisting of gagging, retching, gasping, screaming, crying or moaning, retained consciousness and recollection of events with bilateral jerking activity, emotional displays such as crying during events, the presence of an emotional trigger, and the occurrence of events only in the presence of others. If the examiner can suggest the patient into initiating or stopping seizure activity, a psychogenic seizure is suspected. Incontinence, tongue biting, and self-injury during attacks suggest epilepsy. No feature alone is definitive, but a combination of the features noted above can improve the ability to distinguish psychogenic from epileptic seizures. An elevated serum prolactin level 15–30 minutes after a seizure also suggests epilepsy, but a normal level does not exclude epilepsy. Prolonged EEG-video monitoring is usually necessary for the definitive diagnosis of psychogenic seizures and exclusion of epilepsy. About 10-20% of patients with psychogenic seizures also have epilepsy. The underlying psychopathology may vary remarkably among patients. A history of childhood sexual or physical abuse is common. Depression is also common and is important to identify and treat.

Other psychogenic manifestations that can mimic seizures include panic attacks, dissociative states, and episodic dyscontrol syndrome, a "temper tantrum"-like, impulsively violent behavior pattern seen usually in children and adolescents. Rage attacks are highly unlikely to be epileptic. Ictal or postictal violence is rare and is not usually goal-directed.

LABORATORY AND RADIOLOGICAL INVESTIGATION

Electroencephalography

Laboratory tests cannot substitute for an adequate history and description of events, and they generally provide only supportive evidence for epilepsy. The most sensitive diagnostic test available to help confirm the diagnosis of epilepsy is the EEG. The EEG measures potential differences between points on the scalp or brain in relation to time. "Routine" EEGs are recorded for about 20 minutes. In most forms of epilepsy it is statistically unlikely to record a seizure during a routine EEG; a notable exception is generalized absence seizures, which occur frequently and are easily precipitated by hyperventilation. Patients with epilepsy frequently have EEG abnormalities in-between seizures, called *interictal* abnormalities. Some of these abnormalities, such as *epileptiform* spikes or sharp waves, are specific for epilepsy. Approximately 50% of patients with epilepsy will have a normal first EEG. However, more than 90% will have an abnormal EEG with repeated testing, up to four times, and the use of activation techniques such as sleep, sleep deprivation, hyperventilation, and photic stimulation. The use of sphenoidal electrodes, which record electrical events from the basal temporal region, may also improve the yield of the EEG in select patients. In partial epilepsies, the interictal epileptiform discharges tend to be focal or regional. These discharges generally have a topographic correlation with the epileptogenic zone, the zone from which seizures are generated. Recordings obtained during seizures will generally show a rhythmic discharge. In generalized epilepsies, spikes and sharp waves tend to be generalized and synchronous in the two hemispheres. In generalized absence seizures, the ictal discharge consists of repeated generalized spike-and-slow-wave complexes that typically have a frequency of approximately 3 Hz, but occasionally 2.5–4 Hz. In most other seizure types, the rhythmic discharge has an evolution, generally with spread of activity in the brain and corresponding increase in voltage, followed by eventual decrease in frequency prior to the end of the seizure. Figure 25-1 shows a left temporal spike focus arising from electrodes Sp1, F7, and T7. Figure 25-2 shows the discharge associated with a complex partial seizure. Figure 25-3 shows a generalized absence seizure discharge.

EEG-closed circuit TV (EEG-CCTV) monitoring is a technique that combines prolonged monitoring of the EEG with capture of a clinical seizure on videotape. This technique is expensive, requiring outpatient monitoring for several hours or even inpatient hospitalization on an epilepsy unit. The technique is essential if the routine EEG is either normal or shows only nonspecific abnormalities, and the nature of the "seizures" is unknown. EEG-CCTV monitoring is needed both for identification of the type of epileptic seizure to optimize medical therapy and for diagnosis of psychogenic seizures. It is also important for localization of the seizure focus in order to plan surgical treatment for refractory epilepsy.

Neuroimaging

Making the diagnosis of epilepsy is generally not sufficient in itself. The etiology of epilepsy should always be sought. A structural imaging study of the brain is indicated in new onset epilepsy to identify tumors, malformations, infarcts, and the like, unless the patient clearly has a genetic epileptic syndrome. Magnetic resonance imaging (MRI) is the preferred imaging modality. Computerized tomography (CT) has a lower sensitivity and may miss pathology in the temporal lobes as a result of bone artifact. Figure 25-4 shows an MRI indicating left hippocampal sclerosis. Figure 25-5 shows a right mesial temporal cavernous angioma.

Positron emission tomography (PET) is an imaging technique most commonly used to measure regional cerebral metabolic rates for glucose, by infusion of radiolabelled flurodeoxyglucose (FDG PET). This imaging modality is expensive and often considered a research tool. It is not indicated in the routine evaluation of new onset epilepsy. PET is very useful, however, in localizing the epileptogenic focus in cases of refractory epilepsy, in which

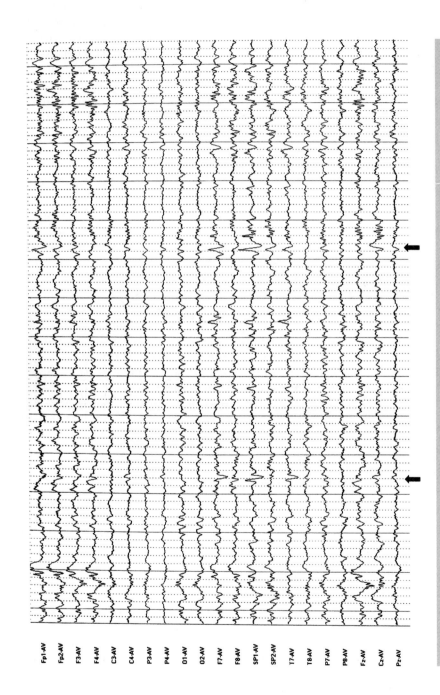

Figure 25-1   *EEG tracing showing a focal, left temporal lobe discharge arising from electrodes Sp1, F7, T7.*

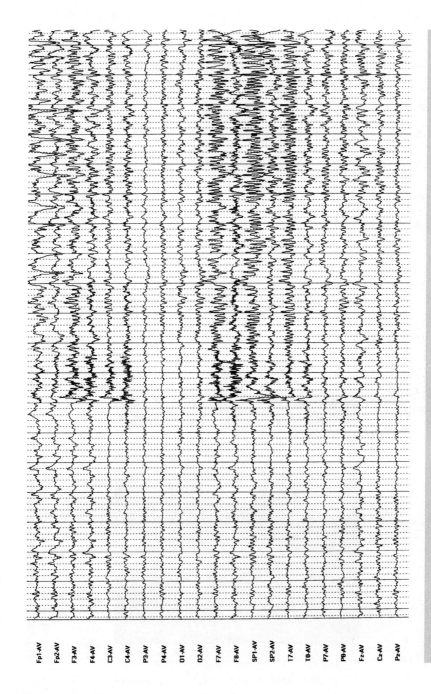

Figure 25-2 **EEG tracing showing a focal left temporal seizure in the same patient above.**

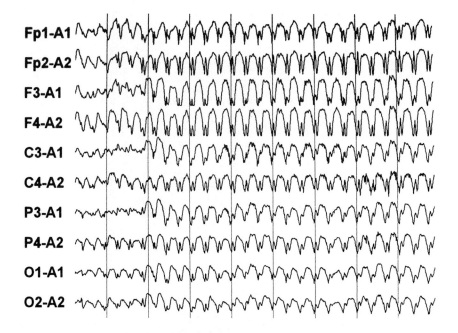

Figure 25-3   **EEG tracing showing a generalized absence seizure discharge.**

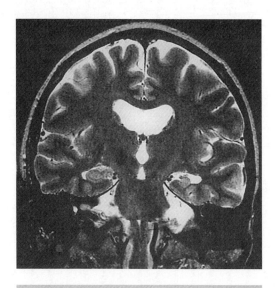

Figure 25-4   **MRI showing left mesial temporal sclerosis.**

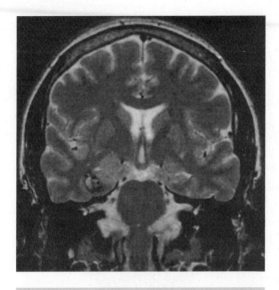

Figure 25-5 **MRI showing a right temporal cavernous angioma.**

surgical therapy is a consideration. The epileptogenic focus is generally hypermetabolic during a seizure, but hypometabolic interictally. Figure 25-6 shows a hypometabolic focus interictally in the left anterior temporal lobe.

Other diagnostic tests

Depending on the specific case, other studies that would help in the diagnosis of a patient with seizures could include a lumbar puncture for the analysis of the cerebrospinal fluid, various metabolic or biochemical blood studies, or genetic testing.

Treatment of the underlying cause

After the diagnosis of epileptic seizures is made, the physician must determine whether or not the etiology requires specific treatment. For example, a brain tumor or an infectious process may need to be treated. In most cases, the etiology of epilepsy does not require specific treatment, such as a small scar or a remote encephalitis. The treatment then is a symptomatic therapy for the seizures.

Medical therapy of seizures

Once the seizure type and the type of epilepsy have been diagnosed, the most effective and safest antiepileptic drug (AED) for that seizure type should be selected, begun at a standard starting dose, in monotherapy. If the seizures are not controlled, the dose can then be increased gradually until seizures

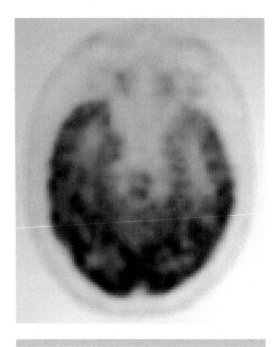

Figure 25-6 **PET image showing a hypo-metabolic focus in the left temporal lobe. This scan was taken during the interictal period.**

stop, or until side effects appear. Serum AED levels can be used to help explain lack of response or adverse experiences, but the clinical response should be the primary guide in treatment. Small AED increments should be used when in the therapeutic range. If side effects occur without seizure control the drug must be returned to a dose that was not associated with side effects, and a second drug must be considered. The second drug is then added with the expectation that the first will be discontinued. Only refractory seizure disorders require polytherapy regimens, and then with only two drugs or rarely three (see discussion below).

The most important standard antiepileptic drugs are: phenytoin (Dilantin), carbamazepine (Tegretol), valproic acid (Depakene, Depakote), ethosuximide (Zarontin), phenobarbital, primidone (Mysoline), and clonazepam (Klonopin). A number of newer agents have also been introduced for the treatment of epilepsy, and we shall discuss these newer drugs after the traditional agents. Phenytoin and carbamazepine are the drugs of choice for partial seizures. Ethosuximide is effective only against generalized absence seizures, whereas phenytoin, carbamazepine, phenobarbital, and primidone are not effective against these seizures. Valproic acid and clonazepam have a wide spectrum of efficacy. Phenobarbital, primidone and clonazepam often are sedating. In addition, tolerance often develops with clonazepam.

There are 9 new antiepileptic drugs, introduced since 1993. Felbamate (Felbatol) has a wide spectrum of efficacy in both partial and generalized seizures. Felbamate is used only in very difficult, refractory cases, because the drug has been associated with aplastic anemia in approximately 1/3000–5000 cases and liver failure in approximately 1/8000 cases. Gabapentin (Neurontin) is indicated as adjunctive therapy for partial-onset seizures. A newer gabapentin-like agent, pregabilin (Lyrica), has recently been introduced. Lamotrigine (Lamictal) has a wide spectrum of efficacy in both partial and generalized-onset seizures. It is approved as adjunctive therapy or monotherapy in partial onset seizures. It has to be introduced very slowly, because of the possible side effect of rash. Topiramate (Topamax) also has a wide spectrum of efficacy and is indicated as primary or adjunctive therapy in both partial and generalized onset seizures. Tiagabine (Gabitril) is effective in partial onset seizures, and is indicated only as adjunctive therapy. Oxcarbazepine (Trileptal) is similar in structure and efficacy to carbamazepine, but is metabolized differently, reducing side effects. It is indicated as monotherapy and adjunctive therapy in partial onset seizures. Levetiracetam (Keppra) and zonisamide (Zonegran) are wide spectrum antiepileptic drugs that are currently approved only for adjunctive therapy of partial onset seizures. Vigabatrin (Sabril) is not approved in the US, but is available worldwide. It is effective in partial-onset seizures, but is also very effective in infantile spasms, a generalized seizure type. It has an associated chronic retinal toxicity resulting in constriction of visual fields. Several older antiepileptic drugs can also be used in patients who do not respond to newer drugs. The effectiveness of some antiepileptic drugs in 3 groups of seizures is outlined in Table 25.5. Several of the antiepileptic drugs have pharmacokinetic and safety advantages over the traditional antiepileptic drugs.

A few other, general principles of antiepileptic treatments should be noted. Idiopathic epilepsies are expected to respond well to medical therapy, whereas cryptogenic and symptomatic epilepsies are more often refractory. Treatment of epilepsy usually implies that the patient has already had multiple seizures. No long-term AED therapy is generally indicated for single provoked seizures, such as seizures caused by a transient metabolic aberration or acute trauma. The risk of seizure recurrence after a single, unprovoked seizure is estimated at 40%. The risk increases with abnormal neurologic status and abnormal EEG. Other factors may also play a role. The decision to give long-term treatment with AEDs should be individualized and made after discussion with the patient, weighing risk of seizure recurrence and risk of treatment. Many experts would not initiate treatment for an isolated,

Table 25-5 **The Antiepileptic Drugs (AEDs) of Choice in Four Groups of Seizures**

		Partial	1ary GTC	G Myoclonic	G Absence
A	Phenytoin	Effective	Effective	Not effective	Not effective
	Carbamazepine	Effective	Effective	Not effective	Not effective
	Valproate	Effective	Effective	Effective	Effective
	Phenobarbital*	Effective	Effective	Not effective	Not effective
	Primidone*	Effective	Effective	Effective	Not effective
	Ethosuximide	Not effective	Not effective	Not effective	Effective
	Clonazepam*	Effective	Effective	Effective	Effective
B	Felbamate**	Effective	Effective	Effective	Effective
	Gabapentin	Effective	Effective	Not effective	Not effective
	Lamotrigine	Effective	Effective	?Effective	Effective
	Topiramate	Effective	Effective	?Effective	?Effective
	Tiagabine	Effective	?	Not effective	Not effective
	Oxcarbazepine	Effective	?Effective	Not effective	Not effective
	Levetiracetam	Effective	Effective	Effective	?Effective
	Zonisamide	Effective	Effective	Effective	?Effective
	Pregabalin	Effective	?	Not effective	Not effective

A. Standard AEDs. B-New AEDs.
*Not indicated as first-line agents because of sedation and other adverse effects.
†Felbamate is not indicated as a first line treatment for epileptic seizures because of risk of aplastic anemia and liver failure.
‡Indicated as adjunctive treatment. Its efficacy as monotherapy is still under investigation.

unproved seizure. On the other hand, a single, delayed post-stroke or post-traumatic brain injury seizure is so likely to recur that most experts would recommend antiepileptic therapy. Another issue is when to discontinue antiepileptic therapy in the seizure-free individual. Once seizures are controlled, therapy must be continued for at least two years. Withdrawal of antiepileptic drug therapy can then be considered, with appropriate restrictions on driving.

   The treatment of status epilepticus is a medical emergency and is discussed in Chapter 23. The treatment of refractory epilepsy brings up a series of additional considerations. Although some epileptic patients fail to respond to medical therapy, there are remediable causes of treatment failure. These include suboptimal or lower than maximum dose treatment, too infrequent dosing, use of drugs that actually aggravate seizures, stress or sleep deprivation, use of alcohol or interfering drugs or illicit substances, poor compliance with medications, incorrect seizure diagnosis, the presence of psychogenic seizures, or an incorrect drug for the patient's seizure type. A video EEG monitoring study may be necessary to ensure that the correct seizure type is being treated. Approximately 36% of patients with epilepsy cannot achieve seizure-freedom. A recent study suggested that 47% of previously untreated patients will become seizure-free with the first AED, but after failing the first AED the chances of seizure freedom drop to 13% with the second AED and 1% with the third. Refractory epilepsy thus can be identified early, and other options can then be considered, especially epilepsy surgery.

Non AED therapy

Patients refractory to medical therapy can be considered for treatment with the ketogenic diet. This very low carbohydrate, low protein and high fat diet treatment is most effective in children with refractory generalized epilepsy.

   The vagus nerve stimulator (VNS) is the first device approved for the treatment of epilepsy. The mechanism of action is not well understood, but its activity appears to be dependent on afferent input to the nucleus of the tractus solitarius. Thalamic activation, activation of the locus ceruleus, and inhibition of the amygdala and hippocampus have been identified to play a role in its activity. VNS is currently approved for the treatment of refractory partial epilepsy, although it does not seem specific for that form of epilepsy. VNS is palliative and is not indicated for patients who are good candidates for resective surgery, who have a good chance of becoming seizure-free.

Surgical therapy

In patients who are truly refractory to medical therapy, surgical treatment can be considered. Table 25.6 lists the surgical procedures performed to treat epilepsy. Focal resection requires precise localization of the epileptic focus. Surgery is most feasible if the region of the focus does not have vital functions, such as language or motor innervation. The best results are typically reported in temporal lobe epilepsy. More than half the patients become seizure-free, and most of the others are markedly improved. Some types of epilepsy are particularly responsive to surgical therapy. These include temporal lobe epilepsy with hippocampal sclerosis and partial epilepsy with focal epileptogenic lesions, such as cavernous angioma, ganglioglioma, or

Table 25-6 **Surgical Treatments for Refractory Epilepsy**

I. Resection of the epileptogenic zone
Temporal focus
Standard en-bloc resection
Tailored resection
Amygdalohippocampectomy
Extratemporal focus
Tailored resection
Hemispherectomy
II. Multiple subpial transections
III. Corpus callosotomy
IV. Stereotactic procedures

dysembryoplastic neuroepithelial tumors (DNET). Seizure freedom can be achieved in 60-80% of these patients.

Multiple subpial transection is a procedure that disconnects horizontal fibers in the cortex without interrupting the vertical functional units. It can be used when the epileptogenic focus involves eloquent cortex, such as the language areas.

Corpus callosotomy is most often performed in two steps starting with a two-thirds anterior corpus callosum section. Complete section may not be necessary. Corpus callosotomy is primarily a palliative procedure, used predominantly in symptomatic multifocal or generalized epilepsy, or if the focus cannot be clearly localized, and the seizures rapidly spread to become bilateral. The best results are in patients with drop attacks. Corpus callosotomy has decreased considerably because of the less invasive use of vagus nerve stimulation, often used in the same groups of patients.

Investigational therapies

Therapies under investigation include new antiepileptic drugs, deep brain stimulation via electrodes in the thalami, subthalamic nuclei, or hippocampi, local brain delivery systems, and intermittent therapy systems such as electrodes activated by early seizure detection techniques. In terms of new drugs, there is promise that drugs can be developed based on identification of specific genetic metabolic defects.

KEY REFERENCES

Britton JW. Antiepileptic drug withdrawal: literature review. *Mayo Clin Proc* 2002;77:1378–1388.

Brodie MJ, Dichter MA. Antiepileptic drugs. *N Engl J Med* 1996;334:168–175.

Browne TR, Holmes GL. Epilepsy. *N Engl J Med* 2001;344:1145–1151.

Chang BS, Lowenstein DH. Epilepsy. *N Engl J Med* 2003;349:1257–1266.

Devinsky O. Patients with refractory seizures. *N Engl J Med* 1999;340:1565–1570.

ILAE Task Force on Classification and Terminology. *Epilepsia* 2001;42:796–803.

Krumholz A, Fisher RS, Lesser RP, et al. Driving and epilepsy. A review and reappraisal. *JAMA* 1991;265:622–626.

LaRoche SM, Helmers SL. The new antiepileptic drugs. Scientific review. *JAMA* 2004;291:605–614.

Sirven JI. Antiepileptic drug therapy for adults: when to initiate and how to choose. *Mayo Clin Proc* 2002;77:1367–1375.

Wiebe S, Blume WT, Girvin JP, et al. A randomized and controlled trial of surgery for temporal-lobe epilepsy. *N Engl J Med* 2001;345:311–318.

Zimmerman RS, Sirven JI. An overview of surgery for chronic seizures. *Mayo Clin Proc* 2003:78:109–117.

ALZHEIMER'S DISEASE, FRONTOTEMPORAL DEMENTIA, AND RELATED DISORDERS

ALZHEIMER'S DISEASE

Introduction

Alzheimer's disease (AD) is the most common dementing illness. Dementia ranks among the most common neurological disorders of older people, and among the most detrimental to the overall health of the population. As many as 5% of people over age 65 have dementia severe enough to interfere with self-care. Surveys of persons over 85 years of age have found an 8% annual incidence and a prevalence of 30–50% of dementia. Over four million persons in the United States are thought to suffer from AD. Dementia accounts for approximately half of the million patients confined to nursing homes in the United States. The economic loss brought about by early retirement and medical and custodial care runs into the billions of dollars. As the population ages, the number of persons suffering from dementia continues to increase; it is estimated that as many as 14 million persons may have dementia by 2050. Dementia decreases life expectancy. Although infrequently cited on death certificates, dementia may represent the fourth or fifth leading cause of death in the United States. Dementia is a source of tragic losses for patients, families, and society as a whole.

Definitions of AD have been published by several professional groups, including the joint conference of the National Institute of Neurological and Communicative Diseases and Stroke-Alzheimer's Disease and Related Disorders Association (NINCDS-ADRDA) in 1984 and by the Diagnostic and Statistical Manual-IV, used by psychiatrists. A slightly modified definition is presented

Table 26-1 **NINCDS-ADRDA Criteria for Probable Alzheimer's Disease**

1. Dementia established by clinical examination and documented by the Mini Mental State or other screening test or neuropsychological testing
2. Deficits in memory and two or more areas of cognition
3. Progressive worsening of memory and other cognitive functions
4. No disturbance of consciousness
5. Onset after age 40, most often after 65
6. Absence of systemic disorders or other brain diseases that could account for the progressive deficits in memory and cognition

in Table 26-1. Note that AD almost always develops in people aged 40 and above, is progressive, and involves memory and at least two other higher cortical function, such as language, praxis, calculation ability, visuospatial functions, gnosis (recognition of objects or people), or executive function. Patients with AD are usually fully alert, unlike the elevated or depressed levels of consciousness seen commonly in delirium. The cognitive dysfunction must be disabling, or sufficient to interfere with activities of daily living, and especially employment status. The final criterion of the definition, absence of another proved cause, implies that a physician has evaluated the patient and performed screening laboratory tests for the diagnosis of dementia.

This evaluation, discussed in Chap. 14, includes blood tests for electrolytes, renal and hepatic function, thyroid function, B_{12} level, sedimentation rate, and a brain imaging study such as a computed tomography (CT) or magnetic resonance imaging (MRI) scan, to exclude other causes of dementia. Laboratory tests recommended for the diagnosis of AD are shown in Table 26-2.

Table 26-2 **Laboratory Tests Recommended by American Academy of Neurology (AAN) 2001 Practice Parameter for Evaluation of Dementia**

1. CBC, electrolytes, glucose, BUN/creat
2. Liver function tests, Thyroid function tests, erythrocyte sedimentation rate (ESR)
3. B_{12} level
4. Depression screening
5. CT or MRI scan

Abbreviations: CBC: Complete Blood Count
                       BUN: Blood Urea Nitrogen

The ultimate diagnosis of AD, of course, depends on neuropathology, usually obtained only at autopsy, but occasionally via brain biopsy in life. If the criteria of Table 26-1 are followed rigorously, the diagnosis of presumed or probable AD correlates at an 80–100% level with a pathologically confirmed diagnosis at autopsy.

Clinical presentation: symptoms and signs

Forgetfulness, or short-term memory loss, is usually the earliest symptom of AD. When asked questions, the patient often turns to a spouse or relative for answers. The patient asks frequently for reminders and tells the same stories over and over. Language and communication remain largely preserved at this early stage, except for memory for names. Mood may be normal or depressed, and the patient often has enough insight to attempt to conceal the deficit. The patient may perform other cognitive functions at a relatively normal level, except that most tasks are performed slowly. It may be difficult to distinguish the patient with early dementia secondary to AD from elderly persons with mild memory loss, out of proportion to age, a condition referred to as *mild cognitive impairment*. Many patients with mild cognitive impairment remain relatively stable over periods of several years, but 12–16% develop dementia each year, a percentage greatly in excess of that of age-matched controls.

As the disease progresses, the memory loss worsens, and other cognitive functions become deficient. Memory loss takes on more malignant forms, such as leaving stove burners on or becoming lost in familiar routes, and the patient may become disoriented to time and place. Syndromes of aphasia, agnosia, and visuospatial impairment may develop. In the case of language, naming is the first affected, but as the disease progresses, comprehension of complex material, reading and writing tasks, and the ability to express a coherent narrative or discourse become impaired. Simple utterances, ability to repeat and read aloud remain intact in most patients. Patients can sometimes mask their deficits with social graces and "cocktail party" conversation, but any discussion of factual information quickly reveals the dementia. The cognitive functions of the right hemisphere also suffer, as depicted in Henry Fonda's character in the film "On Golden Pond," who becomes lost near his lake home. Executive function, or the ability of the patient to plan organized activities and initiate steps leading to a goal, is especially sensitive to dementia. Insight and judgment become impaired as the cognitive deficits progress. Mood tends to be labile, fluctuating from momentary sadness to elation to anger. Some patients have early behavioral alterations, such as agitation, hallucinations, and delusional or paranoid thinking. These behavioral symptoms, along with related problems with activities of daily living such as personal hygiene and bowel and bladder continence, are the most troublesome aspects of dementing illness for caregivers and family, and it is these disorders more than the cognitive deterioration that result in patients being placed in nursing facilities. We speak of the "ABCs" of dementing illness: "A" refers to activities of daily living, "B" to behavior, and "C" to cognition.

Staging of AD is often attempted, using the Mini Mental State Examination (MMSE), where mild cognitive impairment comprises scores of 24–30, mild AD 20–23, moderate AD 10–19, and severe AD <10. There are problems with this formulation, in that the MMSE has a strong education bias, and it does not capture the variability of "focal" syndromes of language disorder, visual-spatial-topographical impairment, or loss of executive function that are highly important to patients' ability to function independently. Nonetheless, some treatment recommendations are based on this staging.

Laboratory testing in Alzheimer's disease

Routine blood and spinal fluid tests are not helpful in the diagnosis of AD, though they rule out other conditions, and even brain imaging studies such as CT and MRI images are of limited help in distinguishing AD from normal aging and mild cognitive impairment. Single photon emission computed tomography (SPECT) and positron emission tomography (PET) scans can detect localized hypometabolism or reduced cerebral blood flow, especially in the parietal lobes on both sides. As will be discussed, apolipoprotein E genotyping may increase the probability of AD in a symptomatic patient. Other new laboratory tests, such as the cerebrospinal fluid (CSF) tau assay and neuronal thread protein, have not been proved reliable (see Chap. 14). These tests are summarized in Table 26-3.

Neuroscientific basis of Alzheimer's disease

Since Alzheimer's seminal case report of presenile dementia in 1907, the neuropathology of the disease has been well established. In the 1960s, however, it was realized that the pathological changes do not differ between the

---

Table 26-3 **Laboratory Tests Not Recommended by AAN 2001 Practice Parameter**

1. Serological test for syphilis (unless evidence)
2. SPECT
3. Genetic testing (e.g., APOE)
4. EEG
5. Lumbar Puncture (unless unusual factors-infection, hydrocephalus, etc.)
6. Uncertain: PET (Medicare approved), other gene markers such as neuronal thread protein, CSF tau

Abbreviation: APOE: Apolipoprotein ε
                 EEG: Electroencephalogram

presenile and senile forms of the disease. The neuropathology of AD involves diffuse atrophy of the cerebral cortex and enlargement of the ventricles, with sparing of the primary motor and sensory areas. Microscopic silver stains reveal loss of neurons and silver-staining *neurofibrillary tangles* in remaining neurons. By electron microscopy the tangles are made up of paired helical filaments, double-stranded microtubular structures not present in normal neurons and composed of aggregations of the microtubular protein, tau. The intercellular space of the cerebral cortex, or neuropil, also contains silver-staining structures called *senile* or *neuritic plaques*. Senile plaques contain a central core of amyloid, surrounded by fragments of neural processes, neurites, or fragments of axons and dendrites,, and glial cells. The exact relationship of the plaques and tangles is not known, and either change by itself is relatively nonspecific, occurring in other diseases and in normal aging. The quantitive degree of plaques and tangles, however, appears to correlate with the degree of dementia. In particular, the deposition of amyloid proteins in the brain appears to be an important part of the pathogenesis of the disorder.

Another important aspect of the pathogenesis of AD involves genetics. The first clue to genetic AD came with the recognition that patients with Down's syndrome, a trisomy of chromosome 21 with mental retardation, is associated with cognitive decline in patients in their late thirties and older; virtually 100% of Down's syndrome patients who live past age 40 have pathological changes of AD in their brains. Three gene loci have now been conclusively linked to early onset, familial AD. All appear to follow autosomal dominant transmission; half of offspring of an affected parent are likely to develop the disease. Chromosome 21 was the first discovered, confirming the link between AD and Down's syndrome. The site on chromosome 21 is closely linked to the amyloid precursor protein gene, supporting the amyloid theory of AD. The other two familial, early onset AD genes, on chromosomes 1 and 14, code for proteins called *Presenilin 1* and *2*. These proteins are also closely involved with the amyloid precursor protein; Presenilin 1 is now known to be one of the secretase enzymes that breaks down the amyloid precursor protein into the A-beta peptide, a 40–42 amino acid peptide that appears to accumulate in the plaques, and also in arteries, and may be toxic to neurons. Many specific mutations of these three AD genes have been reported in families with autosomal dominant AD, but these still represent a very small percentage of the cases of AD. For late onset cases of AD, genetics play a lesser role, and most cases appear sporadic. Even here, however, there is an increased risk of AD with a positive family history. One part of the hereditary risk appears related to the apolipoprotein E gene, located on chromosome 19. Patients with at least one apolipoprotein E4 allele have a much greater chance of developing AD than those with E2 or E3 alleles, and the rare patients with two E4 alleles have a 90% chance of developing AD by age 70. Apolipoprotein E genotyping is available as a laboratory test, one that simply increases the likelihood that a person at risk or with symptoms will turn out to have AD. Most geneticists discourage *presymptomatic* testing of persons at genetic risk for AD, given the lack of specific predictive value and the lack of proved preventive therapy.

Much of the pathogenesis of AD appears to involve amyloid deposition. Transgenic mice with a mutant amyloid precursor protein gene develop neuropathological changes of AD, and a vaccine against amyloid prevents this deterioration. The amyloid deposition also occurs in blood vessels and may be the cause of the ischemic white matter lesions frequently seen on MRI in this disease.

Another area of AD research involves deficiencies in the neurotransmitter, acetylcholine. A consistent neuropathological finding is the presence of neuronal loss in the nucleus basalis of Meynert, a basal forebrain nucleus known to have extensive, cholinergic projections to wide areas of the cerebral cortex. Cholinergic markers are decreased in the brains of patients with AD, and cholinergic ligands used with PET scanning have documented decreased cholinergic binding in life. Repletion of acetylcholine has been a goal of treatment in AD.

Treatment

AD remains an incurable disease, but many attempts have been made to modify its course and symptomatology. The first priority is to find a biological treatment to stop the progression of the disease, or even to restore some lost function. Such curative or *neuroprotective* therapy does not yet exist. The vaccine against the amyloid beta peptide, developed through animal studies, was tested in AD patients in a Phase II trial. Unfortunately, about 10% of the patients came down with an encephalitis-like illness, and the trial was halted. At least one of the patients, who later died, had markedly less amyloid plaque formation in the brain than expected, a result reminiscent of the old joke, "The operation was a success, but the patient died." Hope remains that a more selective or passive vaccine can be developed, and early clinical trials are in progress. Work is also underway to find a pharmaceutical agent that would inhibit the secretase enzyme that breaks down the amyloid precursor protein into its toxic peptide product, or to limit the formation of amyloid by other means.

Other attempts to prevent neuronal loss in AD have been largely disappointing. In one study, vitamin E appeared to slow the progression of AD, but a recent study of mild cognitive impairment did not confirm any benefit with vitamin E. Gingko biloba may have a small symptomatic benefit in AD, but this has not been consistent across trials. Gingko biloba is available in health food stores, not regulated by the Food and Drug Administration (FDA), and it has potentially harmful drug interactions. Estrogen hormones have had a checkered career with regard to AD.

Earlier, retrospective studies suggested that estrogen therapy might be associated with a reduced risk of development of AD, but the more recent Women's Health Initiative showed an increased incidence of cognitive dysfunction, dementia, and also heart attack and stroke. Controlled trials of estrogen therapy in patients with diagnosed AD, moreover, have not shown benefit. Likewise, use of nonsteroidal antiinflammatory drugs (NSAIDs) correlates with a reduced incidence of AD, but no controlled trials have yet supported a protective effect in elderly persons or a treatment effect in patients with established AD. The COX-2 inhibitor Rofecoxib (Vioxx) was taken off the market after trials in patients with AD and colonic polyps, both of which showed an association between the drug and myocardial infarction (MI).

The currently available treatments for AD are symptomatic therapies. The first category would be nonpharmacological, or *cognitive behavioral* therapies. Instructions to caregivers to provide a consistent environment, frequent reminders of the date and place, and other orienting comments, along with gentle correction of errors, all represent behavioral management strategies in AD. Keeping patients at home, in familiar environments, is beneficial for the patients and also reduces costs. The book "The 36 Hour Day," cited in the references, is very helpful to families and caregivers of patients with AD.

Pharmacological therapies are also used to treat behavioral disorders. The cholinesterase inhibitors, to be discussed later, have some beneficial effect on abnormal behaviors. Mild sedatives such as trazodone, antidepressants of the selective serotonin reuptake inhibitor (SSRI) class, and antianxiety agents such as buspirone or antiepileptic drugs such as valproic acid are helpful in controlling agitated behavior and depressed or anxious mood. Use of the benzodiazepine class of minor tranquilizers is generally discouraged in AD, because these drugs interfere with memory and also make patients either somnolent, with increased risk of falling, or paradoxically agitated. Likewise, traditional antipsychotic agents such as haloperidol or phenothiazines are risky in AD patients, because elderly patients are at high risk for extrapyramidal side effects such as parkinsonism and tardive dyskinesia. The atypical antipsychotic agents have been used widely in AD, and most geriatricians, psychiatrists, and neurologists choose them at times, but the FDA has recently issued a warning against use of all atypical antipsychotic drugs in the treatment of patients with AD, because of associated risks of increased coronary and cerebrovascular events, weight gain, and diabetes mellitus. For this reason, AD specialists try to use the other treatments discussed, and save the atypical antipsychotic agents for very refractory patients.

The mainstay of pharmacological treatment for AD is cholinergic therapy. In contrast to the treatment of Parkinson's disease, where precursor therapy with levodopa has been highly successful, precursor therapy in AD

Table 26-4 **Drugs Approved for Therapy of Alzheimer's Disease**

Drug	Mechanism	Dosage	Side Effects
Donepizil (Aricept)	Cholinesterase inhibitor	5–10 mg	Nausea, vomiting, diarrhea, anorexia, occasionally light-headedness, syncope
Rivastigmine (Exelon)	Cholinesterase inhibitor	1.5–6 mg bid	Similar to donepezil
Galantamine (Razadyne, or Razadyne ER)	Cholinesterase inhibitor	4, 8, 12–mg bid Or 8, 16, 24–mg daily	Similar to donepezil
Memantine (Namenda)	N-methyl d-aspartate (NMDA) receptor blocker	10–mg bid	Confusion

with choline or lecithin has not proved effective. Direct-acting cholinergic drugs have likewise not panned out. Acetylcholinesterase inhibitors have proved to be of modest benefit in improving short-term memory in patients with AD. Four anticholinesterase agents are currently on the market; all are FDA approved for mild to moderate AD, and all have side effects involving gastrointestinal toxicity, usually nausea, diarrhea, or anorexia and weight loss. These agents are listed in Table 26-4. Tacrine (Cognex) was the first drug introduced, but its risk of hepatic toxicity, nausea, vomiting, and four-times-per-day schedule of administration made it impractical. Donepizil (Aricept) is a once-a-day acetylcholinesterase inhibitor which has less gastrointestinal toxicity and very rare hepatic toxicity; this drug does not require blood monitoring. Donepizil has proved effective in ameliorating or stabilizing the memory deterioration of AD and in delaying placement of patients in nursing facilities. The drug is given initially as a 5 mg bedtime dose, but the dose should be advanced to 10 mg QHS in most patients. Recently, donepizil has been shown to delay progression to AD in patients with mild cognitive impairment, but this use of the drug has not been approved by the FDA as yet. The gastrointestinal side effects of donepizil are, in most series, the least of any of the anticholinesterase agents. An orally disintegrating tablet is also available. The third approved anticholinesterase drug, rivastigmine or Exelon[R], inhibits both the acetylcholinesterase and butyrylcholinesterase enzymes, a biological change which suggests increased therapeutic effect, but this biochemical difference has not yet been shown to be of clinical importance. The drug tends to cause the most gastrointestinal side effects of the three commonly used agents (excluding tacrine). Rivastigmine requires twice-daily dosing and an escalation from an initial dose of 1.5 mg bid for at least four weeks, to 3 mg bid, to 4.5 mg bid, and finally to 6 mg bid. A recently published head-to-head clinical trial showed modestly increased cognitive effects for rivastigmine as compared to donepizil; the drop-out rate during drug introduction was twice as high with rivastigmine as with donepizil, but toxicity with both agents was similar after the introduction phase. The most recently approved anti-cholinesterase drug, galantamine, has recently been released in a once daily, extended release form; the trade name has changed from Reminyl to Razadyne and Razadyne ER. The once-daily formulation can be given in 8-, 16-, and 24-mg doses. This drug has a reported presynaptic modulating effect that results in more acetylcholine being released, as well as blocking the degradative enzyme, acetylcholinesterase. This effect has not been proved to be biologically important.

In summary, the anticholinesterase drugs provide a symptomatic benefit in patients with AD, but many patients stabilize rather than improve, and patients generally begin deteriorating again by 12–18 months. Nonetheless, these agents appear helpful in keeping patients at home and functioning, at least for a few months or years.

A final pharmacological therapy for AD is the drug memantine (Namenda), a blocker of the NMDA subtype of glutamate receptor. The theoretical basis for use of this drug is that release of excitatory neurotransmitters such as glutamate by dying neurons is thought to overstimulate remaining neurons, leading to cell death, a phenomenon referred to as *excitotoxicity*. Memantine (Namenda) has been shown to have a modest effect in improving cognition in moderate and advanced stages of AD. The drug can be used in monother-apy or added to an anticholinesterase agent. It is started at 5 mg once daily for 1 week, then advanced by 5 mg weekly to a full dose of 10 mg twice daily. The drug may be associated with increased confusion when first introduced, but generally this effect is short-lived, and other side effects are minimal. The drug is being tested for use in early AD patients, but it is not FDA approved except for moderate to advanced stage AD patients.

FRONTOTEMPORAL DEMENTIA, PICK'S DISEASE, AND RELATED CONDITIONS

Introduction

In 1892, in his description of the dementing disease which now bears his name, Arnold Pick emphasized the "focal" nature of the degeneration;

these patients present initially with aphasia or behavioral disorders, suggestive of a localized brain disorder of the frontal or temporal lobes, but
the course is progressive. Pick also described a characteristic, silver-staining,
intracellular inclusion body, now referred to as the *Pick body*. In the current
era, many patients present with atypical dementing illnesses beginning
clinically with temporal or frontal lobe dysfunction, and associated at
autopsy with focal atrophy of the frontal or temporal lobes. Not all of these
patients, however, have Pick bodies. The remaining features, lobar atrophy,
loss of neurons, gliosis, and vacuolation of the neuropil in the affected cortical areas, have been categorized in England under the name *frontotemporal
dementia* (FTD). These patients do not have the typical senile plaques associated with AD, or no more than expected with normal aging. In the United
States, FTD has been considered very uncommon compared to AD, but in
Europe, particularly the Lund-Manchester study, it represents about 10%
of dementia cases.

As in AD, the definitive diagnosis of Pick's disease is by brain biopsy or
autopsy, but a presumptive diagnosis can be made, based on the clinical features and the presence of focal atrophy of the frontal and/or temporal lobes
on one or both sides on brain imaging studies.

Clinical symptoms and signs

The symptoms of frontotemporal dementia are variable, depending on
which lobe of the brain degenerates first. One common presentation is with
aphasia, or progressive language deterioration. In the United States, considerable attention has been devoted to the syndrome of *primary progressive
aphasia*, a progressive loss of language functions, usually with nonfluent
speech. Such patients may remain nondemented, able to function normally
in nonverbal ways, pursuing work if the job permits, continuing hobbies and
artistic expression, remaining independent in self-care. Over time, many
such patients eventually become demented. Other patients with progressive
aphasia have had fluent syndromes, such as the *semantic dementia* described
by Hodges and colleagues. These patients lose the ability to name, or even
to understand words spoken to them. In the United Kingdom, the literature
has emphasized frontal lobe, neurobehavioral deficits, more than language
deficits. Criteria for the diagnosis of FTD are summarized in Table 26-5,
adapted from Neary and Snowden's 1998 review paper.

Laboratory testing

The lobar distribution of Pick's disease should be evident on CT and MRI
scans, if they are examined carefully for this pattern of atrophy. Temporal
lobe atrophy is best seen on coronal MRI scans, as shown in Fig. 26-1. Lobar
degeneration is even more obvious on PET scanning, which makes for a
clear distinction from AD. Figure 26-2 is a PET scan showing bilateral frontal

Table 26-5   *Diagnostic Criteria for Frontotemporal Dementia*

A. Core features
   Insidious onset, gradual progression
   Early decline in interpersonal conduct
   Early emotional blunting
   Early loss of insight
B. Behavioral features
   Decline in personal hygiene, grooming
   Mental rigidity, inflexibility
   Distractibility, impersistence
   Hyperorality, dietary changes
   Perseverative, stereotyped behavior
   Utilization behavior
C. Speech and language
   Aspontaneity, economy (or press) of speech
   Stereotypy of speech
   Echolalia
   Perseveration
   Mutism
D. Physical signs and laboratory tests
   Primitive reflexes
   Incontinence
   Akinesia, rigidity, tremor
   Low or labile blood pressure
   Frontal/temporal atrophy on MRI, PET

hypometabolism in a patient who had progressive aphasia, and then developed uninhibited behavior. Many cases of FTD are familial, and a number of families have had gene mutations demonstrated, largely on chromosome 17. These gene mutations affect the tau gene, leading to the name *taopathies* for this family of conditions. Other cases are negative for tau abnormalities and have ubiquitin staining. FTD is also associated in some patients with motor neuron disease. A separate gene locus, on chromosome 9, has been reported for families with a combination of FTD and motor neuron disease. Another variant of FTD is associated with inclusion body myopathy. The genetic tests for tauopathies and the other variants are not yet routinely available.

Treatment

There is no proved, effective treatment for FTD, or primary progressive aphasia. Although no large, randomized clinical trials have been carried out

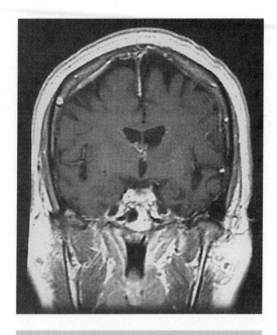

Figure 26-1 **Coronal MRI in Primary Progressive Aphasia.** *MRI of a 62-year-old lady with progressive anomia and nonfluent speech, with preserved ability to perform financial calculations and create spreadsheets.*

in these relatively uncommon conditions, anecdotal experience with use of acetylcholinesterase inhibitors and memantine has been disappointing. SSRI antidepressants may have some effect, at least on the depression that is so often associated with this condition. Dopaminergic agents such as bromocriptine have been tried in cases of nonfluent aphasia secondary to strokes, but anecdotal experience with these drugs in FTD has been disappointing. It is likely that effective treatment will have to await better understanding of the neurobiology and neurochemistry of these conditions.

Course and prognosis

The natural history of FTD is one of gradually progressive disability. Many cases worsen over long periods, sometimes in excess of 10 years; in the early stage, patients may continue to function in terms of memory and ability to perform self-care activities. Some patients develop associated motor neuron disease. At least half of patients diagnosed with FTD eventually develop a full-blown dementia.

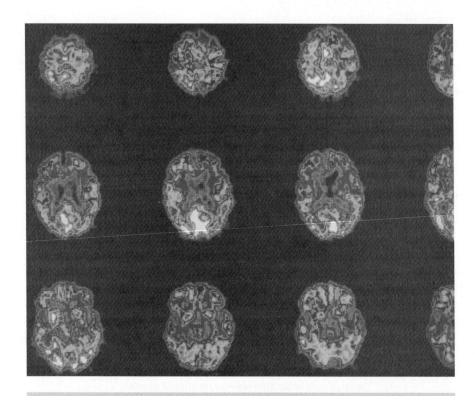

Figure 26-2   **PET scan from a 71-year-old lady who presented with aphasia, then developed behavioral disturbances, disinhibition, and temper outbursts. Note the difference from the PET scan of an Alzheimer's disease patient, Fig. 14-2.**

KEY REFERENCES

Alzheimer's disease and mild cognitive impairment

Bullock R, Touchon J, Bergman H, et al. Rivastigmine and donepizil treatment in moderate to moderately severe Alzheimer's disease over a 2-year period. *Curr Med Res Opin* 2005;21:1317–1327.

Citron M. Strategies for disease modification in Alzheimer's disease. *Nat Rev Neurosci* 2004;5:677–685.

Cummings JL. Alzheimer's disease. *N Engl J Med* 2004;351:56–67.

Kirshner HS. Mild cognitive impairment: to treat or not to treat. *Curr Neurol Neurosci Rep* 2005;5:455–457.

Petersen RC, Thomas RG, Grundman M, et al. Vitamin E and Donepizil for the treatment of mild cognitive impairment. *N Engl J Med* 2005;352:2379–2388.

Rosenberg RN. The molecular and genetic basis of AD: the end of the beginning. *Neurology* 2000;54:2045–2054.

Silverman DHS, Small GW, Chang CY. Positron emission tomography in evaluation of dementia. Regional brain metabolism and long-term outcome. *JAMA* 2001;286: 2120–2127.

Sink KM, Holden KF, Yaffe K. Pharmacological treatment of neuropsychiatric symptoms of dementia. A review of the evidence. *JAMA* 2005;293:596–608.

Wang PS, Schneeweiss S, Avorn J, et al. Risk of death in elderly users of conventional vs. atypical antipsychotic medications. N Engl J Med 2005;353:2335–41.

Wolfe MS. Shutting down Alzheimer's. Sci Am 2006;294:73–79.

Frontotemporal dementia and primary progressive aphasia

Grossman M, Mickanin J, ONishi K, et al. Progressive nonfluent aphasia: language, cognitive, and PET measures contrasted with probable Alzheimer's disease. *J Cog Neurosci* 1996;8:135–154.

Heutink P, Stevens M, Rizzu P, et al. Hereditary frontotemporal dementia is linked to chromosome 17q21–q22: a genetic and clinicopathological study of three Dutch families. *Ann Neurol* 1997;41:150–159.

Hodges JR, Davies RR, Xuereb JH, et al. Clinicopathological correlates in frontotemporal dementia. Ann Neurol 2004;56:399–406.

Hodges JR, Patterson K, Oxbury S, et al. Semantic dementia. Progressive fluent aphasia with temporal lobe atrophy. *Brain* 1992;115:1783–1806.

Hosler BA, Siddique T, Sapp PC, et al. Linkage of familial amyotrophic lateral sclerosis with frontotemporal dementia to chromosome 9q21–q22. *JAMA* 2000;284: 1664–1669.

Kertesz A. Frontotemporal dementia/Pick's disease. *Arch Neurol* 2004;61:969–1971.

Kirshner HS, Tanridag O, Thurman L, et al. Progressive aphasia without dementia: two cases with focal spongiform degeneration. *Ann Neurol* 1987;22:527–532.

Mesulam M-M. Primary progressive aphasia—a language-based dementia. *N Engl J Med* 2003;349:1535–1542.

Neary D, Snowden JS, Gustafson L, et al. Frontotemporal lobar degeneration. A consensus on clinical diagnostic criteria. *Neurology* 1998;51:1546–1554.

PARKINSON'S DISEASE

AND RELATED

DISORDERS

PARKINSON'S DISEASE

Introduction

James Parkinson's original description of the disease that bears his name, from the early nineteenth century, emphasized three cardinal symptoms: tremor, rigidity, and akinesia, or reduced spontaneous movement. These three features are still critically important to our understanding of the disease; many of the other symptoms of Parkinson's disease (PD) can be considered to derive from these cardinal symptoms, including reduced initiative to begin walking, "masked" facial expression, reduced eyeblinking, smaller handwriting, and a speech pattern of soft, rapid, monotonous quality.

PD is second only to Alzheimer's disease (AD) among neurodegenerative conditions. Like AD, it is predominantly a disease of older people, though there are young-onset cases, particularly among the genetic variants of the disease. PD affects about 1% of the population over age 60, roughly doubling in incidence with each additional 5 years of age. About 1 million Americans are affected.

Most cases of PD are *idiopathic*, meaning that the cause is unknown. A search for environmental toxins that might cause the disease has been unsuccessful. Several genes have been found to be associated with PD. The first discovered were mutations in the gene for alpha-synuclein, a component of the Lewy body, the cytoplasmic inclusion body found in the cells of the substantia nigra, and rarely in cortical neurons. Several other genes have been discovered in familial PD; see the review by Feany (2004).

Clinical presentation: symptoms and signs

The most common presenting symptom of PD is resting tremor, a slow, rhythmic shaking of the thumb or hand, disappearing when the patient uses the hand for a voluntary action. The tremor may reemerge when the hand is again at rest, e.g., during walking. This tremor is quite different from the more common "essential tremor" (see Chap. 28), in which the tremor occurs mainly with the arms outstretched or during an action. Occasionally, both types of tremor coexist. Tremor is not present in every case of PD, and is present only intermittently in many patients, but only 10% of cases never have tremor at all. The absence of tremor should make the examiner think of other causes of parkinsonism, which will be discussed later in this chapter.

Other presentations of PD include a "weak," clumsy upper limb, a stiff, painful upper limb, or a gait disorder. Patients are usually not truly weak, but they experience "weakness" related to stiffness of the limb and difficulty initiating movement (*bradykinesia*), with clumsiness of fine movement of the hands and fingers. The gait often becomes affected early, with small steps and difficulty turning, but only later does the full picture emerge of stooped posture, reduced arm swing, shuffling gait, and festination (the patient leans forward, takes faster and faster steps until he or she begins to fall). The examiner can test *postural reflexes* by pulling back on the patient's shoulders from behind; a normal person will quickly make a corrective, backward step and regain balance, whereas the PD patient will lean back and lose balance, falling backward or taking several corrective steps before regaining equilibrium. Other signs include *cogwheel rigidity*, a feeling as if a series of steps occurs as the elbow is flexed and extended, or the wrist is passively moved in a circular fashion. Having the patient move the other arm in a circle tends to bring out cogwheel rigidity. Other symptoms and signs of PD, as mentioned above, include a *masked facies* or reduced facial expression; reduced eyeblinking; a soft voice with rapid, monotonous speech; and small handwriting.

Differential diagnosis

The key difficulty in diagnosing PD is that the examiner has to think of it. Like the diagnosis of hypothyroidism, no single sign is pathognomonic for PD (though unilateral resting tremor comes close); the examiner must think of the diagnosis because of the constellation of symptoms and signs. No laboratory test will make the diagnosis pop into mind.

The differential diagnosis of PD most commonly includes *parkinsonism*, usually a drug- or toxin-induced phenomenon. The most common culprits are dopamine-blocking drugs used for nausea (prochlorperazine, Compazine), for gastroparesis (metoclopramide, Reglan) or for antipsychotic therapy (chlorpromazine, Thorazine; haloperidol, Haldol). Manganese or carbon monoxide poisoning can also cause parkinsonism. Finally, a series of disorders referred to as *parkinsonism-plus* syndromes, some of which will be discussed at the end of this chapter, includes parkinsonism plus other features. These include multisystem atrophy, progressive supranuclear palsy, and corti-cobasal degeneration.

Laboratory and radiological investigation

There is no single laboratory test that confirms the diagnosis of PD. The diagnosis is primarily clinical, based on the symptoms and signs discussed above. Computed tomography (CT) and magnetic resonance imaging (MRI) scans are not sensitive and are mainly useful to exclude other conditions. Investigationally, photon emission tomography (PET) or single photon emission computed tomography (SPECT) imaging with dopaminergic ligands may be useful for early diagnosis, but these tests are not routinely available. Finally, response to medication (therapeutic trial) can confirm the diagnosis of PD.

Treatment

Older medications such as anticholinergic agents (trihexyphenidyl or Artane) may help the tremor but usually do not affect the other manifestations of the disease. Amantadine may also have modest benefit in early stages. These drugs are usually used in mild, early cases, in which the patient has little disability, and the "big gun" therapies are being saved for later need.

The mainstay of treatment for PD, since 1969, has been levodopa, usually given as a combination with carbidopa (under the brand name, Sinemet, or generic levodopa/carbidopa). Carbidopa prevents the decarboxylation of levodopa to dopamine in the periphery, reducing the nausea associated with levodopa, but it does not cross the blood-brain barrier, so the result is more dopamine in the central nervous system (CNS). The most common dose ratio is 25/100, or 25 mg of carbidopa and 100 mg of levodopa. Response to this drug is virtually diagnostic of PD; only about 10% of PD patients fail to respond at all. Treatment failure may indicate that the patient has a different disorder from idiopathic PD. Early side effects are nausea and vomiting, occasionally insomnia or confusion. Dose ratios of 10/100 and 25/250 are also available, as are *controlled release* (CR) preparations of 25/100 and 50/200. The immediate release preparation has a short half-life; early in the course of the disease, patients may respond to twice daily medication, but later there are fluctuations, with early "wearing-off," "on-off," or freezing episodes, and also positive motor signs such as involuntary, restless movements called dyskinesias. When the fluctuations become problematic, use of more frequent dosing or use of the CR preparations may be helpful. These fluctuations may suggest that levodopa is "toxic" to neurons in the basal ganglia, though this concept has not been proved. This possible neurotoxicity, however, is why many experts delay use of levodopa until the disease is beginning to be disabling.

Another approach to the treatment of PD is a family of direct dopaminergic drugs. Four dopaminergic agents, bromocriptine (Parlodel), pergolide (Permax), pramipexole (Mirapex), and ropinirole (Requip) are available. The first two, bromocriptine and pergolide, are ergot drugs, carrying some risk of retroperitoneal fibrosis, and in the case of pergolide, valvular heart disease. The two newer agents, pramipexole and ropinirole, are used predominantly. These drugs do not appear to cause as much motor fluctuations as levodopa, and some studies have even suggested a *neuroprotective* effect in preventing later degeneration. Dopaminergic drugs are not usually as effective as levodopa/carbidopa, however, and even if the physician decides to begin therapy with a dopaminergic agent, addition of levodopa/carbidopa is invariably needed as the disease progresses. In addition, the dopaminergic agents seem to cause more confusion, insomnia, and hallucinations than levodopa/carbidopa, and this side effect is often a major limiting factor in patients with PD who have accompanying dementia.

A few other drugs are used in PD. Two drugs (tolcapone, Tasmar and entacapone, Comtan) inhibit the enzyme catecholamine-O-methyl transferase (COMT), further preventing the metabolism of levodopa and making more dopamine available to the CNS. Tolcapone has largely been abandoned because of liver toxicity, but entacapone can be used in doses of 200 mg with each levodopa/carbidopa dose. A combination of levodopa, carbidopa, and entacapone, Stalevo) is also available in three doses (12.5/50/200, 25/100/200, and 37.5/150/200). A recently introduced agent, apomorphine (Apokyn) can be injected subcutaneously at doses of 0.2–0.6 mg, for immediate effect in patients with "off" or "freezing" episodes. One other enzyme inhibitor, a monoamine oxidase B or MAO-B inhibitor (selegiline, Eldepryl), was originally used in Europe as a minor adjunctive agent in late-stage PD, but it was then investigated as a first-line agent with possible *neuroprotective* effect. Some controversy persists regarding this therapy; most authorities do not accept the evidence for *neuroprotective* effect, and the drug is now used as a less potent, adjunctive agent in advanced PD. Recent research also suggests that Coenzyme Q10 may have a beneficial effect in PD, but this requires confirmation in large clinical trials. Table 27-1 lists the drugs commonly used in PD.

In addition to pharmacological therapy, surgical options have increasingly been attempted in PD. Older approaches involved ablation of structures, including thalamotomy and pallidotomy. These procedures have considerable risk, and currently deep brain stimulation (DBS) with depth electrodes is gaining popularity. These procedures have the advantage that the strength of stimulation can be adjusted, and the stimulator can be turned off if side effects develop. The placement of depth electrodes was first attempted in the thalamus, where there is a definite effect on tremor, but DBS has moved more to the globus pallidus or subthalamic nucleus. Interestingly, DBS in the subthalamic region seems to mimic the effect of levodopa, with reduced tremor, rigidity, and improvement in *bradykinesia*. These therapies do have some risk of brain hemorrhage or infection, so they are generally reserved for patients who are refractory to medical therapy. Finally, transplantation of fetal cells into the basal ganglia has been attempted in PD, but this therapy

Table 27-1 **Drug Therapy of Parkinson's Disease**

Drug	Doses	Usual dosage	Side effects
Trihexiphenidyl (Artane)	1, 2 mg	2 mg tid	Blurred vision, confusion, dry mouth, urinary retention, constipation
Benztropine (Cogentin)	0.5, 1 mg	1 mg bid	Same as for trihexiphenidyl
Amantadine (Symmetrel)	100 mg	100 mg bid	Insomnia, hallucinations, edema, livedo reticularis
Levodopa/ Carbidopa (Sinemet or Sinemet CR)	10/100 25/100 25/250 CR 25/100 CR 50/200	25/100 tid-ii tid Or CR 50/200 tid	Nausea, vomiting, insomnia, confusion/ hallucinations, dyskinesias, hypotension or dizziness
Selegiline (Eldepryl)	5 mg	5 mg bid	Insomnia, nausea, hallucinations, drug interactions
Entacapone (Comtan), or Stalevo (carbidopa, levodopa, entacapone)	200 mg Or 12.5/50/200, 25/100/200, 37.5/150/200	200 mg tid Or Stalevo tid	Used with levodopa/ carbidopa (or in combinations listed), same side effects
Pergolide (Permax)	0.05, 0.25, 1 mg	1 mg tid	Nausea, vomiting, confusion, hallucinations, hypotension, retroperitoneal fibrosis
Pramipexole (Mirapex)	0.125, 0.25, 0.5, 1, 1.5 mg	0.5–1.5 mg tid	Nausea, vomiting, confusion, hallucinations, hypotension
Ropinirole (Requip)	0.25, 0.5, 1, 2, 3, 4, 5 mg	3–8 mg tid	Same as for pramipexole

is considered experimental. In one study, overactivity of the dopaminergic system, with dyskinesias, complicated fetal cell transplantation.

Course and prognosis

As in all neurodegenerative diseases, the course of PD is gradually progressive. There is considerable variability in the rate of progression. Tremor-predominant PD, especially if unilateral, seems to have the most benign prognosis, often progressing slowly over many years before becoming disabling. Older patients with PD often have bilateral rigidity and gait difficulty on presentation, and these patients become disabled over much shorter periods. About half of patients with PD develop mental deterioration, usually taking the form of a fluctuating delirium early on, but later developing into a full-blown dementia. The associated mental changes are very challenging in terms of the treatment of PD, since dopaminergic agents and even levodopa tend to worsen the confusion. Dopamine blocking neuroleptics are generally contraindicated, since they make PD symptoms worse, but occasional use of an atypical neuroleptic agent such as clozapine (Clozaril), risperidone (Risperdal), olanzepine (Zyprexa), or quetiapine (Seroquel) can be helpful. Clozapine is associated with neutropenia and pancytopenia, so weekly complete blood counts are needed. All atypical antipsychotic agents have received a warning from the Food and Drug Administration (FDA) concerning their association with myocardial infarction and stroke. The acetylcholinesterase inhibitor rivastigmine (Exelon) has been approved for treatment of memory loss in patients with PD and dementia.

OTHER EXTRAPYRAMIDAL DISORDERS

Parkinson's disease with dementia

As mentioned earlier in this chapter, about half of patients with PD develop dementia. In some cases, however, cognitive deterioration may predate the development of motor signs such as bradykinesia, tremor, and rigidity. As compared to AD, the course is more fluctuating, with a delirium, characterized by delusional thinking and hallucinations, in addition to the deterioration of memory and other higher cognitive functions. Early hallucinations in a patient suspected of having AD points to the presence of diffuse Lewy body disease, now referred to as *Lewy body dementia*.

The treatment of both Lewy body dementia and PD with dementia involves the same agents for the movement disorder used in PD, but dopamine agonists are usually avoided because of their propensity to aggravate the encephalopathy. A typical antipsychotic agent may be used for the hallucinations and delusions. Anticholinesterase agents used in AD (donepizil, Aricept; rivastigmine, Exelon; and galantamine, Razadyne) also appear to improve memory function in patients with PD with dementia and Lewy body dementia; as mentioned above, rivastigmine is FDA approved for this indication.

Progressive supranuclear palsy

Progressive supranuclear palsy (PSP) is a relatively rare disease, made famous by the actor, Dudley Moore. Patients have Parkinson-like symptoms of rigidity and bradykinesia, but they rarely have tremor, and the posture is often more in extension at the neck than in flexion, as in PD. The most characteristic symptom is loss of conjugate eye movements, usually beginning with reduced downward gaze, then upgaze, and only late in the course affecting horizontal eye movements. The inability to look down, combined with the extended posture of the neck, leads to frequent falls and difficulty walking down steps, early symptoms of the disease. The eye movement abnormality is not always evident early in the disease, leading to confusion with PD. Dysarthria and dysphagia are often severe in this condition, as compared to PD. The patient may have a wide-open-eyed expression, sometimes referred to as a "look of perpetual astonishment." Later in the course, midbrain atrophy may be visualized on MRI scanning.

The treatment of PSP is problematic. Some patients may benefit from levodopa/carbidopa or dopamine agonists in terms of the Parkinson-like symptoms, but many patients do not respond. The remainder of the management is supportive, including speech and physical therapy, adaptive equipment such as walkers, antidepressants, and botulinum toxin (Botox) for dystonia.

Multiple system atrophy

This disorder is defined clinically by combinations of three areas of symptomatology: parkinsonism, usually without tremor; dysautonomia, especially orthostatic hypotension, with abnormalities of sweating, erectile dysfunction, and neurogenic bladder; and ataxia. Presenting symptoms may involve any one of the three components, or combinations of two or all three. Dysarthria and dysphagia are also frequent problems. This disorder comprises at least three diagnoses made in the past on the basis of partial presentations: striatonigral degeneration for the parkinsonism, olivopontocerebellar atrophy (OPCA) for the ataxia, and Shy-Drager syndrome for the dysautonomia. The diagnosis is made primarily on clinical grounds, but the MRI scan may show hypointensity of the putamen on T2-weighted images, sometimes surrounded by a hyperintense rim. Associated cortical and cerebellar atrophy develop over time.

The treatment of multiple system atrophy (MSA) involves levodopa/carbidopa for the parkinsonism, autonomic treatments such as fludrocortisone (Flurinef) or midodrine (ProAmatine) for the orthostatic hypotension, and physical therapy for the ataxia.

Corticobasal degeneration

Corticobasal degeneration is another neurodegenerative disease that can resemble PD. Patients often have rigidity, bradykinesia, and gait instability, but usually no tremor. In addition, many patients have disproportionate difficulty with one upper limb, resembling ideomotor apraxia. Many patients also have dysarthria, apraxia of speech, or aphasia, sometimes progressing to muteness and difficulty swallowing. The diagnosis is primarily clinical. MRI scans may be normal in early stages or show asymmetric frontoparietal atrophy. PET scanning may show focal, central hypometabolism (pre- and post central gyri). The neuropathology involves ballooned cortical neurons with achromasia, or loss of the nuclear chromatin, especially in the motor cortex.

The treatment of corticobasal degeneration, like all of the *Parkinson-plus* syndromes, is limited. Levodopa and dopamine agonists usually help the Parkinsonism only modestly. Again, physical therapy, adaptive equipment, antidepressant therapy, and Botulinum toxin for dystonia amount to most of the supportive care that can be offered.

Huntington's disease

Huntington's disease (HD) is an autosomal dominantly inherited movement disorder, known to the medical community since George Huntington's land-mark description in 1872, and a subject of popular interest since the folk musician Woody Guthrie developed the illness. It usually has onset in midlife, though adolescent onset cases occasionally occur (*Juvenile HD*). The sexes are equally affected. The disease often begins with either a movement disorder, involving involuntary choreiform movements, or a behavioral dis-order, with features of depression, changes in personality, impaired concen-tration and memory, loss of initiative and frontal "executive function" deficits, and finally dementia. The movement disorder often begins with "piano-playing" choreiform movements of the fingers, facial twitching, or adventitious movements during gait. Juvenile onset cases sometimes pre-sent with Parkinsonian rigidity rather than chorea. The eye movement examination in HD patients may show loss of saccadic movements in fol-lowing a target, a deficit portrayed in the novel "Saturday" by Ian McEwan.

The genetics of the disease have recently been fully elucidated. HD is one of the *trinucleotide repeat* disorders, in this case extra CAG repeats in a gene locus on chromosome 4. The severity of the disease, as well as younger age at onset, correlates with the number of such repeats. A genetic test for CAG repeats in the *huntingtin* gene can be obtained as a blood test to confirm the diagnosis in an affected individual; testing of presymptomatic offspring of HD patients should not be done except in the context of a Genetics program with extensive counseling. The exact link between the abnormal gene and the neuropathological effects is still a matter of research, but presumably the overproduction of the huntingtin protein has toxic effects leading to cell death. The pathology, as in so many neurodegenerative disorders, involves premature cell death of neurons, in this case in small neurons of the striatum and globus pallidus. Levels of the inhibitory neurotransmitter GABA are especially low, but other transmitters may also be affected. Magnetic reso-nance (MR) imaging in HD is useful in detecting the early atrophy of the caudate nuclei, with dilatation of the frontal horns of the lateral ventricles.

Treatment of HD is limited. Dopamine blocking agents such as haloperi-dol (Haldol) may reduce the involuntary movements, and antidepressants may aid in treating the emotional disturbance. Surgical approaches to HD are being investigated.

Wilson's disease

S.A.K. Wilson first described this genetic disorder in 1912. This disease resembles some of the other neurodegenerative diseases discussed in this chapter, in that it begins in young people (usually under age 40) with combinations of tremor, dystonia and movement disorders, parkinsonism, dysphagia and dysarthria, and psychiatric and cognitive symptoms. Keys to the diagnosis are abnormal liver function tests or cirrhosis, and episodes of hemolysis. In general, the liver abnormalities precede the neurological symptoms, but the liver dysfunction can be asymptomatic or consistent with a prior episode of *hepatitis*. The disorder is now known to result from an abnormality of copper metabolism, with copper deposition in the liver, brain, eyes, and other organs. The diagnosis is made by the neurological abnormalities, combined with abnormal liver function tests, elevated 24-hour urinary excretion of copper, and low serum ceruloplasmin. Slit lamp examination of the eyes may disclose Kayser-Fleischer rings along the cornea. Liver biopsy may occasionally be necessary for diagnosis. MRI scans may disclose cavitary lesions in the putamen and globus pallidus (dark on CT imaging, dark on T1-weighted MRI, and bright on T2-weighted MRI).

Wilson's disease is essential to diagnose early, in that the disease is much more treatable than most of the neurodegenerative diseases. Copper binding agents such ad D-penicillamine, given in doses of 1–2 g/day in four divided doses, or Trientine prevent further copper accumulation in the brain and liver. Treatment must be initiated as soon as possible, before irreversible changes have occurred. Liver transplantation is occasionally necessary for patients with severe cirrhosis.

KEY REFERENCES

Parkinson's disease

Christine CW, Aminoff MJ. Clinical differentiation of Parkinsonian syndromes: prognostic and therapeutic relevance. *Am J Med* 2004;117:412–419.

Eskandar EN, Cosgrove GR, Shinobu SA. Surgical treatment of Parkinson's disease. *JAMA* 2001;286:3056–3059.

Feany MB. New genetic insights into Parkinson's disease. *N Engl J Med* 2004;351:1937–1940.

Freed CR, Greene PE, Breeze RE, et al. Transplantation of embryonic dopamine neurons for severe Parkinson's disease. *N Engl J Med* 2001;344:710–719.

Lang AE, Lozano AM. Parkinson's disease. First of two parts. *N Engl J Med* 1998;339:1044–1053.

Lang AE, Lozano AM. Parkinson's disease. Second of two parts. *N Engl J Med* 1998;339:1130–1143.

Miyasaki JM, Martin W, Suchowersky O, et al. Practice parameter: initiation of treatment for Parkinson's disease: an evidence-based review: report of the Quality

Standards Subcommittee of the American Academy of Neurology. *Neurology* 2002;58:11–17.

Nutt JG, Wooten GF. Diagnosis and initial management of Parkinson's disease. *N Engl J Med* 2005;353:1021–1027.

Schapira AH, Olanow CW. Neuroprotection in Parkinson disease. Mysteries, myths, and misconceptions. *JAMA* 2004;291:358–364.

Suchowersky O, Reich S, Perlmutter J, et al. Practice Parameter: diagnosis and prognosis of new onset Parkinson disease (an evidence-based review): report of the Quality Standards Subcommittee of the American Academy of Neurology. *Neurology.* 2006;66:968–75.

Suchowersky O, Gronseth G, Perlmutter J, et al. Practice Parameter: neuroprotective strategies and alternative therapies for Parkinson disease (an evidence-based review): report of the Quality Standards Subcommittee of the American Academy of Neurology. *Neurology.* 2006;66:976–82.

The Deep-Brain Stimulation for Parkinson's Disease Study Group. Deep-brain stimulation of the subthalamic nucleus or the pars interna of the globus pallidus in Parkinson's disease. *N Engl J Med* 2001;345:956–963.

Lewy body dementia

Aarsland D, Perry R, Brown A, et al. Neuropathology of dementia in Parkinson's disease: a prospective, community-based study. *Ann Neurol* 2005;58:773–776.

Bonanni L, Thomas A, Onofrj M. Diagnosis and management of dementia with Lewy bodies: third report of the DLB consortium. *Neurology* 2005;65:1863–72.

Cummings JL. Lewy body diseases with dementia: pathophysiology and treatment. *Brain Cogn* 1995;28:266–280.

Emre M, Aarsland D, Albanese A, et al. Rivastigmine for dementia associated with Parkinson's disease. *N Engl J Med* 2004;351:2509–18.

Poewe W. Treatment of dementia with Lewy bodies and Parkinson's disease dementia. *Mov Disord* 2005;12(Suppl. 12):S77–S82.

Progressive supranuclear palsy

Daniel SE, deBruin VM, Lees AJ. The clinical and pathological spectrum of Steele-Richardson-Olszewski syndrome (progressive supranuclear palsy): a reappraisal. *Brain* 1995;118:759–770.

Litvan I, Campbell G, Mangone CA, et al. Which clinical features differentiate progressive supranuclear palsy (Steele-Richardson-Olszewski syndrome) from related disorders? A clinicopathological study. *Brain* 1997;120:65–74.

Multisystem atrophy

Jaros E, Burn DJ. The pathogenesis of multiple system atrophy: past, present, and future. *Mov Disord* 2000;15:784–788.

Wenning GK, Colosimo C, Geser F, et al. Multiple system atrophy. *Lancet Neurol* 2004;3:93–103.

Wenning GK, Tison F, Shlomo B, et al. Multiple system atrophy: a review of 203 pathologically proven cases. *Mov Disord* 1997;12:133–147.

Mark MH. Lumping and splitting the Parkinson Plus syndromes: dementia with Lewy bodies, multiple system atrophy, progressive supranuclear palsy, and cortical-basal ganglionic degeneration. *Neurol Clin* 2001;19·607–627.

Corticobasal degeneration

Bergeron C, Pollanen MS, Weyer L, et al. Unusual clinical presentations of cortical-basal ganglionic degeneration. *Ann Neurol* 1996;40:893–900.

Gibb WRG, Luthert PJ, Marsden CD. Corticobasal degeneration. *Brain* 1989;112: 1171–1192.

Litvan I, Cummings JL, Mega M. Neuropsychiatric features of corticobasal degeneration. *J Neurol Neurosurg Psychiatry* 1998;65:717–721.

Huntington's disease

Furtado S, Sucherowsky O. Huntington's disease: recent advances in diagnosis and management. *Can J Neurol Sci* 1995;22:5–12.

Martin JB. Huntington's disease: new approaches to an old problem. *Neurology* 1984;34:1059–1072.

Walling HW, Baldassae JJ, Westfall TC. Molecular aspecits of Huntington's disease. *J Neurosci Res* 1998;54:301–308.

Wilson's disease

Brewer GJ, Yuzbasiyan-Gurkan V. Wilson's disease. *Medicine* 1992;71:139–164.

El-Youssef M. Wilson disease. *Mayo Clin Proc* 2003;78:1126–1136.

ESSENTIAL TREMOR

INTRODUCTION

Tremor is an oscillatory movement of a body part, usually with a regular periodicity. As discussed in Chap. 5, tremor is further described according to the position or activity in which it occurs, and the amplitude and frequency of the movements. Of the three categories of tremor introduced in Chap.5, resting, postural, and action or intention tremor, essential tremor is almost entirely a postural tremor, though when severe it may have a small resting component, and it typically continues into intentional movements.

SYMPTOMS AND SIGNS

Essential tremor typically begins in the hands and fingers, with the arms outstretched, with tremor persisting into skilled actions. The tremor is of small amplitude and rapid frequency. In some patients, the voice and the head and neck are also tremulous. As discussed in Chap. 5, many factors can aggravate a normal, physiological tremor; essential tremor represents the presence of tremor in the absence of these aggravating factors. Essential tremor is usually inherited as an autosomal dominant trait.

DIFFERENTIAL DIAGNOSIS

The differential diagnosis of essential tremor includes the other two categories, resting tremor and intention tremor, as well as other causes of primarily postural tremor. Resting tremor is most commonly seen in Parkinsonís disease (PD). The diagnostic difficulty relates to the occasional presence of both resting and action tremor in the same patient. If the patient also has cogwheel rigidity, a stooped posture, and a small-stepped gait, the examiner should have no difficulty identifying the diagnosis as PD. If the patient has predominantly tremor, as often occurs in early PD and in essential tremor, the diagnosis can be more difficult. Time will usually tell, but therapeutic trials of dopaminergic agents for PD (see Chap. 26) or drugs used in essential tremor may provide diagnostic information.

With regard to other causes of a postural or action tremor, hyperthyroidism and alcohol withdrawal come up as frequent causes of tremor of this type. Adrenergic states such as extreme anxiety or fear should be evident, but occasionally a pheochromocytoma can secrete epinephrine and norepinephrine spontaneously. Pharmacological agents can aggravate tremor, especially adrenergic agents such as beta-agonists used for asthma. The medication list of a patient with presumed essential tremor should therefore be reviewed, including any herbal or "natural food" substances, especially "energy" or "power" formulations which may contain sympathomimetic agents. The presence of a family history is always important in supporting the diagnosis of essential tremor. Finally, postural tremor can accompany other neurological disorders. As mentioned in Chap. 5, patients with torticollis and other dystonias may have associated *dystonic tremor* , which can resemble essential tremor, except that the distribution is usually most severe in the muscles affected by the dystonia (such as head and neck tremor in torticollis, or "writing tremor" in writer's cramp). Orthostatic tremor, discussed in Chap. 5, may represent a form of essential tremor. Tremors can also develop in distal muscle groups of limbs affected by peripheral neuropathy. In this case, essential tremor would not be diagnosed unless a more widespread tremor emerged. Postural tremor can occur in the context of other neurological diseases, including PD (see above) and spinocerebellar degenerations (Roussy-Levy syndrome), Wilsonís disease, and others. These conditions are diagnosed based on the pattern of neurological abnormalities in all of the neurological systems. Essential tremor should involve the presence of a postural tremor, in the absence of other neurological signs, unless the patient coincidentally suffers from another neurological disease.

The third type of tremor, intention tremor, is not usually confused with essential tremor, because the ataxia of the limbs and/or trunk is obvious, in addition to the tremor on skilled actions. Ataxia implies a condition of the cerebellum or its connections, and not a pure essential tremor.

LABORATORY TESTING

Like all movement disorders, essential tremor is diagnosed mainly by the clinical findings, in this case a postural tremor, the absence of another cause, and a positive family history. A careful history and physical examination is necessary to establish these findings. Brain imaging is rarely indicated, unless other neurological signs complicate the diagnosis. Laboratory testing to exclude hyperthyroidism, and in some cases drug screens, or urinary catecholamine testing for pheochromocytoma, are appropriate. Electrodiagnostic testing (electromyogram/nerve conduction velocity (EMG/NCV) can be used to detect peripheral neuropathy, if suspected. Needle studies of muscle groups during tremor can help distinguish a postural tremor from a resting tremor, but such testing is used primarily as a research tool.

TREATMENT

Once other causes of tremor have been eliminated, the treatment of essential tremor is fairly straightforward. Exaggerated physiologic tremors are generally treated by removal of the offending drug or condition, if possible. Alcohol often diminishes essential tremor, a phenomenon which has made alcoholics of some tremor sufferers. Beta-blockers such as propranolol are also quite effective in doses of 20–160 mg daily, though with undesirable side effects of lethargy, bradycardia, and hypotension. These agents are usually effective, and in my own experience it is best to use short-acting agents such as propranolol, and permit the patient to time the doses just before activities in which the reduction of tremor is essential. Public speakers or actors, for example, may take propranolol approximately 30 minutes before a scheduled performance. The barbiturate drug primidone also has some benefit in essential tremor, with the principal side effect of drowsiness. The drug can be given as a small dose, such as 50 mg, repeatedly during the day, or a larger dose, such as 250 mg, at bedtime. Recently, clinical trials with the antiepileptic drugs gabapentin (Neurontin) and topiramate (Topamax) have shown benefit in essential tremor, though these agents have not been specifically approved by the Food and Drug Administration (FDA) for essential tremor. For the most severe and disabling tremors, surgical thalamotomy has been used, usually greatly diminishing tremor on the contralateral side of the body. Bilateral thalamotomy carries risks such as muteness or very soft voice and changes in appetite. Deep brain stimulation electrodes in the thalamus have also been successful in reducing essential tremor. These treatments, again, should be reserved for severe, disabling tremors.

COURSE AND PROGNOSIS

The course of essential tremor is generally slowly progressive over time. Many patients live decades with essential tremor. The presence of essential tremor by itself does not presage the development of other neurological disabilities.

KEY REFERENCES

Louis ED. Essential tremor. *N Engl J Med* 2001;345:887–891.

Louis ED. Essential tremor. *Lancet Neurol* 2005;4:100–110.

Lyons KE, Pahwa R. Deep brain stimulation and essential tremor. *J Clin Neurophysiol* 2004;21:2–5.

Sullivan KL, Hauser RA, Zesiewicz TA. Essential tremor. Epidemiology, diagnosis, and treatment. *Neurologist* 2004;10:250–258.

MULTIPLE SCLEROSIS AND OTHER DEMYELINATING DISEASES

INTRODUCTION

Multiple sclerosis (MS) is known as the "crippler of young adults," a neurological disease with a typical age of onset between 20 and 40, and with a female to male predominance of about 1.5–2:1. The epidemiology of MS also involves a geographic distribution, in which the disease is more common in colder climates and rare in tropical countries. There are likely genetic factors as well, and this may account for the very highest incidence and prevalence in Scandinavia and the Scottish islands, the Shetlands and Orkneys.

Clinically, the disease usually begins with acute exacerbations, or attacks, followed by periods of remission, when the symptoms improve. This "relapsing-remitting" pattern of disease is the hallmark of MS.

MS is defined pathologically by the presence of demyelinating *plaques* in the white matter of the central nervous system (CNS), including the brain, optic nerves, and spinal cord. These plaques contain inflammatory cells, including plasma cells, and gliosis (*sclerosis*). Larger plaques involve not only demyelination, or breakdown of the myelin sheath, but also loss of axons. Current research in MS indicates that axonal loss occurs early in the disease and likely accounts for the development of permanent neurological deficits.

CLINICAL PRESENTATION: SYMPTOMS AND SIGNS

MS usually has its onset in young adults, though occasional cases begin in childhood or at more advanced ages. The most common presentation is an acute exacerbation or "attack," which can take many forms. One of the most common is *optic neuritis*, an inflammation of the optic nerve of one eye, with acute loss of visual acuity, often a central scotoma in the visual field, and pain on moving the eye. On examination, visual acuity is reduced, there may be a central visual field defect or scotoma, the afferent pupillary light reflex may be less than the consensual one (*afferent pupillary defect*), and the optic fundus may show either swelling of the optic nerve head (*papillitis*) or a normal nerve head acutely, followed by the development of optic atrophy, or pallor and whiteness of the optic disc (*retrobulbar neuritis*). Optic neuritis is not always a harbinger of MS; follow-up studies have differed widely on the recurrence rate and later development of MS in patients with optic neuritis, varying from as little as 17% to as high as almost 90%.

Another common initial symptom of MS is *acute transverse myelitis*, an inflammation of the spinal cord. Here, the symptoms most typically involve weakness and numbness below a specific spinal level, often with bowel and bladder involvement as well. Transverse myelitis, like optic neuritis, can represent an attack of MS, or an isolated symptom of unknown cause, perhaps related to a viral infection.

Other symptoms of MS can be extremely variable. Weakness or numbness on one or both sides, dizziness, ataxia, double vision, and loss of visual acuity in one eye would all be common symptoms, but this is certainly not an all-inclusive list. In addition, patients with MS often feel a sense of fatigue in association with attacks of the disease and report worsening of symptoms in association with a rise in body temperature, from taking a hot bath, being outside on a hot day, or having a fever from an infection.

There are many less common presentations of MS. Many patients complain of memory loss, and numerous studies have documented deficits in memory and executive function related to MS. In general, these deficits reflect widespread lesions in the cerebral white matter. Syndromes of cognitive loss in MS usually do not reach the level of a dementia, but occasionally patients with very advanced disease do become demented. Depression is also very common in patients with MS, more so than in other chronic diseases such as rheumatoid arthritis. Pain is not a cardinal symptom of MS, but case series have shown that pain is very common in MS. Pain can take the form of back pain, related to pressure on lumbar discs in patients with asymmetric weakness in the legs and an abnormal gait pattern; *dysesthetic* pain, related to areas of numbness and sensory loss; and severe facial pain, resembling the idiopathic syndrome of tic douleureux (see Chap. 17).

Perhaps the most important characteristic of MS presentations is the temporal profile. Most patients with MS present with acute exacerbations, with remissions between attacks. Some attacks are associated with complete recovery, but some leave residual disability. Over time, the patient often accumulates deficits and disabilities. The pattern of exacerbations and remissions often continues for many years. Later in the course, however, many patients develop a *secondary progressive* pattern of disease, in which the deficits gradually worsen, with or without exacerbations. These two patterns, relapsing-remitting and secondary progressive, are the most common forms of MS. Occasionally, patients have a slowly progressive form of the disease from the start. This *primary progressive* pattern of MS accounts for less than 10% of the patients and more commonly involves men, often of middle age. Rarely, patients present with a progressive disorder and then have exacerbations, a form called *relapsing-progressive*.

Some MS experts also speak of *benign multiple sclerosis*, meaning a subgroup of patients who never become disabled by the disease. According to some experts, *benign MS* can be diagnosed in a patient with relapsing-remitting MS, in whom no disabling attack occurs within the first 10 years. Not all authorities agree, and there is no guarantee that such a patient might not have a severe attack of MS in the future.

DIFFERENTIAL DIAGNOSIS

Many of the symptoms of MS, described above, are nonspecific. As already mentioned, optic neuritis or transverse myelitis can occur in isolation, and many such patients never develop MS. These syndromes are often of unknown cause, but many are likely viral.

Other diseases may also mimic attacks of MS. Vascular disease, such as stroke, can occasionally cause localized lesions in the CNS with similar symptoms of weakness, numbness, diplopia, dizziness, or ataxia. Isolated optic nerve lesions can be vascular, as in the syndromes of ischemic optic neuropathy or giant cell (temporal) arteritis (see Chap. 9).

Other infectious or inflammatory diseases can also mimic MS. Sarcoidosis is known for producing inflammatory lesions in the nervous system. Many patients with sarcoidosis will show pulmonary involvement, which would not be part of MS, and sarcoidosis can cause syndromes of meningitis, uveitis, or VII cranial nerve palsies in presentations not typical for MS. Similarly, collagen vascular diseases such as systemic lupus erythematosus, Sjögren's syndrome, and Behçet's disease can produce close copies of MS attacks.

LABORATORY AND RADIOLOGICAL INVESTIGATION

The first task in diagnosis of MS is to characterize the clinical history and neurological examination findings. Laboratory tests are useful only in confirming a clinical suspicion of MS and are prone to misinterpretation if not considered as an adjunct to clinical diagnosis. In fact, the most recent International Panel on the Diagnosis of Multiple Sclerosis emphasized that no single clinical feature or laboratory test is sufficient for the diagnosis of MS. The most important aspect is the demonstration of dissemination of lesions in both time and space (different locations in the central nervous system white matter). The clinical criteria for diagnosis of clinically definite MS are shown in abbreviated form in Table 29-1. Is there a history of multiple attacks in time and of involvement of different locations of the CNS, attributable to the CNS white matter? Are there objective signs on neurological examination of more than one such lesion? For example, if a patient has a history of loss of vision in one eye and a more recent attack with weakness and stiffness of one leg, documentation of reduced visual acuity, an afferent pupillary defect, a central scotoma, and optic nerve pallor would serve to document one lesion in the optic nerve. If the same patient had weakness and increased reflexes in one leg, evidence of a second lesion would be present. In this case, the criteria for multiple, objectively documented CNS white matter lesions would be met, and the patient would be diagnosed with *clinically definite MS*.

Table 29-1 **Diagnostic Criteria for Multiple Sclerosis (From McDonald WI, et al., Ann Neurol 2001;50:121–127)**

Clinical Presentation	Additional Data Needed for MS Diagnosis
≥2 or more attacks; objective clinical evidence of ≥2 lesions	None
≥2 or more attacks; objective clinical evidence of 1 lesion	Dissemination in time by MRI, or ≥2 MRI lesions and positive CSF, or await further clinical attack in a different CNS site
1 attack; objective clinical evidence of ≥2 lesions	Dissemination in time by MRI, or second clinical attack
1 attack; clinical evidence of 1 lesion (monosymptomatic, clinically isolated syndrome)	Dissemination in space by MRI, or ≥2 MRI lesions and positive CSF and dissemination in time by MRI, or second clinical attack
Slowly progressive syndrome suggestive of MS	Positive CSF and ≥9 T2 MRI lesions in brain or 4–8 brain lesions and 1 spinal cord lesion, or ≥2 lesions in spinal cord, or abnormal visual evoked potential plus 4–8 MRI lesions or <4 brain lesions and 1 spinal cord lesion and dissemination in time by MRI, or continued progression for one year

If the history suggested two attacks involving different areas, but the neurological examination documented only one lesion, the diagnosis would be *clinically probable MS*. If the history suggested only one lesion, such as optic neuritis or tranverse myelitis, the diagnosis would be *clinically possible MS*. A single, progressive disorder such as progressive myelopathy would also qualify as *possible MS*.

Once the clinical diagnosis is made, confirmatory laboratory testing should be obtained. The magnetic resonance imaging (MRI) scan is extremely helpful in MS, because it detects the plaques of MS. If a plaque is acute, or recent, it may enhance with contrast agents such as gadolinium. MS plaques occur mainly in the white matter, often in a periventricular location, at right angles to the ventricles. Occasionally, optic nerve inflammation can be detected with MRI. MRI can also be done of the spinal cord to look for intramedullary lesions.

Spinal fluid analysis is also very helpful in the diagnosis of MS. Nonspecific findings such as increased mononuclear cells and elevated protein are consistent with, but not diagnostic of, MS. The most characteristic spinal fluid finding in MS is evidence of increased CNS gamma globulin formation, tested by electrophoresis with oligoclonal bands of abnormal gamma globulin, or an increased IgG-to-albumin ratio, as compared to that in the serum. Similar changes in gamma globulins can occur in other inflammatory or infectious diseases of the CNS, but in a context of symptoms suggestive of MS, these changes can confirm the diagnosis.

Finally, *evoked response* electroencephalographic tests can be used to uncover clinically undocumented lesions in patients with MS. The most commonly used is the visual evoked response (VER). A delay in the P100 wave of the VER can detect a clinically silent optic neuritis, or evidence of a past attack for which the physical examination does not provide objective evidence. The brainstem auditory evoked response (BAER) can likewise detect brainstem lesions, and the somatosensory evoked response (SSER) can detect posterior column lesions in the spinal cord. These tests can be used to support a diagnosis of "laboratory-supported" probable or definite MS.

TREATMENT

The treatment of MS is divided into three separate categories: symptomatic treatments, acute interventions, and preventive therapies.

Symptomatic treatments

Symptomatic treatments for MS are many. The principal symptoms requiring treatment include fatigue, spasticity, pain syndromes, bladder and bowel dysfunction, depression, and cognitive deficits. Many MS patients complain of fatigue, some only during exacerbations and others quite chronically. Treatments for fatigue include recognition of the symptom, frequent rest periods, and drug therapy with amantadine, modafinil (Provigil), stimulants such as methylphenidate (Ritalin), or 4-aminopyridine. Modafinil has had some evidence supporting benefit, but the available studies have differed on the degree of benefit. For spasticity, medications include baclofen, administered either orally or via a spinal pump, tizanidine (Zanaflex), or occasionally a benzodiazepine such as clonazepam. For neuropathic pain, gabapentin (Neurontin), pregabilin (Lyrica), amitriptyline (Elavil), or carbamazepine (Tegretol), all have had some success, though this remains a difficult problem for many patients. Headaches are often treated similarly to migraines (see Chap. 30). Patients who are depressed, a common symptom in MS, often benefit from selective serotonin reuptake inhibitors (SSRIs) such as fluoxetine (Prozac), sertraline (Zoloft), paroxetine (Paxil), excitalopram (Lexapro), or others. Finally, many patients with MS experience difficulty with short-term memory and related cognitive deficits. No specific treatment has been approved for this indication, but the anticholinesterase drugs used in Alzheimer's disease (see Chap. 26) have been used both anecdotally and investigationally.

Acute treatment

Acute intervention for a disabling attack of MS usually involves corticosteroids. The most common method of administering high dose steroid therapy quickly is to infuse intravenous methylprednisolone either once daily at a dose of 1000 mg, or in divided doses. The duration of treatment is not well agreed upon; three days may suffice for a mild attack, but a full week may be given in some instances. Based on treatment trials in optic neuritis, high dose methylprednisolone actually delays the development of full-blown MS, whereas lower dose, oral corticosteroid therapy such as oral prednisone seems to increase progression to MS. Most MS experts therefore recommend steroid therapy only via an intravenous course of 3–5 days, unless an oral dose is used to taper after an intravenous course.

Preventive treatment

The third aspect of MS treatment is the progression of further attacks and, thereby, the accumulation of disability. Four agents are Food and Drug Administration (FDA) approved for prevention of attacks and disability in patients with relapsing-remitting MS. Three of the four are interferons: Betaseron (interferon-1-beta), injected every other day as a subcutaneous dose; Avonex (interferon-1-alpha), injected intramuscularly once weekly; and Rebif (interferon-1-alpha), injected subcutaneously three times weekly. Betaseron and Rebif involve larger doses of interferon and may have more potent effects, but Avonex is more convenient for patients. Finally, glatiramer acetate (Copaxone) is a peptide of amino acids that may alter the immune response against myelin. Copaxone must be injected subcutaneously every day, but it has fewer side effects in terms of local injection reactions and flu-like symptoms, which frequently follow interferon injections. All four drugs have been shown to reduce the number of exacerbations, the accumulation of disability, and also the appearance of new MRI lesions. Most MS experts recommend initiation of therapy as soon as the diagnosis is clear. Recent clinical trials have supported benefit of treatment in patients with early symptomatic MS, such as patients with only one attack or those with one attack and MRI or CSF evidence of MS.

A new, monthly administered, intravenous agent called Tysabri was withdrawn from the market because of the development of the disease progressive multifocal leukoencephalopathy in a few MS patients who took the drug in combination with beta-interferon 1A (Avonex), and also in a patient treated for Crohn's disease. The drug is being reintroduced as monotherapy for MS, however, because of its impressive efficacy and because the PML cases occurred mainly in patients on combination therapy. An oral agent to prevent exacerbations or recurrent attacks would be an extremely welcome addition to the MS armamentarium. One promising new agent called fingolimod has recently been reported to decrease new MRI lesions, but further clinical trials will be required before the drug is approved for treatment of MS.

Patients with secondary progressive MS tend to worsen gradually, and evidence that the interferon agents and glatiramer acetate prevent this progression is limited. Patients who are still experiencing acute exacerbations are generally continued on treatment. Antibodies against the interferons may reduce the efficacy of the drug, and commercial assays for such antibodies are available. Finally, chemotherapy agents have long been administered for patients with slowly progressive MS symptoms. One agent, mitoxantrone (Novantrone), has been approved for use in this group. The drug is administered by intravenous infusion every 3 months, and the duration of therapy is limited to 3 years by the risk of cardiotoxicity. Older chemotherapy agents such as cyclophosphamide (Cytoxan), azathioprine (Imuran), or methotrexate are occasionally used, especially in patients with rapidly progressive disease. For very fulminating cases, plasma exchange and intravenous immunoglobulin are occasionally prescribed.

Course and prognosis

As discussed above, patients with MS have widely differing courses, a few with *benign MS* characterized by only occasional, nondisabling attacks, the majority with exacerbating and remitting, more disabling symptoms. Of the relapsing-remitting group, the majority eventually develops progressive disease (*secondary progressive MS*). A few have progressive disease from the start.

Recent research has suggested that progressive disability relates to axonal loss, rather than to inflammatory/demyelinating lesions, and that such axonal loss occurs early in the disease. Some MS authorities believe that this makes it especially important to initiate disease-modifying treatment early in the course.

The precise cause of MS is not understood. A large body of research has supported an abnormality of the immune system, and it is likely that inherited factors related to the immune response govern susceptibility to MS. MS is an *autoimmune disease*, in which there is evidence of activated lymphocytes and plasma cells within the lesions of MS, evidence of antibody production in the spinal fluid oligoclonal bands, and similarity to animal models in which an immune response is raised to myelin or its component proteins. There is also epidemiological evidence, however, that MS is not entirely a genetic disease, and that some environmental factor or factors are also important. Infections have always been suspected as triggers of MS in persons who are genetically susceptible. In the past, various infections have been implicated, including measles, canine distemper virus, herpes viruses, and Chlamydia pneumoniae. Recent studies have found a high percentage of antibodies to the Epstein-Barr virus, the virus of infectious mononucleosis, in children with MS. The exact cause of MS, however, remains elusive, and a cure for the disease will likely await a more complete elucidation of the causative factors and pathogenesis of the disease.

KEY REFERENCES

Coyle PK, Hartung H-P. Use of interferon beta in multiple sclerosis: rationale for early treatment and evidence for dose- and frequency-dependent effects on clinical response. *Multi Scler* 2002;8:2–9.

Freedman M S, Thompson EJ, Deisenhammer F, et al. Recommended standard of cerebrospinal fluid analysis in the diagnosis of multiple sclerosis. A consensus statement. *Arch Neurol* 2005;62:865–870.

Frohman E, Phillips T, Kokel K, et al. Disease-modifying therapy in multiple sclerosis: strategies for optimizing management. *Neurologist* 2002;8:227–236.

Goodin DS, Frohman EM, Garmany GPJ, et al. Disease modifying therapies in multiple sclerosis: report of the Therapeutics and Technology Assessment Subcommittee of the American Academy of Neurology and the MS Council for Clinical Practice Guidelines. *Neurology* 2002;58:169–178.

Hunter SF, Weinshenker BG, Carter JL, et al. Rational clinical immunotherapy for multiple sclerosis. *Mayo Clin Proc* 1997;72:765–780.

Jacobs LD, Beck RW, Simon JH, et al. Intramuscular interferon beta-1a therapy initiated during a first demyelinating event in multiple sclerosis. CHAMPS Study Group. *N Engl J Med* 2000;343:898–904.

Kappos L, Antel J, Comi G, et al. Oral fingolimod (FTY720) for relapsing multiple sclerosis. *N Engl J Med* 2006;355:1124–40.

Kroencke DC, Lynch SG, Denney DR. Fatigue in multiple sclerosis: relationship to depression, disability, and disease pattern. *Mult Scler* 2000;6:131–136.

Kuhlmann T, Lingfeld G, Bitsch A, et al. Acute axonal damage in multiple sclerosis is most extensive in early disease and decreases over time. *Brain* 2002;125: 2202–2212.

Levin LI, Munger KL, Rubertone MV, et al. Multiple sclerosis and Epstein-Barr virus. *JAMA* 2003;289:1533–1536.

Lucchinetti CF, Rodriguez M. The controversy surrounding the pathogenesis of the multiple sclerosis lesion. *Mayo Clin Proc* 1997;72:665–678.

McDonald WI, Compston A, Edan G, et al. Recommended diagnostic criteria for multiple sclerosis: guidelines from the International Panel on the Diagnosis of Multiple Sclerosis. *Ann Neurol* 2001;50:121–127.

Noseworthy JH, Lucchinetti C, Rodriguez M, et al. Multiple sclerosis. *N Engl J Med* 2000;343:938–952.

Polman CH, O'Connor PW, Havrdova E, et al. A randomized, placebo-controlled trial of natalizumab for relapsing multiple sclerosis. *N Engl J Med*. 2006;354:899–910.

Rao SM, Leo GJ, Bernardin L, et al. Cognitive dysfunction in multiple sclerosis. I. Frequency, patterns, and prediction. *Neurology* 1991;41:685–691.

Rao SM, Leo GJ, Ellington L, et al. Cognitive dysfunction in multiple sclerosis. II. Impact on employment and social functioning. *Neurology* 1991;41:692–696.

Trapp BD, Peterson J, Ransohoff RM, et al. Axonal transaction in the lesions of multiple sclerosis. *N Engl J Med* 1998;338:278–285.

MIGRAINE AND RELATED
HEADACHE SYNDROMES

INTRODUCTION

Migraine headaches are an extremely common disorder, occurring in approximately 15% of all women and 6% of men. Migraine is the most common headache syndrome, also a major cause of lost work productivity, suffering, and expense to society.

SYMPTOMS AND SIGNS

Migraine is generally known for the severity of headache, the presence of a throbbing, pulsating quality of headache, often a unilateral distribution, and the association with nausea and often vomiting. As we shall see, not all of these features need to be present for a headache to be diagnosed as a migraine. Likewise, many but not all migraine headaches are preceded by an "aura," or anticipatory symptoms.

Classifications of migraine have changed in recent years. The first distinction is between migraine with aura, formerly called *classical migraine*, and migraine without aura, formerly called *common migraine*. The aura is most commonly visual, especially positive phenomena such as zigzag lines, shimmering lights, or fortification spectra, less commonly a visual field defect or scotoma. Other, less common auras involve neurological symptoms such as paresthesias on one side of the body, or even such stroke-like symptoms as weakness (hemiplegic migraine), confusion or aphasia (acute confusional migraine), or diplopia (basilar or ophthalmoplegic migraine). Rarely, a typical migraine episode may be followed by persistent neurological deficits such as hemiparesis or visual field defects; this condition is called *migrainous stroke*. Migraine may actually have as many as four phases: (1) a prodrome, usually of vague malaise; (2) the aura; (3) the headache phase; and (4) the postdrome, or fatigue that follows a migraine attack. The headache itself is usually but not always throbbing and pounding, and it is more often unilateral than bilateral. Other, very characteristic symptoms associated with migraine headaches are nausea, vomiting, photophobia, and phonophobia. Table 30-1 lists criteria for the diagnosis of migraine.

The precise cause of migraine remains enigmatic. We know from cerebral blood flow and positron emission tomography (PET) studies that a wave of ischemia, or *oligemia* begins at the back of the brain at the onset of the aura of a typical migraine, continuing into the headache phase. In the past, the aura was thought to be associated with vasoconstriction, the headache with vasodilatation, but this model of migraine is now known to be an oversimplification. Neuronal firing in serotonergic pathways in the brain is thought to be the primary event in migraine, and the vascular changes are secondary.

Table 30-1 **International Headache Society (HIS) Diagnostic Criteria for Migraine with and without Aura**

Without aura:
At least five attacks fulfilling the following:
  Headache lasting 4–72 hours
  Headache has $\geq$2 of the following characteristics:
  -   Unilateral site
  -   Pulsating quality
  -   Moderate or severe intensity
  -   Aggravation by physical activity
$\geq$1of the following during headache:
  -   Nausea and/or vomiting
  -   Photophobia or phonophobia
At least one of the following:
  -   History, physical and neuro examinations do not suggest 2° headache
  -   History and/or examination suggests 2°, but lab investigations excluded
  -   2° headache is present, but migraines do not occur for the first time in
      association
With aura:
At least two attacks with $\geq$ $^{3}/_{4}$ of the following:
  -   One or more reversible aura symptoms
  $\geq$1 aura symptom develops gradually over >4 min or $\geq$2 aura sx in succession
  No aura symptom lasts >60 minutes
  Headache follows aura with pain-free interval of <60 minutes (or begins before or
  during aura)

DIFFERENTIAL DIAGNOSIS

The principal differential diagnosis of migraine is with the more serious causes of headache, discussed in Chap. 16. Migraine has overlap with other headache syndromes such as cluster, analgesic rebound, and chronic daily headaches.

TREATMENT

The treatment of migraine includes nonpharmacological management, abortive or acute therapy, and preventive or prophylactic therapy. Non-pharmacological treatment includes avoidance of substances that seem to trigger migraine, such as chocolate or caffeine, relaxation therapy, and various forms of psychotherapy, biofeedback, and physical therapy techniques. Abortive therapy involves medications taken when a migraine attack first begins. For mild to moderate headaches, a simple nonsteroidal anti-inflammatory drug such as naproxyn (in doses ranging from 220 mg to 550 mg) or a combination of aspirin and acetaminophen (Exedrin Migraine) can be effective. Multiple other analgesic combinations are available. For more severe headaches, two classes of agents have proved effective. The first is the triptans, of which the first was sumatriptan (Imitrex), now available by injection, nasal spray, and pill. Six other triptans are now on the market for abortive use in migraine. These agents are listed in Table 30–2. Differences among the triptans are mainly in the half-life, of which one, frovatriptan, is longer-acting than all of the others and particularly well suited for long, gradually developing migraines such as menstrual migraines. Most of the others are shorter–acting and more useful for very sudden attacks. Triptans are thought to work by stimulating specific serotonin receptors in the brain. The other class of abortive agents for migraine is the ergotamines. Earlier

Table 30-2   *Triptan Drugs for Migraine*

Generic name	Brand name	Half-life	Doses (oral only)
Sumatriptan	Imitrex	2.5 hours	25, 50, 100 mg
Zolmitriptan	Zomig	3 hours	2.5, 5 mg
Naratriptan	Amerge	6 hours	1, 2.5 mg
Rizatriptan	Maxalt	2–3 hours	5, 10 mg
Eletriptan	Relpax	4 hours	20, 40 mg
Almotriptan	Axert	3–4 hours	6.25, 12.5 mg
Frovatriptan	Frova	26 hours	2.5 mg

ergotamines have been largely abandoned because of the vasoconstriction they cause, but the drug dihydroergotamine is still in use. This drug activates serotonin receptors in a way similar to that of the triptans, but patients may respond better to one or the other agent. Dihydroergotamine is available by injection (0.5 mg or 1 mg intramuscularly) or by nasal spray, under the trade name Migranol. Occasionally, migraines are so severe that narcotic analgesics are needed for abortive treatment. This treatment should be reserved for reliable patients with relatively infrequent headache episodes, because of the risk of drug dependency or "rebound" headaches (see below).

In general, migraines can be treated with abortive agents alone if they occur once or twice monthly, or less frequently. For headaches occurring more frequently, prophylactic treatment is usually indicated. There are a number of alternative drugs to choose. The first drug approved for migraine prevention was propranolol (Inderal), a beta-blocker. This drug is effective in doses of 40–160 mg daily, but side effects such as lethargy, bradycardia, and hypotension are common. Several other beta-blockers have also been shown to be effective in preventing migraines, including atenolol (Tenormin), metoprolol (Toprol, Lopressor), nadolol (Corgard), and timolol (Blocadren). The next class of agents applied to migraine was the calcium channel blockers, particularly verapamil, which can be given in doses from 80–480 mg daily. This drug less often causes lethargy as compared to propranolol, but it can also cause bradycardia, hypotension, and also peripheral edema and constipation. The other "old-fashioned" migraine remedy is a low-dose tricyclic antidepressant such as amitriptyline (Elavil), in doses of 10–50 mg at bedtime. Side effects such as dry mouth, sedation, and weight gain limit the use of this agent. Elderly patients are particularly sensitive to the anticholinergic side effects. Newer migraine prophylactic agents are drugs originally introduced as antiepileptic agents. These include valproic acid (Depakote), gabapentin (Neurontin), topiramate (Topamax), lamotrigine (Lamictal), and levetiracetam (Keppra). Of these, only valproic acid and topiramate have Food and Drug Administration (FDA) indications for migraine; treatment with the others should be considered "off-label." These drugs are often effective in preventing migraines. Topiramate appears particularly effective, and its side effect profile is generally favorable. Weight loss is an often desirable side effect, whereas paresthesias, difficulty thinking of words, and kidney stones are negative side effects. The other antiepileptic drugs, many of which have received only limited testing in migraine, are discussed in Chap. 25, on epilepsy.

A rare migraine syndrome is *status migrainosus* , continuous or repeated bouts of migraine headache, not interrupted by headache-free periods. This syndrome is often confused with the analgesic rebound headache, to be discussed below. True status migrainosus requires treatment, often in the hospital. The pattern can be stopped with use of dihydroergotamine on an every 8-hour schedule either intravenously or intramuscularly or intravenous valproic acid (Depacon).

CLUSTER HEADACHE

Cluster headache can be considered a variant of migraine. Cluster headaches are briefer than migraines, and more localized, generally involving the periorbital area. They are usually unilateral, periorbital, very sharp and severe in pain quality, and sometimes associated with autonomic symptoms such as tearing of the eye, runny nose, and nasal congestion. Cluster headaches often occur at a stereotyped time, such as awakening at 2 a.m. or 3 a.m. with severe headache pain. Patients with cluster headache often state that they cannot stand the pain, and they frequently get up and pace, whereas migraine patients more often want to lie down in a quiet, dark place.

The term "cluster" refers to the temporal clustering of the headache episodes. Patients may have daily cluster headaches for days or weeks, then the headaches may remit for months or even years.

Many treatments have been tried for cluster headaches. Acute, abortive therapies include oxygen inhalation, triptans, dihydroergotamine, and narcotic analgesics. A short course of corticosteroids, such as prednisone 100 mg daily for 5 days, may help to stop the cluster. Verapamil has been used along with corticosteroids to prolong the effect. Many of the other migraine prophylactic agents discussed above have also been used in cluster headaches, with variable success. Lithium carbonate is occasionally effective for refractory, chronic cluster headaches. In the past, the chronic ergot agent methysergide was used in the treatment of both cluster and migraine headaches, but complications such as limb ischemia and retroperitoneal fibrosis have led to the near obsolescence of this drug.

CHRONIC DAILY HEADACHE

The last category of headache that we shall discuss, chronic daily headache, is actually a mixture of headache types. In headache clinics, chronic daily headaches are often the most common category of new patients. Traditionally, these headaches were considered to be "tension headaches". In the past, the cause of tension headache was thought to be prolonged contraction of muscles in the forehead and the back of the head, and these headaches were even called *muscle contraction headaches*. Most authorities now believe that the evidence for muscle contraction as the cause of tension headaches is weak, and the old term has come back into use. Exactly how chronic anxiety and depression cause headache is unclear, but these are certainly major etiological factors in chronic daily headaches. Tension and anxiety also aggravate migraine headaches. The most common pattern is for a *migraineur* to awaken with headache on the morning after a stressful period.

Other causes of chronic daily headaches include some of the headache syndromes discussed in Chap. 16, including temporal arteritis, cervical spondylosis, Chiari malformation, hydrocephalus, idiopathic intracranial hypertension, venous sinus thrombosis, and even brain tumors and abscesses. For this reason, a careful history and examination are essential in all patients.

The last, and perhaps most common cause of chronic daily headache is the *rebound headache* syndrome, also called *transformed migraine* or *analgesic-associated headache*. The fact that daily use of analgesic agents, including such seemingly harmless drugs as acetaminophen (Tylenal) or ibuprofen (Motrin, Advil), are associated with chronic daily headaches, is beyond dispute, though the exact mechanism is debated. One common way that I explain this phenomenon to patients is that each time an analgesic is taken the headache severity diminishes, but the headache does not go away completely. The headache will then build up, and the patient again takes the analgesic, leading to another cycle of partial relief and gradual build-up of headache. Soon the patient is, paradoxically, taking daily pain medications yet having daily headaches. The headache simply does not go through its spontaneous evolution and disappearance, but rather the pain is prolonged for days, weeks, months, or even years. Patients continue to take the analgesics because each dose seems to produce relief, yet obviously the treatment is unsuccessful. In addition, once the analgesic rebound pattern is established, no other preventive treatments for headaches work effectively. The headache may start as a migraine, or there may be occasional, severe, migraine-like episodes within a chronic daily headache pattern, in which case the term *transformed migraine* is appropriate. Sometimes the analgesic rebound headache arises after a head injury, when analgesics are prescribed for the acute headache and then continued indefinitely. Sometimes tension headache, the other common cause of chronic, daily headaches, is a part of the pathophysiology of rebound headache; not all analgesic rebound headaches are migraine-related. Migraineurs seem more predisposed to develop analgesic rebound headache, sometimes with only relatively light use of analgesics. I have seen patients develop analgesic rebound headache after being prescribed analgesic agents for another problem, such as osteoarthritis. The treatment of analgesic rebound headache is problematic, in that the patient must be persuaded to stop the frequent use of analgesics, and this will often result in worsening of the headaches before they get better. Sometimes the use of a prophylactic agent such as amitriptyline, topirimate, or gabapentin may help get the patient over this period of increased headache, and those who persevere may be rewarded by excellent long-term resolution. Occasionally, a pattern of occasional migraines will reemerge, and these can then be treated successfully with either abortive or prophylactic medications.

KEY REFERENCES

Bartleson JD. Treatment of migraine headaches. *Mayo Clin Proc* 1999;74:702–708.

Cady R, Dodick DW. Diagnosis and treatment of migraine. *Mayo Clin Proc* 2002;77: 255–261.

Ducros A, Denier C, Joutel A, et al. The clinical spectrum of familial hemiplegic migraine associated with mutations in a neuronal calcium channel. *N Engl J Med* 2001;345:17–24.

Ferrari MD. Migraine. *Lancet* 1998;351:1043–1051.

Ferrari, MD, Roon KI, Lipton RB, et al. Oral triptans (serotonin 5-HT$_{1B/1D}$ agonists) in acute migraine treatment: a meta-analysis of 53 trials. *Lancet* 2001;358:1668–1675.

Goadsby PJ. The pharmacology of headache. *Prog Neurobiol* 2000;62:509–525.

Goadsby PJ, Lipton RB, Ferrari MD. Migraine—current understanding and treatment. *N Engl J Med* 2002;346:257–270.

Kaniecki R. Headache assessment and management. *JAMA* 2003;289:1430–1433.

Kirshner HS. Management of headache. In: Parris WCV, ed. *Contemporary Issues in Chronic Pain Management*. Chap. 13. Boston, MA: Kluwer Academic Publishers; 1991:203–220.

Mathew NT, Kurman R, Perez F. Drug induced refractory headache—clinical features and management. *Headache* 1990;30:634–638.

Mathew NT, Loder E. Evaluating the triptans. *Am J Medicine* 2005;118 (Suppl. 1): 28S–35S.

Schwartz BS, Stewart WF, Simon D, et al. Epidemiology of tension-type headache. *JAMA* 1998;279:381–383.

Silberstein SD. Practice parameter: evidence-based guidelines for migraine headache (an evidence-based review). *Neurology* 2000;55:754–762.

Warner JS. Rebound headaches—a review. *Headache Q* 1999;10:207–219.

BELL'S PALSY

INTRODUCTION

Bell's palsy refers to an idiopathic paralysis of cranial nerve VII, the facial nerve, as described by Sir Charles Bell in the nineteenth century. To the present time, we do not understand the cause of Bell's palsy, though most experts favor a viral etiology. Herpes simplex virus is considered the most likely viral cause, but the link has never been proved. Herpes viruses are known to lie dormant in nerve ganglia and then activate, producing symptoms in the distribution of the nerve. Bell's palsy is extremely common, occurring in as many as 20–30 cases/100,000 of population per year, often in young, healthy people.

CLINICAL PRESENTATION: SYMPTOMS AND SIGNS

Bell's palsy refers to a paralysis of the face on one side. Many patients complain that the face feels "numb," even "like novocaine," and yet careful sensory testing usually reveals entirely normal perception of light touch and sharp/dull stimuli. The facial weakness often begins around the mouth, raising confusion with an upper motor neuron facial paralysis, as in a stroke. The weakness often worsens over a few days, frequently resulting in a virtually complete facial palsy. The peripheral nature of the facial palsy is obvious when the paralysis is severe, such that patient cannot elevate the eyebrow, nor wrinkle the forehead, nor close the eye completely. The face may droop to the point that the patient drools out of the affected side of the mouth. Speech is not usually much affected, except for labial consonants such as the "m" and "p" sounds. Some patients note hyperacusis, or excessive loudness of sounds, because a branch of the VII nerve supplies the stapedius muscle, which dampens sounds. Hearing is otherwise unaffected by Bell's palsy, but some patients complain of ear pain on the ipsilateral side. Taste is frequently affected on the anterior two-thirds of the tongue. Patients frequently do not notice the taste loss, since foods and liquids are exposed to both sides of the tongue, but careful testing of perception of salty and sweet solutions with a Q-tip on the tongue serves to indicate taste involvement on the ipsilateral side A deficit in taste helps to confirm the diagnosis of Bell's palsy, since the taste fibers accompany the facial nerve only from the point of exit from the pons to the splitting off of the chorda tympani in the middle ear; the taste fibers then travel to the tongue with the lingual branch of the XII nerve.

During recovery from Bell's palsy, partial movement of the facial muscles usually returns. Two physical examination findings can document reinnervation. The first is *synkinesis*, or the simultaneous contraction of muscles around the mouth and around the eye. For example, the patient will have a mouth twitch every time the eye blinks. Synkinesis implies that surviving neurons of the facial nerve are supplying both the orbicularis oculi and the lower facial muscles, a sign of reinnervation. The second sign is *crocodile tears*, or lacrimation upon smelling or tasting food, implying that the salivary and lacrimal glands are also innervated by the same nerve fiber.

DIFFERENTIAL DIAGNOSIS

The most common differential diagnoses for Bell's palsy are a central facial weakness or another, non-idiopathic cause of a peripheral facial palsy. With regard to stroke, a facial palsy predominantly involving the lower face should always raise concern about a central palsy. A mild, partial peripheral VII palsy can be hard to distinguish from a central lesion, but complete sparing of the eyebrow and forehead should be considered suspicious for a central VII paresis. This could be part of stroke, a brain tumor, brain abscess, or other central nervous system lesion. Other clues to the presence of a central facial palsy include associated sensory loss and lack of taste involvement.

With regard to peripheral facial palsies, many other etiologies come into the differential diagnosis. One of the most common is a Herpes zoster infection of the geniculate ganglion and ear, or Ramsay-Hunt syndrome. This syndrome is much more likely to have associated, severe pain in the ipsilateral ear, and often vesicles can be visualized in the external ear canal and pinna. Hearing may also be affected, and vertigo occasionally results from involvement of the vestibular portion of the VIII nerve. The prognosis of Ramsay-Hunt syndrome is less good than that of idiopathic Bell's palsy, and early treatment with an antiviral drug such as valacyclovir (Valtrex) plus prednisone is usually indicated.

Many other causes of peripheral facial palsy have been reported. Facial palsy can occur as a mononeuropathy, likely on a vascular basis, in patients with diabetes or hypertension. Lyme disease can affect the facial nerve in the second phase of the illness. Human immunodeficiency virus (HIV) also causes facial palsies, as can inflammatory conditions such as sarcoidosis and

Sjögren's syndrome. Lesions in the brainstem, as in tumors, multiple sclerosis plaques, or strokes can affect the facial nerve, usually in the fibers descending from the facial nerve nucleus. Other brainstem signs will often accompany a facial palsy of brainstem origin, though taste will usually not be affected, since the taste fibers leave the facial nerve to join the tractus solitarius after they enter the brainstem. Lesions of the VIII nerve, even if large, do not usually cause obvious facial weakness, though surgery to remove an acoustic neuroma sometimes results in facial palsy. Compressive lesions lower down, such as a parotid tumor or trauma at the level of the stylohyoid foramen, where the nerve exits the skull, can affect the facial nerve. Note that taste will not be affected in lesions at this location, since they affect the facial nerve distal to the splitting off of the chorda tympani fibers. Recently, an intranasal flu vaccine appeared to be associated with an increased incidence of Bell's palsy.

LABORATORY AND RADIOLOGICAL INVESTIGATION

If a patient has a typical Bell's palsy, no laboratory investigation is necessary. If there is any question about a brainstem or central lesion, a magnetic resonance imaging (MRI) of the head can be done. In many cases, swelling or inflammation can be visualized in the facial nerve on MRI. This, of course, is an expensive test to confirm what is usually an obvious diagnosis. If there is a question of Herpes zoster oticus or Ramsay-Hunt syndrome, careful inspection of the ear canal for vesicles is useful, and antibody titers can be obtained. Electromyogram/nerve conduction velocities (EMG/NCVs) of the facial nerve can be performed to assess the degree of denervation that has developed in the facial nerve distribution. This can be useful for prognostic purposes; extensive denervation augurs an incomplete recovery.

TREATMENT

Idiopathic facial palsy (Bell's palsy) has a relatively benign prognosis, but treatment may speed the recovery. Prednisone has been used since the 1960s, as summarized in the paper by Adour (1972). Corticosteroids probably have to be given within the first 1–3 days of the paralysis to have much effect. I prescribe prednisone at 60 mg daily for 4–5 days, 40 mg for 4–5 days, and 20 mg for 4–5 days. Others use more rapid steroid tapering doses, as in a Medrol Dosepak. Patients with diabetes, or older people, may have increased likelihood of adverse steroid effects compared to healthy, younger people. Antiherpetic agents such as acyclovir or valacyclovir (Valtrex) may also speed recovery, though this is not as solidly backed by evidence as the steroid effect. Valtrex 1000 mg three times daily for 5–7 days seems a reasonable course. Decompression of the facial nerve was formerly favored by otolaryngologists, but virtually no evidence supports this surgery. Electrical stimulation of the nerve has likewise not been proved beneficial. These treatment recommendations are very similar to those published in a practice guideline of the American Academy of Neurology. Protection of the eye with a patch at night and eye drops or lubricants is an important aspect of treatment, since patients can develop corneal ulcers and have permanent loss of vision, as a result. If a facial palsy does not recover or is caused by inadvertent surgical trauma, as in an acoustic neuroma resection, a graft of the XII cranial nerve to the VII nerve can lead to some recovery of function in the facial muscles.

COURSE AND PROGNOSIS

Most patients with Bell's palsy recover well, even without specific treatment. At least 70% of patients recover completely, and 80–90% have substantial improvement. Elderly patients and those with diabetes are less likely to recover completely than young, healthy patients.

KEY REFERENCES

Adour KK, Ruboyianes JM, Von Doersten PG, et al. Bell's palsy treatment with acyclovir and prednisone compared with prednisone alone: a double-blind, randomized, controlled trial. *Ann Otol Rhinol Laryngol* 1996;105:371–378.

Adour KK, Wingerd J, Bell DN, et al. Prednisone treatment for idiopathic facial paralysis (Bell's palsy). *N Engl J Med* 1972;287:1268–1272.

Gilden DH. Bell's palsy. *N Engl J Med* 2004;351:1323–1331.

Grogan PM, Gronseth S. Practice parameter: steroids, acyclovir, and surgery for Bell's palsy (an evidence-based review): report of the Quality Standards Subcommittee of the American Academy of Neurology. *Neurology* 2001;56:830–836.

Murakami S, Hato N, Horiuchi J, et al. Treatment of Ramsay-Hunt syndrome with acyclovir-prednisone: significance of early diagnosis and treatment. *Ann Neurol* 1997;41:353–357.

Mutsch M, Zhou W, Rhodes P, et al. Use of the inactivated intranasal influenza vaccine and the risk of Bell's palsy in Switzerland. *N Engl J Med* 2004;350:896–903.

CARPAL TUNNEL
SYNDROME

INTRODUCTION

Carpal tunnel syndrome (CTS) is the most common of the *entrapment neuropathies*, neuropathies caused by pressure or repetitive injury to a peripheral nerve. CTS develops from pressure on the median nerve in the carpal tunnel at the wrist. It is associated with repetitive use of the hands, as in factory workers, women who sew or stitch shoes and boots, and in the current era people who type repetitively on a computer.

CLINICAL PRESENTATION: SYMPTOMS AND SIGNS

The first symptoms of CTS are usually pain and tingling, or paresthesias, in the median distribution of the hand, including the palm, the thumb, index, and middle fingers, and the median half of the ring finger. These sensory symptoms are exacerbated by prolonged wrist flexion or repetitive use. In some patients, the pain and paresthesias seem to go above the wrist, into the forearm or upper arm. Objective sensory loss, however, should be confined to the median distribution of the hand. Sensory symptoms often wake the patient from sleep, presumably because the wrist flexes during sleeping postures. If the CTS is not treated, motor weakness in the distribution of the median nerve can follow, with poor opposition of the thumb and atrophy of the thenar eminence of the hand. The weak muscles are primarily the opponens pollicis and abductor pollicis brevis muscles.

Provocative tests, as part of the physical examination, are useful in the bedside diagnosis of CTS. Tinel's sign, or electric shocks radiating into the median nerve territory in response to tapping over the volar side of the wrist, is characteristic of CTS. A second provocative test is Phalen's sign, or aggravation of symptoms with prolonged (30–60 second) flexion of the wrist to 90°.

DIFFERENTIAL DIAGNOSIS

The diagnosis of CTS is usually straightforward, based on the symptoms, with sensory loss in the median nerve territory and positive Tinel's and Phalen's signs. Ulnar compression at the elbow should produce paresthesias more in the ulnar distribution of the hand, with a positive Tinel's sign at the elbow. A brachial plexopathy causes weakness in a brachial plexus distribution, usually involving more proximal muscles of the arm. Brachial plexopathies usually cause weakness without much sensory loss, an opposite pattern to that of CTS. Compressive brachial plexopathies are usually painful. Nerve root syndromes, such as a cervical disk at C5-6 may present with pain radiating down from the neck, into the arm, with weakness of the biceps and other muscles, and with sensory loss in the forearm and thumb, but never an isolated, median nerve territory numbness and weakness.

Perhaps a more problematic differential diagnosis is that between CTS and a more generalized neuropathy. Diabetic patients, for example, seem to be more sensitive to pressure on individual nerves, because of their underlying diabetic peripheral neuropathy. Diabetics thus develop CTS with only minimal compression or nerve injury, and in general they have a worse prognosis for recovery after treatment. Other neuropathies can also present with focal symptoms suggestive of CTS.

Another differential diagnosis is that between CTS as an individual nerve entrapment syndrome and CTS as part of a multiple *overuse* or *repetitive strain* syndrome. Patients such as factory workers often have combinations of symptoms suggestive of CTS, ulnar nerve entrapment at the elbow, brachial plexus symptoms perhaps related to thoracic outlet syndrome, and cervical radiculopathy. In these patients, too, surgical treatment for CTS will not solve the entire problem.

LABORATORY AND RADIOLOGICAL INVESTIGATION

As in so many of the diagnoses discussed in this book, the diagnosis of CTS should first be made by the history and physical examination, with the provocative tests of Tinel's and Phalen's signs. If there is doubt, an electromyogram/nerve conduction velocity (EMG/NCVs) study (see Chap. 38) is the best test for objective verification of CTS, and it also excludes the involvement of other, single nerves, an underlying peripheral neuropathy, or a cervical radiculopathy. Occasionally, early in CTS, the patient has only paresthesias, and the NCVs may not yet show a delay across the carpal tunnel, and EMG may not detect denervation changes in the median-innervated muscles. Clinical suspicion of CTS from the history and physical examination should still make CTS the probable diagnosis. If there is doubt about the diagnosis, magnetic resonance imaging (MRI) studies of the cervical spine can exclude a cervical radiculopathy.

Patients with a multiple nerve, repetitive strain syndrome may or may not have objective evidence of CTS on EMG/NCVs. In this population, MRI and cervical spine films often show nothing more than mild degenerative joint disease.

TREATMENT

The first level of treatment for CTS is to counsel the patient to avoid any pressure on the median nerve at the wrist. Proper, "ergonomic" work postures, such as supports for the wrist in people who work at computers, may help to minimize the symptoms. If the symptoms are fully developed, the next stage of treatment is a wrist splint, which holds the wrist in a neutral position. Most patients benefit from wearing the splint to bed at night, so that the wrist cannot flex during sleep. This treatment alone will often suffice. Nonsteroidal anti-inflammatory drugs may also provide some relief. If splinting alone does not control the symptoms adequately, a steroid injection into the wrist may be helpful, though care must be taken not to increase the degree of compression of the median nerve. If all of these measures fail, the patient should be referred to an orthopedic hand surgeon for carpal tunnel decompression surgery. For those few patients who still complain of neuropathic pain even after surgical decompression, nonsteroidal anti-inflammatory drugs and drugs for neuropathic pain such as gabapentin (Neurontin) or pregabilin (Lyrica) may also be of some benefit.

KEY REFERENCES

Andersen JH, Thomsen JF, Overgaard E, et al. Computer use and carpal tunnel syndrome: a 1-year follow-up study. *JAMA* 2003;289:2963–2969.

D'Arcy CA, McGee S. Does this patient have carpal tunnel syndrome? *JAMA* 2000;283:3110–3117.

Dawson DM. Entrapment neuropathies of the upper extremities. *N Engl J Med* 1993;320:2013–2018.

Dawson DM, Hallett M, Wilbourn AJ. *Entrapment Neuropathies*. 3d ed. Philadelphia: Lippincott Williams & Wilkins; 1999.

Gerritsen AA, de Vet HC, Scholten RJ, et al. Splinting vs surgery in the treatment of carpal tunnel syndrome: a randomized controlled trial. *JAMA* 2002;288:1245–1251.

Gerritsen AA, de Krom MC, Struijs MA, et al. Conservative treatment options for carpal tunnel syndrome: a systematic review of randomised controlled trials. *J Neurol* 2002;249:272–280.

Katz JN, Simmons BP. Carpal tunnel syndrome. *N Engl J Med* 2002;346:1807–1812.

Rempel DM, Harrison RJ, Barnhart S. Work-related cumulative trauma disorders of the upper extremity. *JAMA* 1992;267:838–842.

Schrijver HM, Gerritsen AA, Strijers RL, et al. Correlating nerve conduction studies and clinical outcome measures on carpal tunnel syndrome: lessons from a randomized controlled trial. *J Clin Neurophysiol* 2005;22:216–221.

Stevens JC, Beard CM, O'Fallon WM, et al. Conditions associated with carpal tunnel syndrome. *Mayo Clin Proc* 1992;67:541–548.

PERIPHERAL

NEUROPATHIES

Karl Misulis, MD, PhD

INTRODUCTION

Peripheral neuropathies are among the most common causes of referral to neurologists, yet most can be diagnosed and treated by any physician. The most common cause of peripheral neuropathy is diabetes mellitus (DM). A multitude of other conditions is associated with peripheral neuropathy.

The term peripheral neuropathy means damage to the peripheral nervous system rather than the central nervous system. Neuropathies can be classified by: (1) the location of the neuropathy; (2) the type of pathology of the nerve; (3) whether the neuropathy affects motor nerves, sensory nerves, or both; and (4) the time course or chronicity of the neuropathy.

The *location* of the lesion means that the neuropathy may affect single or multiple nerves. The classification of neuropathies by location divides them into: (1) *mononeuropathy*, (2) *mononeuropathy multiplex*, and (3) *polyneuropathy*.

Mononeuropathy denotes damage to one peripheral nerve. The most common mononeuropathy is carpal tunnel syndrome (CTS), affecting the median nerve at the wrist (Chap. 32). Other common mononeuropathies are peroneal neuropathy producing foot drop, ulnar neuropathy producing weakness of many intrinsic muscles of the hand, and radial neuropathy causing wrist drop.

Mononeuropathy multiplex denotes multiple mononeuropathies. Patients with DM and a few other diseases can develop a predisposition to multiple mononeuropathies which can present with involvement of almost any combination of individual nerves. One example would be ulnar neuropathy plus median neuropathy plus a thoracic radiculopathy. This clinical presentation is seldom due to anything else but DM.

Polyneuropathy denotes involvement of virtually all of the nerves, especially the distal nerve distributions. The longest nerves typically manifest the most prominent symptoms. Numbness of the feet, with some involvement of the hands is typical, often referred to as a *stocking-glove distribution*.

The *pathology* of the nerve lesion refers the type of damage. There are five fundamental types of damage to the peripheral nerves: (1) *mechanical damage*, (2) *vascular damage*, (3) *axonal degeneration*, (4) *neuronal degeneration*, and (5) *demyelinating neuropathy*.

Mechanical damage includes compression and infiltration of the nerve. Compression neuropathies include entrapment neuropathies such as CTS or ulnar neuropathy at the elbow. Compression need not be sustained to produce damage, as with peroneal palsy or radial palsy.

Vascular damage is characterized by ischemic damage to one or more nerves. Severe peripheral vascular disease can produce ischemic damage to peripheral nerves, giving symptoms of distal polyneuropathy. Infarction of a single peripheral artery branch can produce damage to a single nerve. This usually occurs when there is arterial interruption by trauma.

Axonal degenerations are characterized by degeneration of the motor and/or sensory axons. This is the most common pathology of neuropathies and includes most diabetic neuropathies.

Neuronal degenerations are those in which the cell bodies degenerate, with resultant death of the axon. Motor neuron degenerations are most common and include amyotrophic lateral sclerosis (ALS) and spinal muscular atrophy (SMA).

Demyelinating neuropathies are often immune-mediated. Acute inflammatory demyelinating polyradiculoneuropathy (AIDP or Guillain-Barŕe syndrome) is the most common demyelinating neuropathy. Chronic inflammatory demyelinating polyradiculoneuropathy (CIDP) is a progressive or relapsing demyelinating neuropathy, a more chronic form of AIDP.

The *chronicity* of a neuropathy refers to the duration of the symptoms. Neuropathies can be divided by duration into: (1) *acute neuropathies*, with onset within a few days; (2) *subacute neuropathies*, with onset within 2–4 weeks; and (3) *chronic neuropathies*, with onset more than 1 month prior to presentation, usually many months.

The chronicity of a peripheral neuropathy narrows the differential diagnosis. Acute neuropathies include trauma with compression or section of the nerve. AIDP is also an acute neuropathy, although it can be present in a subacute fashion. Chronic neuropathies include diabetic neuropathy, CIDP, and most other neuropathies with etiologies other than trauma.

MOTOR, SENSORY, OR BOTH

Peripheral nerves are motor, sensory, or both. The symptoms and signs depend on whether motor or sensory involvement is clinically significant, as well as the distribution of the neuropathy. Most causes of peripheral neuropathy affect both motor and sensory nerves, but proper classification can narrow the differential diagnosis significantly.

CLINICAL PRESENTATION: SYMPTOMS AND SIGNS

Symptoms

The distribution of the symptoms depends on the location of the peripheral nerve pathology. Single nerve lesions have localized symptoms. Polyneuropathies affect the limbs diffusely, usually with a distal predominance.

Motor symptoms include: (1) weakness, (2) fatigue, (3) cramps, and (4) muscle twitches.

Sensory symptoms include: (1) numbness, (2) pain, (3) alteration of sensation, and (4) loss of coordination (sensory ataxia).

MOTOR SYMPTOMS

Weakness is a common complaint with mononeuropathies and polyneuropathies. Patients may report a wider extent of weakness than is found on examination, e.g., a patient may report weakness of all of the muscles of the forearm, but the formal examination shows only wrist and finger extensor weakness, as in radial nerve palsy; because these muscles stabilize the wrist, weakness is perceived to be in this whole part of the limb.

Fatigue is distinguished from weakness, in that fatigue leads to weakness only with repeated effort. Fatigue is a common complaint in patients with neuropathies, even when there is no perceptible weakness on formal examination.

Cramps are muscle contractions that can be seen in some normal patients and in patients with neuropathies or some myopathies. Cramps can be nocturnal, with exercise, or unassociated with a precipitating activity.

Muscle twitches, or fasciculations, are a common complaint and can be seen in patients with neuropathies, motor neuron diseases (MNDs) such as ALS, and in some normal patients. Often, educated patients are concerned that muscle twitches indicate ALS; fortunately, most muscle twitches are benign.

SENSORY SYMPTOMS

Numbness means loss of sensation. Patients with peripheral neuropathy often have an increased threshold for sensory stimulation, meaning that a higher degree of stimulation is required for the patient to perceive it.

Pain is common with neuropathy and is usually located in the distribution of the sensory disturbance. Pain can be of various types, depending on the pathology. Damage to small axons often produces burning pain, whereas damage to large axons often produces sharp, stabbing, or shooting pain. All of these painful sensations relate to pathology in the nerves themselves, rather than to nociception of a true painful stimulus, and hence they are referred to as neuropathic pain.

Alteration of sensation is common, though patients may not volunteer this symptom, and the examiner must ask about it. Patients may misperceive dull stimuli as sharp or tingling. The term *paresthesia* is an abnormal spontaneous sensation, whereas *dysesthesia* refers to abnormal perception of a stimulus with a tingling character (see Chap. 17). These active sensory symptoms may coexist with numbness; the threshold to perceive a sensory stimulus may be elevated, but once a stimulus exceeds the threshold the sensation may seem hyperacute, with tingling, pins and needles, or burning character.

Loss of coordination is an uncommon complaint in patients with neuropathy, but it may be found on examination. Patients may exhibit clumsiness and have difficulty with walking, especially at night, when the loss of visual cues worsens the gait instability. Another term for this incoordination, caused by reduced sensory function, is sensory ataxia.

Signs

Motor signs include: (1) weakness, (2) fatigue, (3) cramps, and (4) fasciculations.

Sensory signs include: (1) sensory loss, (2) hyperpathia, (3) hyporeflexia, and (4) sensory ataxia.

MOTOR SIGNS

Weakness is determined by testing proximal and distal muscles. Weakness must always be appreciated by comparison with other muscle groups. Patients with focal weakness have normal strength in other muscles. Patients with distal weakness have normal proximal strength by comparison, just as patients with proximal weakness (usually a muscle disorder) have normal distal strength by comparison. Patients with generalized weakness, on the other hand, can be classified as weak only in comparison to the examination of a normal patient of the same age and build.

The strength examination must be focused according to the findings (see Chap. 2). A totally normal screening examination, including testing of muscles reported abnormal on history is sufficient. Note that the screening examination may miss some disorders, such as radial palsy, but the complaints should trigger detailed examination of extensor muscles of the wrist, fingers, and elbow, in addition to more detailed examination of muscles innervated by the median and ulnar nerves.

Weakness is classified according to the medical research council (MRC) scale (Table 33-1). This is a standard scale in use by most medical schools and hospitals. Muscles to be examined in a screening examination may include hand grip (finger flexors), elbow flexion (biceps), shoulder abduction (deltoid), foot dorsiflexion (tibialis anterior), knee extension (quadriceps), and hip flexion (iliopsoas).

Table 33-1 **MRC Strength Examination**

- 5 = normal strength
- 4 = weak but able to move the muscle against a resistance
- 3 = able to move the muscle against gravity but not against resistance
- 2 = able to move the muscle but not against gravity
- 1 = able to contract the muscle but not move the limb
- 0 = no visible contraction

Fatigue is a symptom that is difficult to demonstrate unless profound. In the absence of frank weakness, fatigue is seldom due to peripheral neuropathy and is more suggestive of a neuromuscular transmission abnormality such as myasthenia gravis.

Cramps are felt by the patient but are not always visible during examination. They are usually elicited by exercise of an affected muscle, and they may produce a visible contraction, indenting the muscle. Cramps are usually painful. Cramps can occur in patients without neuromuscular disease, so their presence is not pathologic in the absence of other findings.

Fasciculations are perceived by the patient as muscle twitches. They may appear during the examination as brief, twitching movements of the muscles under the skin. They are easiest to see in thin patients and are more prominent in selected muscle groups, especially the gastrocnemius. Fasciculations in the absence of other abnormalities on examination or testing are not abnormal; these are termed *benign fasciculations*. In patients with weakness, fasciculations can suggest motor neuron dysfunction, although they are not in themselves diagnostic of ALS.

SENSORY SIGNS

Sensory loss refers to an increased threshold for detection of a sensory stimulus. Sharp sensation with disposable wire or a broken Q-tip is most commonly used; needles are not needed and should not be used on successive patients. The patient usually reports that the sharp stimulus does not feel sharp, although absolute anesthesia is uncommon. The distribution of the sensory loss aids in the diagnosis. Patients with mononeuropathy or mononeuropathy multiplex will have one or more focal areas of altered sensory threshold. In polyneuropathy, the sensory deficit is most prominent in the distal extremities (*stocking-glove* distribution). The legs are typically affected prior to the arms, which may be asymptomatic at the time of presentation.

Hyperpathia is pain perceived with a non-noxious stimulus. A firm touch may cause pain. Patients often consider this a paradox; there is an increased sensory threshold, but when sensation is perceived it is painful.

Sensory ataxia is incoordination that is not due to motor or cerebellar dysfunction, but rather due to defective sensory input to the brain and spinal cord. The impaired coordination may resemble cerebellar ataxia.

Hyporeflexia refers to decreased tendon reflexes caused by loss of the sensory feedback from the muscles.

TYPES OF NEUROPATHIES

Symptoms and signs differ depending on the type of neuropathy. As mentioned above, neuropathies are divided into five fundamental pathologies: (1) axonal degenerations, (2) demyelinating neuropathies, (3) neuronal degenerations, (4) vascular neuropathies, and (5) mechanical damage. Mechanical and vascular neuropathies are usually focal, whereas most of the others are generalized.

Axonal polyneuropathies

Axonal neuropathies are the most common neuropathies. Many are related to systemic diseases, others are idiopathic or inherited. Symptoms and signs are usually motor and sensory, with the sensory symptoms predominating.

Nerve conduction studies (NCS) (see Chap. 38) show little change in maximal conduction velocity, indicating that the myelin sheaths are relatively intact, but with more severe involvement, conduction velocities can be mildly slow. Electromyography (EMG) shows chronic denervation with long-duration symptoms. Active denervation is seen with rapid progression of the disorder. If a lumbar puncture is performed, the findings in patients with axonal neuropathy are usually normal, except for occasional, mildly elevated cerebrospinal fluid (CSF) protein levels.

The differential diagnosis for axonal neuropathy is large, but some of the more important are: (1) diabetic polyneuropathy; (2) idiopathic polyneuropathy; (3) inherited neuropathies; and (4) toxic neuropathies, such as those due to chemotherapy agents or lead.

Demyelinating polyneuropathies

Demyelinating neuropathies are characterized by damage to the myelin sheath with relative preservation of the axon. With severe demyelination, there can be damage to the axons as well. Causes of demyelinating neuropathy are often autoimmune or inherited. Some of the most important demyelinating neuropathies are: (1) acute inflammatory demyelinating polyradiculoneuropathy (AIDP), (2) chronic inflammatory demyelinating polyradiculoneuropathy (CIDP), and (3) Charcot-Marie-Tooth disease (CMT).

AIDP and CIDP are discussed below. CMT is a family of hereditary neuropathies, in most of which demyelination is prominent. CMT is not common, but a family history should be sought in all patients with neuropathy, especially in patients with neuropathy without a defined cause.

NCS shows slowing of conduction which can be distal and/or proximal. EMG shows no denervation, unless the demyelination is long-standing and/or severe. On lumbar puncture, the CSF shows elevated protein in most patients with active demyelinating neuropathy; neuromuscular specialists use CSF analysis to monitor the activity of demyelinating neuropathies.

Neuronal degenerations

Neuronal degenerations are characterized by pathology of the nerve cell body, with secondary degeneration of the axon, resembling a pure-motor axonal neuropathy. Degenerations of the motor neurons are called motor neuron diseases (MNDs). MNDs are distinguished from axonal neuropathies by the absence of sensory involvement, involvement of proximal as well as distal muscles (axonal neuropathies are mainly distal), and other associated features, such as the prominence of fasciculations and muscle cramps and the involvement of the tongue.

The most important MNDs are: (1) ALS, (2) spinal muscular atrophy (SMA), and (3) primary lateral sclerosis (PLS).

Vascular neuropathies

Vascular neuropathies are caused by ischemia to a nerve or nerves. Some diabetic mononeuropathies, such as a diabetic III nerve palsy, are caused by occusion of the small arteries of the vasa nervorum, causing focal ischemia to the nerve. Vasculitic diseases, such as polyarteritis nodosa and rheumatoid arthritis, can cause neuropathy in multiple nerve distributions.

Mechanical neuropathies

Mechanical neuropathies include: (1) direct trauma, (2) stretch injuries, and (3) entrapment or compression neuropathies.

Direct trauma is damage to the nerve from transient compression or section. The damage can be of three basic types: neurapraxia, axonotmesis, and neurotmesis. *Neurapraxia* involves damage to the axons, but without severing of the nerve. There is loss of function distal to the lesion, but the prognosis is generally good, since the axons can repair themselves to some extent. Recovery is good, but often incomplete. *Axonotmesis* involves damage to the axon with preservation of the supporting tissues, usually resulting from more severe compression. The prognosis and speed for recovery are less favorable, but patients can have substantial improvement, since the axons can regrow along the neural sheath. *Neurotmesis* is severing of the nerve, including axons and supporting tissues. Neurotmesis is usually due to penetrating trauma such as a knife or bullet. The prognosis for recovery is poor, since in humans peripheral nerve regeneration is very limited. Repair of the nerve sheath by microsurgical techniques can offer improved recovery, but reinnervation is not assured. Transient compression producing nerve damage is common with the radial nerve (*Saturday night palsy*) and peroneal nerve.

Stretch is usually from trauma in which a limb is distracted. The supporting tissues are able to stretch better than the axons, so stretch injuries are often in the axonotmesis category. If the stretch is mild, neurapraxia can result, allowing rapid improvement. Recovery from significant stretch injury is often incomplete and very protracted because of the proximal nature of the lesion. Common types of stretch injury are seen with upward or downward pulling of the arm. Downward distraction of the arm results in stretch of the upper aspect of the brachial plexus, supplied by C5 and C6 nerve roots. Patients have weakness especially of the deltoid and biceps, affecting arm flexion and abduction. Upward motion of the arm produces stretch of the lower brachial plexus, with resultant weakness of muscles innervated by the C8 and T1 nerve roots. This is a common injury in motorcycle accidents. Other nerve stretch injuries can occur with dislocation of almost any joint.

Entrapment is ongoing compression of a nerve in a susceptible region. The cause may be partly developmental and partly environmental, meaning that patients may have a susceptible anatomy, such as a small carpal tunnel, perhaps made smaller by weight gain or pregnancy, but also provocative activity such as repetitive use of a computer. Common entrapment neuropathies include the median nerve at the wrist (CTS) and ulnar nerve near the elbow (cubital tunnel syndrome). Release of the entrapment is often needed to allow improvement and cessation of progression of the deficit.

DIFFERENTIAL DIAGNOSIS

Types of peripheral neuropathy

For the purpose of differential diagnosis, it is helpful to begin with a simplified classification of neuropathies into the following categories: (1) acute versus subacute versus chronic, (2) axonal versus demyelinating versus neuronal, and (3) sensory versus motor versus both. With correct classification of the neuropathies, the differential diagnosis can be significantly narrowed. For example, an acutely developing demyelinating neuropathy with both sensory and motor involvement is likely AIDP. On the other hand, a chronic neuronal degeneration producing only motor involvement is most likely a motor neuron degeneration such as ALS.

Alternatives to peripheral neuropathy

MYOPATHY

Myopathy refers to inflammation or degeneration of skeletal muscle. Myopathy is distinct from neuropathy, but it must be considered in the differential diagnosis of neuropathies which have mainly motor symptoms and signs. Most myopathies (see Chap. 34) are associated with proximal weakness, whereas most neuropathies affect distal muscles. Sensory loss and loss of reflexes also favor neuropathy.

NEUROMUSCULAR TRANSMISSION ABNORMALITIES

Weakness is the most common complaint of patients with disorders of neuromuscular transmission. Although these conditions are much rarer than neuropathies, they have to be considered when patients report weakness without sensory complaints. Important neuromuscular transmission disorders include: (1) myasthenia gravis, (2) Lambert-Eaton myasthenic syndrome, and (3) botulism. These disorders can be difficult to diagnose, but all have as their hallmarks a fatiguing weakness, usually starting in the ocular and facial muscles in myasthenia gravis, in the limbs in Lambert-Eaton syndrome, and with autonomic signs as well as bulbar weakness in botulism (see Chap. 35). Neuropathies are not associated with dramatic fatigue in strength testing, and they involve distal muscles and may also affect sensation and reflexes.

MOTOR NEURONOPATHIES

Motor neuron diseases (MNDs) are included in the differential diagnosis of peripheral neuropathies, although the only pure motor peripheral neuropathy is multifocal motor neuropathy (MMN). MMN is a pure-motor neuropathy, usually painless, and associated with severe slowing or conduction block on nerve conduction studies. This neuropathy is important to diagnose because it has a much better prognosis than MND, and it may respond to immunomodulatory treatments. MNDs typically produce symptoms of upper and/or lower motor neuron dysfunction. The important entities are: (1) ALS, (2) SMA, and (3) PLS. MNDs are diagnosed by finding signs of upper and/or lower motor neuron dysfunction in the absence of sensory symptoms and with no other structural or functional cause, such as diabetes, spinal stenosis, stroke, and vitamin B_{12} deficiency, to name just a few. Luckily, most of these other conditions produce both motor and sensory symptoms.

LABORATORY AND RADIOLOGICAL INVESTIGATION

Laboratory studies used for the evaluation of peripheral neuropathy begin with NCS and EMG. This is a two-part single test which helps to identify and characterize peripheral neuropathies. If the electrophysiologic testing confirms the diagnosis of neuropathy, other tests are indicated depending on the type.

Screening tests for peripheral polyneuropathy might include: (1) EMG and NCS; (2) blood studies, including complete blood test (CBC), creatine kinase (CK), thyroid function tests, vitamin B_{12} level, folic acid level, erythrocyte sedimentation rate (ESR), and antinuclear antibody (ANA); and (3) if there is a risk of heavy metal exposure, a 24-hour urine for lead, mercury, arsenic, and thallium.

NCS and EMG

NCS is measurement of conduction of compound motor and sensory action potentials from peripheral nerves.

Motor nerve conduction study is performed by stimulation of a mixed (motor and sensory) nerve and recording from electrodes overlying a muscle. By stimulating at two points along the course of the nerve and recording the two compound motor action potentials (CMAPs), the conduction velocity can be calculated by dividing the distance between the two stimulating sites by the time difference between the CMAPs. There are standard values for NCV and amplitude of the CMAP. In general, NCV is more important for interpretation than CMAP amplitude.

Sensory nerve conduction study is performed by stimulation of the sensory portion of a peripheral nerve and recording from the same nerve proximal to the stimulation site. The conduction velocity is calculated directly by dividing the distance between the stimulating and recording sites by the latency of the sensory nerve action potential (SNAP). There are normal values for sensory NCV and SNAP amplitude. In general, the NCV is more important for interpretation than the SNAP amplitude.

Electromyography EMG is performed by recording directly from muscles, using a small electrode which is part of a needle. The needle electrode is inserted directly into the muscle, and recordings are made at rest and during voluntary contractions. Normally, there is no electrical activity at rest, and there are well-formed triphasic motor unit potentials (MUPs) with voluntary activation. The MUPs are the compound action potentials created by activation of a group of muscle fibers by electrical discharge of a single motor axon.

Interpretation of the NCS and EMG is complex but can be summarized by the following guidelines: (1) slowing of NCV indicates a defect in myelin, such as a demyelinating neuropathy; (2) denervation changes on EMG indicate a defect in the axon, such as an axonal neuropathy; (3) slowing of one segment of a single nerve indicates a mononeuropathy, suggesting nerve entrapment; (4) slowing of NCV of multiple nerves indicates a polyneuropathy.

Nerve and muscle biopsy

Nerve biopsy is needed for only a small percentage of patients with peripheral neuropathy. The main use is for patients with suspected inflammatory neuropathies, such as CIDP or vasculitis, rarely for infections such as leprosy or protein depositions such as amyloidosis.

Muscle biopsy is performed mainly when the differential diagnosis includes myopathy. The most common findings are inflammatory myopathy (polymyositis and dermatomyositis) and muscular dystrophies.

Imaging

Imaging is rarely performed for peripheral neuropathy. Polyneuropathy is not associated with focal, structural lesions, with the exception of a paraneoplastic neuropathy associated with a malignant tumor.

Mononeuropathy is usually related to predictable compression at the carpal tunnel (median nerve), fibular head (peroneal nerve), or another, similar area. Rarely, a mononeuropathy may be due to tumor infiltration or compression, which can be visualized on MRI or computed tomography (CT).

Analytical laboratory

Blood and urine analysis is commonly performed for patients with neuropathy.

BLOOD

Numerous blood studies can be performed for patients with peripheral neuropathy. Some of these are: (1) serum immunoelectrophoresis (SIEP) or immunofixation for paraproteins; (2) hemoglobin A1C to detect diabetes; (3) B_{12} level for pernicious anemia; (4) folic acid level; (5) human immunodeficiency virus (HIV) screening for patients at risk; and (6) antinuclear antibody (ANA), extractable neuronal antibody ENA, ANCA (antinuclear cytoplasmic antibody, both the p- and c-types), erythrocyte sedimentation rate (ESR), and C' reactive protein (CRP) for autoimmune or inflammatory disorders. Blood studies are not always needed if the cause of the neuropathy is obvious, as in diabetics or patients who have received chemotherapy. However, the clinician must be vigilant for other causes of neuropathy.

Special analyses for specific neuropathies are available as *neuropathy panels* on a commercial basis; these panels of tests are less expensive to perform than long lists of individual studies. Such panels include examinations for paraneoplastic antibodies and antiganglioside neuropathies.

URINE

Routine urinalysis is not of much value in the evaluation of patients with peripheral neuropathy. Twenty four-hour urine for heavy metals can be ordered if there is a suspicion of a heavy metal-induced neuropathy. Urine tests for porphobilinogen can detect the rare neuropathies related to porphyria.

Top 10 peripheral neuropathies

DIABETIC NEUROPATHY

Diabetic neuropathy is the most common neuromuscular disorder seen in neurologic practice. Almost every patient with diabetes eventually develops peripheral neuropathy. Most patients have loss of sensation but do not have pain sufficient to need treatment. Many patients, however, develop neuropathic pain with burning and/or shooting pain.

Diabetic neuropathy can be divided into several specific types: (1) distal, small-fiber neuropathy; (2) diabetic polyradiculopathy, also called *proximal diabetic neuropathy* or *diabetic amyotrophy*; (3) sensorimotor polyneuropathy; (4) diabetic mononeuropathy; (5) mononeuritis multiplex.

The polyneuropathies are commonly painful and can produce burning pain along with sensory loss in the feet. With progression, the hands may be involved.

Mononeuropathy develops in many patients and is often superimposed on a polyneuropathy. The ulnar nerve is commonly affected, producing weakness of the intrinsic muscles of the hand and decreased sensation on digits 4 and 5 of the hand. Bilateral ulnar neuropathy is common in DM. Cranial nerves can also be involved, most commonly the III nerve, but occasionally the IV, VI, or VII nerves.

The diagnosis of diabetic neuropathy depends on a history of DM, or the presence of laboratory markers of DM on a screening evaluation, such as an elevated fasting glucose, elevated hemoglobin A1C, or abnormal glucose tolerance test. The neuropathy may precede the diagnosis of diabetes, so vigilance for later development of DM is warranted.

The treatment of diabetic neuropathy is largely symptomatic, though tight glucose control may prevent worsening of the neuropathy. Tricyclic antidepressants, a new antidepressant drug duloxetine (Cymbalta), and a few anticonvulsant drugs are helpful in reducing neuropathic pain in patients with diabetic neuropathy. Foot care is needed; the loss of foot sensation predisposes the diabetic patient to injury with development of serious infections.

AIDP

AIDP is also known as Guillain-Barré syndrome (GBS). AIDP is caused by autoimmune-mediated damage to the myelin sheath. The diagnosis should be suspected when there is a combination of acute to subacute onset of weakness and areflexia. The first symptom is often tingling and fatigue, leading to many misdiagnoses of psychogenic illness, yet as the disease progresses the weakness becomes far more profound than the sensory dysfunction. An ascending pattern of weakness is most common, but many variations occur on this theme. A minority of patients have pain, either in the limbs or in the back. The examination shows weakness with decreased reflexes. The tendon reflexes are depressed in almost all cases and usually become totally absent over time. Increased tendon reflexes are not expected and should lead to suspicion of a spinal or cerebral cause for the weakness.

The diagnosis of AIDP is supported by NCSs which show slowing of nerve conduction velocity. The NCSs, however, may not become abnormal until a few days into the illness. EMG is initially normal, but with prolonged and severe weakness can show denervation. CSF shows increased protein with no cellular response.

The treatment is supportive, with close monitoring of pulmonary function tests (see Chap. 23); some patients require mechanical ventilation. Recovery is hastened by immune suppression by intravenous immunoglobulin (IVIG) or plasma exchange. Corticosteroids are of no value.

CIDP

CIDP is an autoimmune demyelination of the peripheral nerves which has a more indolent course than AIDP and may be progressive or have episodic exacerbations. The immunology of CIDP is different from that of AIDP. The symptoms are weakness and sensory change which is generalized, although it may be asymmetric. Dysesthesias are common.

The examination shows weakness with sensory loss, most prominent distally. Tendon reflexes are often decreased and may be absent. There are no corticospinal tract signs. NCS shows demyelinating polyneuropathy. EMG may show denervation with prolonged duration of symptoms.

The treatment of CIDP involves immune modulation, but the approach differs from AIDP; while steroids are of no benefit for AIDP, they are of significant benefit for many patients with CIDP. IVIG and plasma exchange are also used for patients with CIDP. Chemotherapeutic agents are also sometimes used in refractory cases, with mainly anecdotal evidence of benefit.

MECHANICAL NEUROPATHIES

Mechanical neuropathies are due to pressure or stretch of an area of peripheral nerve at a sensitive location or entrapment at selected areas. The most important compressive neuropathies are: (1) carpal tunnel syndrome, median nerve entrapment at the wrist; (2) ulnar nerve compression at the elbow; (3) radial nerve compression in the upper arm; (4) peroneal nerve compression at the fibular neck.

CTS is the most common entrapment neuropathy (see Chap. 32). Ulnar neuropathy produces sensory loss on the ulnar aspect of the palm and dorsal aspect of the hand, but not into the forearm. Digits 5 and the ulnar half of 4 are affected. Weakness of the ulnar-innervated intrinsic muscles of the hand is often seen. Pain in the elbow region radiating down the arm is common. The examination shows tenderness in the ulnar groove (Tinel's sign), sensory loss in a distal ulnar-nerve distribution, and often weakness of the interossei.

Radial compression at the upper arm is often seen in alcoholics who fall asleep with an arm over the back of a chair while intoxicated, hence the name *Saturday night palsy*. The depth of sleep, decreased tone, and immobility cause radial nerve compression, most prominent at the spiral groove. The most prominent symptom and sign is a *wrist drop*. Patients often complain of weakness of the entire arm, because the lack of radial stabilization prevents full use of the median- and ulnar-innervated muscles, particularly wrist and finger flexion. Examination shows the radial weakness with loss of wrist and finger extension. The wrist and finger flexors may seem weak, because the wrist goes into flexion with attempted contraction; when the examiner stabilizes the wrist, strength of the wrist and finger flexors appears normal.

Peroneal compression at the fibular neck is commonly seen with prolonged bed rest, where the peroneal nerve is compressed by bed railings. Weakness and immobility predispose to the peroneal compression. The symptoms involve weakness of the foot extensors, or *foot drop*, along with numbness on the top of the foot which is often not noticed. Examination shows weakness of the tibialis anterior with preservation of the gastrocnemius and other posterior tibial-innervated muscles. The diagnosis is supported by a NCS showing impaired conduction across the fibular neck.

AMYOTROPHIC LATERAL SCLEROSIS (ALS)

ALS is a neuronal degeneration affecting both upper and lower motor neurons. There is no alteration of sensation. The cause is unknown, although genetic and environmental factors may play a role. The symptoms include weakness, usually noted first in the hands and arms, with the legs affected later. Occasionally, the disease can present with weakness in the legs or in the bulbar muscles. Coordination difficulty and frank weakness are typical. Muscle twitching is often noted, and if not reported by the patient should be asked about. Muscle cramps are common. There are no sensory symptoms, although patients may report the sensory complaints from the twitching and cramps. The signs of ALS include weakness, again most prominent in the arms, with the intrinsic muscles of the hands most severely affected. Wasting of the interossei is often obvious at presentation. Upper motor neuron degeneration produces increased reflexes and upgoing plantar responses. The hallmark of ALS is the presence of both upper and lower motor neuron signs (spastic tone, hyperreflexia and wasting, fasciculations) in the same limb. Fasciculations may be noted in the arms, legs, and/or tongue. While fasciculations are not always pathologic and not specific for ALS, the presence of tongue fasciculations with limb weakness and upper motor neuron signs is very suspicious for this disease. Dysarthria is common with advancement of the disease. Visual changes are absent.

The diagnosis of ALS is predominantly clinical. NCSs are normal. EMG shows widespread denervation with involvement of proximal and distal muscles. The finding of upper motor neuron signs is required for security of the diagnosis of ALS. Imaging is normal.

The treatment of ALS is symptomatic. Anticonvulsants such as phenytoin are used for bothersome fasciculations, although most patients do not need to be treated. Riluzole (Rilutek) appears to slow the progression of the disease, increasing average survival by about 3 months, but some specialists believe that the modest benefit is not worth the expense and adverse effects.

B$_{12}$ DEFICIENCY AND OTHER NUTRITIONAL NEUROPATHIES

Vitamin B$_{12}$ deficiency is usually due to impaired absorption rather than due to nutritional deficiency. Rarely, vegans can take so little B$_{12}$ in their diets that they develop B$_{12}$ deficiency, but the more common causes are the disease pernicious anemia, in which the vitamin cannot be absorbed, or patients who have had small bowel resections or have loss of gastric acid. B_{12} deficiency can result in macrocytic anemia, although not all patients develop hematologic abnormalities, and neurologic manifestations may predate the hematologic manifestations.

Neurologic complications of B_{12} deficiency include polyneuropathy, ataxia, and corticospinal tract findings which would suggest CNS changes. There may also be mood changes and encephalopathy, formerly referred to as *megaloblastic madness*. The history is usually of weakness, ataxia, and/or confusion. The examination shows findings commensurate with the neurologic lesion(s), and can include: (1) dementia; (2) corticospinal tract findings with hyperreflexia and upgoing plantars; (3) peripheral neuropathy with sensory loss and paresthesias (some of which may be attributable to degeneration of the posterior columns of the spinal cord); and (4) sensory ataxia affecting both limb coordination and gait. Tendon reflexes may sometimes be decreased despite corticospinal tract dysfunction because of the polyneuropathy. In addition, visual loss occurs rarely.

The laboratory diagnosis of vitamin B_{12} deficiency starts with a reduced B_{12} level in the serum. Measurement of methylmalonic acid levels is of even greater sensitivity. MRI is not diagnostic, but may show some abnormalities on T2-weighted imaging of the spinal cord.

The treatment of B_{12} deficiency is by replacement with injections; oral replacement has been long thought to be ineffective, but recently some success has been reported with large-dose oral B_{12} replacement, on the order of 1000 mcg daily. The prognosis is good, in that there is likely to be significant improvement after B_{12} replacement.

Other vitamin deficiencies are less likely to produce polyneuropathy and are not discussed here in detail. The most important is thiamine; patients with thiamine deficiency associated with alcoholism are predisposed to polyneuropathy in addition to cognitive disturbance and cerebellar ataxia. Neuropathy can also be seen in patients with pellagra, a deficiency of niacin (vitamin B_3) and often other B vitamins, as well as the amino acid tryptophan, and in pyridoxine (B_6) deficiency. Pyridoxine deficiency develops in patients on the antituberculous drug isoniazid, and this drug is now routinely supplemented with oral pyridoxine.

CHEMOTHERAPY NEUROPATHY

Chemotherapy is well recognized to produce peripheral neuropathy. Polyneuropathy is the most prominent manifestation, although mononeuropathies can develop. Chemotherapeutic agents which are especially likely to produce polyneuropathy are vincristine, cisplatin, paclitaxel, and etoposide, although other agents have also been reported to produce neuropathy as well.

Chemotherapy neuropathy can progress for a few months after cessation of the drug. Subsequently, the neuropathy can significantly improve.

Treatments for neuropathic pain are often needed. There is no treatment available to improve recovery.

AIDS NEUROPATHY

HIV is associated with peripheral neuropathy of various types. Among these are: (1) immune-mediated neuropathy resembling AIDP or CIDP, (2) cytomegalovirus (CMV) polyradiculitis, and (3) Herpes zoster or *shingles*.

HIV screening is not part of the evaluation of most patients with neuropathy, although this should be considered, especially in patients with HIV risk factors, those with herpes zoster, and those with painful sensory neuropathy without an obvious cause.

Treatment for the HIV is required, but it does not have a clear effect on the neuropathy. Treatments for neuropathic pain are required for many patients.

FAMILIAL NEUROPATHIES

Familial neuropathies can be demyelinating or axonal. Inheritance can be dominant or recessive. There may be other associated symptoms including central neurologic dysfunction. The general clue to the identification of a familial neuropathy is onset early in life, as well as a history of similar neuropathies in other family members. Hereditary sensory motor neuropathy (HSMN) is the general abbreviation given for the most common type of hereditary neuropathy. CMT is the prototypic HSMN. CMT is divided into four categories: (1) CMT-1, an autosomal dominant neuropathy with hypertrophy of nerves and both sensory and motor findings; (2) CMT-2, autosomal dominant neuropathy of usually pure motor type, without nerve hypertrophy; (3) CMT-3, autosomal recessive neuropathy, also called Dejerine-Sottas disease, or a sporadic neuropathy with hypertrophic changes; and (4) CMT-4, autosomal recessive neuropathy with onset in childhood.

In addition, there are many other hereditary neuropathies, which are less common and less important for routine practice, including the hereditary sensory autonomic neuropathies (HSAN). These neuropathies are suspected by the clinical appearance, including the appearance of autonomic signs such as orthostatic hypotension, and the absence of other causes identified on laboratory study.

PARANEOPLASTIC NEUROPATHY

Polyneuropathy is commonly seen in patients with cancer, usually due to chemotherapy or radiation therapy. Direct nerve infiltration is uncommon. A rare cause is paraneoplastic neuropathy, where antibodies induced by a tumor result in polyneuropathy or other neurologic complication. Panels of tests for paraneoplastic antibodies are available commercially.

Treatment of peripheral neuropathies

The treatment of peripheral neuropathy is either disease-modifying or symptomatic. Disease-modifying treatment can result in symptomatic improvement, provided that the neurons can regenerate.

DISEASE-MODIFYING TREATMENT

Disease-modifying treatment is available for only a small minority of causes of neuropathy. Treatments can include nutritional supplementation, immune-modulating therapy, or anti-infective treatment. Nutritional supplementation is beneficial mainly for patients with B_{12} deficiency, rarely for patients with pellagra (B_3) or pyridoxine (B_6) deficiency, such as that associated with isoniazid. Isolated deficiency of any other vitamin is unlikely to produce peripheral neuropathy. Immune-modulating therapy is used for patients with autoimmune neuropathies. Options for immune treatment include: (1) corticosteroids; (2) IVIG; (3) plasma exchange, or plasmapheresis; and (4) chemotherapeutic agents. AIDP is treated with IVIG or plasma exchange. Corticosteroids are not helpful for AIDP, and chemotherapeutic agents are not used. CIDP can be managed with any of these treatments. Corticosteroids and IVIG are most commonly used, although chemotherapeutic agents have been employed as steroid-sparing agents. MMN is usually treated with IVIG, although cyclophosphamide may also be helpful; corticosteroids have not shown benefit.

SYMPTOMATIC TREATMENT

Symptomatic treatment of peripheral neuropathies includes treatment for neuropathic pain, cramps, and fasciculations. There is no pharmacological treatment for sensory loss or weakness.

Neuropathic pain

Neuropathic pain is treated by medications and physical means. Some of the classes of treatment, as discussed in Chap. 17, are: (1) anticonvulsants; (2) antidepressants, especially amitriptyline and duloxetine (Cymbalta); (3) analgesics, including both narcotic and non-narcotic agents; and (4) anesthetic agents.

Anticonvulsants include carbamazepine (Tegretol), classically used for patients with sharp, shooting pains, as in trigeminal neuralgia; gabapentin (Neurontin); pregabilin (Lyrica); topiramate (Topamax); lamotrigine (Lamictal); and levetiracetam (Keppra).

Many of these agents are not specifically approved for treatment of neuropathic pain. Anticonvulsants are used mostly for lancinating pain and dysesthesias. These are large-axon symptoms which are particularly susceptible to anticonvulsant treatment.

Antidepressants are among the most powerful treatments for neuropathic pain. They not only help the pain, itself, but also can help depressive symptoms which frequently accompany chronic pain. Of the antidepressants, tricyclic antidepressants TCAs are generally thought of as more effective, followed by selective serotonin and neuroepinephrine reuptake inhibitors (SSNRIs) and selective serotonin reuptake inhibitors (SSRIs). While there are multiple agents used, the most commonly used agents are amitriptyline (Elavil) and duloxetine (Cymbalta). Antidepressants are commonly used in combination with anticonvulsants and/or analgesics.

Analgesics are required for some patients with neuropathic pain. Routine use of narcotic analgesics should be minimized. Nonopioid agents are commonly used at night when neuropathic pain disturbs falling asleep. Opiate analgesics are used if patients do not respond to nonopioid agents including anticonvulsants and antidepressants. Of the opioid analgesics, sustained-release agents generally are preferred over immediate release agents because of their effectiveness and lesser abuse potential. Among the agents used for neuropathic pain are: (1) acetamenophen (Tylenal); (2) propoxyphene with or without acetaminophen (Darvon or Darvocet); (3) sustained release oxycodone (Oxycontin); (4) sustained release morphine (MS Contin); (5) tramadol (Ultram); (6) hydrocodone preparations (Lortab, Vicodin); (7) codeine preparations (Tylenal #3); and (8) fentanyl transdermal patch (Duragesic). When opioid analgesics are used, prescriptions should be provided by only one practitioner, and doses and amounts should be monitored. Patients must be counseled about the risk of addiction.

Local anesthetics are used for some patients with neuropathic pain. Lidoderm patches are helpful in patients with very localized pain, as in postherpetic neuralgia. The patches can be applied in the anatomic distribution of the pain.

NONPHARMACOLOGICAL TREATMENTS

Nonpharmacological treatments include: (1) physical therapy, (2) relaxation therapies of various types, (3) transcutaneous electric nerve stimulation (TENS), (4) infrared light therapy, and (5) magnetic stimulation. Physical therapy helps to maintain use of affected limbs and improve strength. Infrared (Anodyne) therapy has been found to be very effective for patients with foot pain due to diabetic neuropathy. Other causes of neuropathy also appear to respond to infrared therapy. Although expensive, the freedom from adverse effects makes this a good option for many patients. TENS and magnetic stimulation have both been found effective for some patients with neuropathic pain. Magnetic stimulation is performed in a variety of ways with peripheral treatments including static and pulsed magnetic fields. Transcranial magnetic stimulation is also being studied, though this should not be considered part of routine therapy.

Cramps and fasciculations

Cramps are due to repetitive discharge of muscle fibers which can be due to electrical transmission between damaged motor axons. Patients with damage to the peripheral nerves may have cramps, though these can also be seen in some myopathies. Cramps are treated by many of the same anticonvulsants used for neuropathic pain.

Fasciculations are spontaneous single discharges of motor axons, which can occasionally be seen in some normal patients, in the *benign cramp and fasciculation* syndrome; in peripheral neuropathies with denervation; and in MNDs, including ALS. Fasciculations are seen in some patients without any complaints. Patients may be aware of the fasciculations especially in the calves. The twitching can be felt by some patients. Fasciculations are also treated with anticonvulsants as listed above, though phenytoin (Dilantin) is particularly helpful for many patients. Fasciculations usually do not require treatment.

COURSE AND PROGNOSIS

Peripheral neuropathy is a chronic condition, but the prognosis depends on the etiology. Some general predictions follow: (1) idiopathic, axonal polyneuropathy gradually worsens, though it is usually not disabling; patients may have distal weakness and sensory loss, but it does not spread throughout the body; (2) AIDP worsens over days to 3–4 weeks, then stabilizes, then improves, usually leaving only mild distal weakness and numbness, with depressed distal reflexes; (3) CIDP is a progressive or relapsing disorder which improves with immune-modulating treatment; and (4) mononeuropathies may improve if there is not severe persistent nerve compression; if compression persists, there may be progressive sensory and motor loss.

KEY REFERENCES

Aring AM, Jones DE, Falko JM. Evaluation and prevention of diabetic neuropathy. *Am Fam Physician* 2005;71(11):2123–2128.

Briani C, Brannagan TH, Trojaborg W, et al. Chronic inflammatory demyelinating polyneuropathy. *Neuromusc Disord* 1996;6:311–325.

Bromberg MB. An approach to the evaluation of peripheral neuropathies. *Semin Neurol* 2005 Jun;25(2):153–159.

Burns TM, Ryan MM, Darras B, et al. Current therapeutic strategies for patients with polyneuropathies secondary to inherited metabolic disorders. *Mayo Clin Proc* 2003;78:858–868.

Chance PF, Fischbeck KH. Molecular genetics of Charcot-Marie-Tooth disease and related neuropathies. *Hum Mol Genet* 1994;3:1503–1507.

Chemali KR, Tsao B. Electrodiagnostic testing of nerves and muscles: when, why, and how to order. *Cleve Clin J Med* 2005 Jan;72(1):37–48.

DeJonghe B, Sharshar T, Lefaucheur J-P, et al. Paresis acquired in the intensive care unit. A prospective multicenter study. *JAMA* 2002;288:2859–2867.

Harden RN. Chronic neuropathic pain. Mechanisms, diagnosis, and treatment. *Neurologist* 2005;11(2):111–22.

Lacomis D, Petrella JT, Giuliani MJ. Causes of neuromuscular weakness in the intensive care unit: a study of ninety-two patients. *Muscle Nerve* 1998;21:610–617.

Lewis RA. Chronic inflammatory demyelinating polyneuropathy and other immune-mediated demyelinating neuropathies. *Semin Neurol* 2005;25(2):217–228.

Lupski JR, Chance PF, Garcia CA. Inherited primary peripheral neuropathies. Molecular genetics and clinical implications of CMT1A and HNPP. *JAMA* 1993;270:2326–2330.

Mendell JR, Sahenk Z. Painful sensory neuropathy. *N Engl J Med* 2003;348:1243–1255.

Plasma Exchange/Sandoglobulin Guillain-Barre Syndrome Trial Group. Randomised trial of plasma exchange, intravenous immunoglobulin, and combined treatments in Guillain-Barŕe syndrome. *Lancet* 1997;349:225–230.

Ropper AH. The Guillain-Barŕe syndrome. *N Engl J Med* 1992;326:1130–1136.

Ropper AH, Gorson KC. Neuropathies associated with paraproteinemia. *N Engl J Med* 1998;338:1601–1607.

Singleton JR. Evaluation and treatment of painful peripheral polyneuropathy. *Semin Neurol* 2005 Jun;25(2):185–195.

MYOPATHIES

Gerald M. Fenichel, MD

INTRODUCTION

Skeletal muscle is the largest organ system of the body. Skeletal muscle disorders may be either genetic or acquired. Genetic disorders encompass disturbances of structural proteins (dystrophies), disturbances of the energy of contraction, and disturbances of ion channels. Acquired disorders are mainly inflammatory.

PROXIMAL MUSCULAR DYSTROPHIES

Most muscular dystrophies have a childhood onset, but they may occur at all ages. Characteristic of each dystrophy is a molecular defect causing abnormal protein formation. The protein may be absent, in part or in whole. Each dystrophy therefore has variable phenotypic expression. In most dystrophies, the underlying molecular abnormality involves structural proteins.

Dystrophin deficiency

The responsible gene for dystrophin is located on the short arm of the X chromosome. Most cases are associated with a detectable deletion or duplication of segments within the gene. Whether the deletion is in frame or out of frame determines whether dystrophin is absent from the muscle or present in a reduced, altered form. The former is associated with the severe *Duchenne* form (Duchenne muscular dystrophy, DMD), while the latter causes the milder *Becker* form (Becker muscular dystrophy, BMD).

DUCHENNE MUSCULAR DYSTROPHY

Boys with DMD are usually normal at birth. During the first years, proximal weakness in the legs causes difficulty rising from the ground and climbing stairs. Tightness is noted in muscles that cross two joints in the legs (the iliotibial bands and the heel cords) causing toe walking and an unsteady gait.

351

Progression of weakness is relentless, and the ability to walk is lost by 8–10 years of age. Now, with prednisone therapy, bracing, reconstructive surgery, and physical therapy, the average age of wheelchair confinement is 12.2 years. Cardiomyopathy is invariable and, without treatment, death occurs by age 20.

Laboratory diagnosis of DMD involves clinical features, an elevated creatine kinase (CK), and myopathic electromyographic (EMG) changes. The serum concentration of CK is 10,000 IU or higher. EMG is usually no longer necessary, since a genetic test is available; the simplest confirmatory test is blood deoxyribonucleic acid (DNA), which confirms a deletion in the dystrophin gene. When a deletion is not detectable, muscle biopsy establishes the absence of dystrophin.

The management of the DMD patient includes physical therapy, bracing, scoliosis surgery, pharmacological therapy for heart failure, and prednisone. Prednisone improves muscle strength and function when started early. The beneficial effect lasts for at least 3 years.

BECKER MUSCULAR DYSTROPHY (BMD)

BMD shares all the characteristics of the severe, DMD form but has a milder course. Onset of weakness appears in the first decade, but some patients present as late as age 40. A frequent complaint, and sometimes the only symptom, is leg cramps. In many, the cardiomyopathy is more disabling than the weakness. Cardiac transplantation is then an option.

Laboratory diagnosis is similar to that of DMD. Serum CK concentrations are not elevated as high as in DMD. Diagnosis is either by showing a mutation in the dystrophin gene or reduced quantity or size of dystrophin on muscle biopsy. Therapy is similar to the measures for DMD, but often started later and done less aggressively.

Other limb-girdle dystrophies

Defects in other muscle proteins produce phenotypes similar to DMD and BMD. Because proximal muscles are involved more than distal muscles, the name *limb-girdle muscular dystrophies* (LGMDs) is used. LGMDs transmitted by autosomal dominant inheritance are designated LGMD type 1 and those by autosomal recessive inheritance as LGMD type 2. Autosomal recessive LGMD is more common than autosomal dominant LGMD.

Congenital muscular dystrophies

The congenital muscular dystrophies (CMDs) are a group of disorders that are usually present at birth with severe hypotonia and weakness. All are autosomal recessive traits and have some associated central nervous system dysfunction, especially mental retardation. Joint contractures at birth are prominent. Approximately half of occidental cases are associated with deficiency of the protein *merosin*. The most common form of CMD in Japan is Fukuyama type CMD secondary to deficiency of fukutin-related protein.

Characteristic of *the Walker-Warburg syndrome* and *Muscle-Eye-Brain disease* is the combination of muscular dystrophy, lissencephaly (a smooth, non-gyrated appearance to the cerebrum), cerebellar malformations, and severe retinal and eye malformations.

Emery-Dreifuss dystrophy (Emerin deficiency)

The inheritance of the most common form of Emery-Dreifuss muscular dystrophy (EDMD) is as an X-linked, recessive disease. Wasting and weakness occur in the upper arms, shoulders, and anterior compartment muscles of the legs. Contractures of the elbows, the posterior neck, the paraspinal muscles, and the Achilles tendons are early features. Conduction block caused by atrial paralysis is associated with cardiac arrhythmias and sometimes sudden death. DNA studies confirm the diagnosis. Most patients require a cardiac pacemaker at an early age.

Facioscapulohumeral dystrophy

Inheritance of facioscapulohumeral dystrophy (FSHD) is as an autosomal dominant trait. The genetic abnormality is a deletion in a 3.3 kB repeating sequence on chromosome 4q35. The severity of illness is in relationship to the deletion size. FSHD varies in severity even within the same family. Phenotypes vary from mild facial weakness to total paralysis of the face and limbs requiring wheelchair confinement during childhood. Onset is usually in adolescence. The most severe form of FSHD occurs in infancy. The face is passive and expressionless, and limb weakness is severe. Deafness and Coats' disease, an oxidative vascular degeneration of the retina, are associated. DNA studies establish the diagnosis. Treatment is supportive.

Distal muscular dystrophies

Several muscle dystrophies have a predominantly distal pattern of weakness. Such myopathies are relatively uncommon and are often mistaken for hereditary or acquired neuropathies or for motor neuron disorders. However, a serum CK concentration greater than 500 IU/L indicates a myopathic process.

MYOTONIC DISORDERS

Myotonia is difficulty of muscle relaxation after contraction. It may occur as an associated symptom of a muscular dystrophy or as part of a channelopathy.

Myotonic dystrophy

MYOTONIC DYSTROPHY TYPE 1

Myotonic dystrophy Type 1 (DM 1) is an autosomal dominant trait characterized by muscle wasting and weakness, myotonia, and multisystem abnormalities, including cardiomyopathy or cardiac arrhythmias, mild mental retardation, excessive daytime sleepiness, cataracts, and endocrine dysfunction. The genetic abnormality is a cytosine-thymine-guanine (CTG) trinucleotide repeat. The number of repeats correlates with severity of disease. The typical picture is one of distal weakness of all limbs. Facial weakness includes the masseter, temporalis, and sternocleidomastoid muscles ("hatchet-faced" appearance). Weakness may affect proximal muscles as well. With time, dysphonia and dysphagia are noted. Myotonia can be demonstrated by sharp percussion of the thenar muscle with a reflex hammer or by asking the patient to squeeze your hand. Percussion of the thenar eminence produces abduction of the thumb, which gradually relaxes and allows the thumb to return to resting. After squeezing the examiner's hand, the patient has difficulty letting go. Myotonia is worse in cold weather.

The diagnosis of myotonic dystrophy is predominantly clinical; this is a diagnosis, like Parkinson's disease, that the physician has to think of, upon seeing the patient, to diagnose; the diagnosis will not "pop out" by doing a systematic examination. EMG may confirm myopathic features and myotonia. DNA analysis establishes the diagnosis. Supportive treatment includes footdrop braces, mexiletine for myotonia, and modafinil for hypersomnolence.

Congenital myotonic dystrophy

Newborns of myotonic mothers have the largest number of CTG repeats and have severe disease. The main features are severe hypotonia, respiratory insufficiency, facial paralysis, failure to thrive, and mental retardation. Frequent respiratory infections are the rule.

MYOTONIC DYSTROPHY TYPE 2 (DM 2) OR PROXIMAL MYOTONIC MYOPATHY (PROMM)

DM2 affects proximal rather than distal muscles. Transmission is also by autosomal dominant inheritance. Cataracts occur but endocrine and cardiac disturbances are less common than in DM1. Muscle stiffness and pain usually begin in adult life. The prognosis is relatively good. Molecular diagnosis is available.

CHANNELOPATHIES

The clinical syndromes associated with ion channel abnormalities are usually myotonia, periodic paralysis, or both.

Calcium-channel abnormalities

FAMILIAL HYPOKALEMIC PERIODIC PARALYSIS

Familial hypokalemic periodic paralysis (FHPP) is an autosomal dominant trait. Onset of symptoms is in the second decade. During an attack, serum potassium may fall as low as 1.5 mEq/L, but weakness is noted at higher concentrations. The initial symptoms are a sense of heaviness in the legs or back. Proximal weakness follows. Distal weakness may also occur. Attacks last for several hours, but strength then returns completely. Attacks vary in severity and frequency and may occur several times per week to a few per year. A carbohydrate load often precipitates an attack. The clinical features plus the decreased concentration of serum potassium establish the diagnosis. Molecular genetic testing is available. An acute attack is treated by administration of 5–10 g of oral potassium. Acetazolamide is useful for prophylaxis.

Secondary hypokalemic paralysis

Secondary causes of hypokalemic periodic paralysis include thyrotoxicosis, renal or adrenal failure, overuse of potassium-depleting diuretics, and renal tubular acidosis.

Sodium-channel abnormalities

HYPERKALEMIC PERIODIC PARALYSIS (POTASSIUM-SENSITIVE PERIODIC PARALYSIS)

The main symptom of hyperkalemic periodic paralysis is weakness provoked by potassium exposure. Myotonia may be associated but is not prominent. Inheritance is as an autosomal dominant trait. Onset is in early childhood. Rest after exercise provokes an attack. Weakness develops rapidly. Exercise early in the course may abort an attack. Light attacks are characterized by fatigue and mild weakness, lasting less than an hour. During severe attacks, the patient is unable to arise from the chair or the bed.

Secondary hyperkalemic periodic paralysis

Hyperkalemia may cause weakness in disorders other than familial hyperkalemic periodic paralysis. The difference between secondary hyperkalemic periodic paralysis and genetic hyperkalemic periodic paralysis is that higher concentrations of potassium are required in secondary hyperkalemic periodic paralysis to cause weakness. Renal failure and potassium-retaining diuretics are causes of secondary hyperkalemic periodic paralysis.

PARAMYOTONIA CONGENITA

Paramyotonia congenita is the combination of hyperkalemic periodic paralysis and myotonia of the face, eyes, tongue, and hand muscles. Paramyotonia of the face causes stiffness of expression and narrowing of the palpebral fissures. Repeated exercise makes myotonia worse. Cold exposure worsens myotonia and causes muscle weakness. The clinical features and molecular diagnosis establish the diagnosis. Treatment is not required.

MYOTONIA FLUCTUANS

Myotonia fluctuans is a dominantly inherited trait. The characteristic features are muscle stiffness exacerbated by exercise or potassium ingestion. Bouts of stiffness characterize the onset in adolescence. The stiffness affects extraocular, bulbar, or limb muscles. It improves by loosening up the limb, as in myotonia congenita, but muscles become stiff after or during exercise. Weakness, unlike paramyotonia congenita, is not a part of the disorder. Abnormalities in exon 22 and exon 14 of the sodium channel gene are responsible. Mexiletine or acetazolamide are effective therapeutic agents.

Potassium-channel abnormalities

ANDERSEN'S SYNDROME

The features of Andersen's syndrome are periodic paralysis, cardiac arrhythmias, and dysmorphic features. Inheritance is autosomal dominant. The onset of paralysis is during the first two decades. Attacks are associated with either high or low serum potassium concentrations. Dysmorphic features may include wide-spaced eyes, low-set ears, a small chin, clinodactyly of the fifth finger, and syndactyly of the toes. Cardiac involvement includes prolongation of the QT interval, ventricular tachycardia, and fatal cardiac arrest.

Chloride-channel abnormalities

MYOTONIA CONGENITA

Both a dominant and a recessive form of myotonia congenital exist. The dominant form is usually milder than the recessive form. Myotonia is worse when sitting or when cold and relieved by activity. All muscles are involved, including the face and the tongue. In addition, particularly in the recessive form, muscular hypertrophy may be pronounced ("little Hercules" syndrome). Mexiletine relieves myotonia in some patients.

METABOLIC MYOPATHIES

Disturbances in providing energy for contraction cause exercise intolerance, cramps, and myoglobinuria. The three main categories of metabolic myopathies are disorders of carbohydrate metabolism, disorders of lipid metabolism, and disorders of mitochondria. Intramuscular carbohydrate stores are the initial energy source for muscle contraction. As exercise continues, blood supply to muscle increases, delivering glucose and lipids from other body stores. No effective treatment for metabolic myopathies is available.

Disorders of carbohydrate metabolism

MYOPHOSPHORYLASE DEFICIENCY

Muscle phosphorylase exists in two forms: phosphorylase a, the active form and phosphorylase b, the inactive form. Phosphorylase b kinase catalyzes the conversion of the inactive form to the active form. Abnormalities of activation result in absence of phosphorylase activity and exercise intolerance. Inheritance of myophosphorylase deficiency is an autosomal recessive trait.

Young children with myophosphorylase deficiency are unable to keep up with peers. Adolescents experience fatigue and pain within minutes of initiating exercise. The cramping pain may last for several hours. Needle electromyography of the cramped muscle is electrically silent. Microscopic examination of the muscle biopsy specimen shows increased glycogen in subsarcolemmal blebs and muscle fiber necrosis. Histochemical staining for myophosphorylase is absent, and biochemical assay of enzyme activity shows significant reduction.

Other enzyme deficiencies

Similar clinical syndromes result from deficiencies in other enzymes that support glycolysis. These are phosphofructokinase (PFK) deficiency, phosphoglycerate kinase deficiency, phosphoglycerate mutase deficiency, and lactate dehydrogenase deficiency. Transmission of phosphoglycerate kinase deficiency is by X-linked inheritance, whereas all of the others are autosomal recessive traits.

Disorders of lipid metabolism

CARNITINE PALMITOYL TRANSFERASE (CPT) DEFICIENCY

Fatty acids become increasingly important after 20–30 minutes of endurance exercise, and they are the major energy suppliers after 1 hour. CPT links carnitine to long-chain fatty acids, to transport the fatty acid across the mitochondrial membrane from outside to inside (CPT-I), and then unhooks carnitine after transport (CPT-II). CPT-I deficiency causes a systemic disorder of infants. CPT-II deficiency, an autosomal recessive trait, causes exercise intolerance and myoglobinuria.

The onset of symptoms in CPT deficiency is usually after age 20. The first episode of weakness and myoglobinuria occurs after strenuous exercise, especially in cold weather and a period of fasting. Biochemical analysis of the muscle reveals the deficiency of CPT.

CARNITINE DEFICIENCY MYOPATHY

Carnitine influences the balance between free coenzyme A (CoA) and acylated CoA in the mitochondria and transfers long-chain fatty acids across the mitochondrial membrane under the action of the enzyme CPT. Most carnitine deficiencies are secondary to a defect in another enzyme system, a mitochondrial disorder, or a systemic disease. Carnitine deficiency is more likely to produce a slowly progressive proximal weakness rather than exercise intolerance, cramps, and myoglobinuria. Treatment with oral l-carnitine is not always successful.

MITOCHONDRIAL MYOPATHIES

Several defects in respiratory chain function cause mitochondrial myopathies. Muscle is rarely the only organ affected. Other organ involvement includes the brain, eye, heart, and kidney. Skeletal muscle involvement usually produces a progressive proximal myopathy and exercise intolerance. Severe mitochondrial diseases cause lactic acidosis. Histochemistry of affected muscle usually shows *ragged-red fibers*. Treatment of most mitochondrial disorders is limited to managing lactic acidosis.

CONGENITAL MYOPATHIES

Congenital myopathies are genetic disorders presenting at birth with hypotonia and areflexia. The weakness tends to be nonprogressive or only slowly progressive. Unlike dystrophies, the serum concentration of creatine kinase is either normal or only modestly elevated. Muscle biopsy is critical to diagnosis. The basis for differentiating individual disorders is their muscle histology.

CENTRAL CORE DISEASE

Central core disease is an autosomal dominant trait. Malignant hyperthermia and central core disease coexist in some families. The affected newborn is hypotonic and may have congenital hip dislocation. Motor milestones are delayed. Examination reveals diffuse limb and face weakness. Tendon reflexes are hypoactive. Associated skeletal abnormalities include pes cavus and a high-arched palate. Muscle biopsy is diagnostic. Cross-section reveals type 1 fiber predominance with central cores of myofibrillary disorganization. Specific treatment is not available.

NEMALINE MYOPATHY

Nemaline myopathy is genetically and clinically heterogeneous. Both dominant and recessive forms exist. Most common is congenital hypotonia, slow progression of facial and limb weakness, and scoliosis. Cardiomyopathy may be associated. A severe infantile variety is fatal. Such newborns have profound hypotonia and respiratory failure. Muscle biopsy reveals small, rod-like particles in muscle fibers. Treatment is supportive.

CENTRONUCLEAR OR MYOTUBULAR MYOPATHY (MTM)

The terms *centronuclear* or *myotubular myopathy* (MTM) encompass a group of disorders in which muscle fibers containing central nuclei resemble the myotube stage in muscle development. The severe infantile form is X-linked and characterized by extraocular, facial, and limb weakness. It is fatal from respiratory failure. One other X-linked and two autosomal forms also exist. Laboratory studies show normal or slightly elevated serum CK concentrations, and a characteristic muscle histology in which the center of muscle fibers contains a large, plump nucleus. Like other congenital myopathies, type 1 fibers predominate.

CONGENITAL FIBER-TYPE DISPROPORTION MYOPATHY

Children with congenital fiber-type disproportion myopathy are floppy at birth and diffusely weak. The face and neck are involved. Contractures of the heel cords and congenital hip dislocation are common. Weakness remains throughout life. Type 1 fibers are smaller but more numerous than type II fibers. Autosomal dominant inheritance occurs in approximately 40% of cases.

INFLAMMATORY MYOPATHIES

Inflammatory myopathies are either secondary to an underlying immune-mediated disorder or an infectious process. Polymyositis and dermatomyositis are examples of immune-mediated disorders, whereas several viruses, bacteria, and parasites cause infectious myositis.

DERMATOMYOSITIS

Dermatomyositis results from a humeral attack on muscle capillaries. It is the most common form of myositis in children. Dermatomyositis in adults is often associated with an underlying malignancy. In childhood dermatomyositis, the onset of rash is usually coincident with the onset of muscle weakness. A purplish discoloration of the skin appears over the cheeks and eyelids that blanches with pressure. The rash spreads over the body, affecting the extensor surfaces of the limbs. Soft-tissue calcification may occur with disease progression. Weakness is symmetrical, affecting proximal more than distal muscles, and may be painful.

The diagnosis is primarily by CK testing and muscle biopsy; EMG testing and magnetic resonance (MR) imaging of muscle are also helpful. The serum CK concentration is elevated but is not always proportional to disease activity. The characteristic histological feature is *perifascicular atrophy*, small myofibers surrounding normal-sized fibers deeper in the fascicle. The fibers around the edge of the fascicles are the watershed region of blood supply.

The treatment of childhood dermatomyositis begins with high-dose steroids, and usually there is some response. Other types of immunosuppressive drugs, such as methotrexate, are often required. High-dose intravenous pooled human immunoglobulin (IVIG 2 g/kg/day over 2–5 days) improves functional ability and strength.

POLYMYOSITIS

Polymyositis occurs mainly in adults, usually between the ages of 40 and 60 years, and it is slightly more frequent in women than in men. Systemic symptoms at onset include malaise, fever, and anorexia. The weakness is more proximal than distal and often associated with muscle aching but not pain. Extraocular and bulbar muscles are usually not involved, but dysphagia may be associated. Tendon reflexes are hypoactive or even absent in weak muscles. Other organ involvement includes Raynaud's phenomenon, cardiac conduction defects, cardiomyopathy, and interstitial pneumonitis and fibrosis.

The diagnosis of polymyositis is similar to that of dermatomyositis. The serum CK concentration is roughly proportional to disease severity. Muscle biopsy reveals inflammatory cells composed of predominantly T-lymphocytes and macrophages. The pathology, showing attack on muscle fibers by cytotoxic T-cells, is different from that of dermatomyositis, in which humoral antibodies attack the muscle capillaries. Corticosteroids or immunosuppressive agents treat the disease. The disease relapses and remits when treated with immunosuppressive agents or corticosteroids. The 5-year survival rate is 66%.

INCLUSION BODY MYOSITIS

Inclusion body myositis (IBM) is the most common myopathy beginning after 50 years of age. It is much more common in men than in women and causes distal weakness of the limbs. The deep finger flexors are first affected. Early weakness occurs in the quadriceps and anterior tibial muscles. Muscle atrophy and weakness is often asymmetrical. Progression is slow but unrelenting, causing severe disability. Facial weakness and dysphagia occur in one-third of patients.

The clinical features suggest the diagnosis, and muscle biopsy is confirmatory. Muscle histology reveals endomysial inflammation, fiber size variation, macrophage invasion of nonnecrotic muscle fibers, and characteristic *rimmed* vacuoles. IBM is unresponsive to prednisone and other immunosuppressive therapies. A rare variant is associated with frontotemporal dementia (see Chap 26).

KEY REFERENCES

Adams C. Myotonic dystrophy. In: *GeneClinics: Medical Genetic Knowledge Base* [database online]. Seattle, WA: University of Washington; updated 14 August 2001. Available at http://www.geneclinics.org.

Amato AA, Barohn RJ. Idiopathic inflammatory myopathies. *Neurol Clin* 1997;15: 615–648.

Barohn RJ, Amato AA, Sahenk Z, et al. Inclusion body myositis: explanation for poor response to therapy. *Neurology* 1995;45:1302–1304.

Gordon E, Hoffman EP, Pegoraro E. Congenital muscular dystrophy overview. In: *GeneClinics: Medical Genetic Knowledge Base* [database online]. Seattle, WA: University of Washington; updated 2 January 2004. Available at http://www.geneclinics.org.

Kleopa KA, Barchi RL. Genetic disorders of neuromusuclar ion channels. *Muscle Nerve* 2002;26:299–325.

North N. Nemaline myopathy. In: *GeneClinics: Medical Genetic Knowledge Base* [database online]. Seattle, WA: University of Washington; updated 25 November, 2002. Available at http://www.geneclinics.org.

Korf BR, Darras BT, Urion DK. Dystrophinopathies. In: *GeneClinics: Medical Genetic Knowledge Base* [database online]. Seattle, WA: University of Washington; updated 24 March, 2004. Available at http://www.geneclinics.org.

Ryan MM, Schnell C, Strickland CD, et al. Nemaline myopathy: a clinical study of 143 cases. *Ann Neurol* 2001;50:312–320.

Saperstein DS, Amato AA, Barohn RJ. Clinical and genetic aspects of distal myopathies. *Muscle Nerve* 2001:24:1440–1450.

MYASTHENIA GRAVIS AND OTHER NEUROMUSCULAR JUNCTION DISORDERS

Gerald M. Fenichel, MD

MYASTHENIA GRAVIS

Myasthenia gravis (MG) is the most common disorder of the neuromuscular junction. The usual cause is an immunological abnormality. Some childhood-onset cases are caused by genetic abnormalities.

Clinical features

The usual initial features are ptosis, diplopia, or both. Dysfunction of other bulbar muscles or limb weakness present as the initial feature in only 10% of cases. Weakness fluctuates, usually least in the morning and worse after prolonged muscle use. Weakness remains restricted to the ocular muscles (*ocular myasthenia*) in 10% of patients. Most patients with MG develop generalized weakness during the first year after onset.

Asymmetrical weakness of several extraocular muscles in both eyes is typical. The pupillary responses, however, are normal. The prominent features are medial rectus palsy, ptosis, and weakness of eye closure. Oropharyngeal muscle weakness causes dysphonia, dysphagia, and altered facial appearance. The characteristic facial appearance of myasthenic patients includes drooping of the corners of the mouth and an incomplete smile.

Weakness may affect any trunk or limb muscle, but some are more often affected than others. Neck flexors are usually weaker than neck extensors, and the deltoids, triceps, extensors of the wrist and fingers, and ankle dorsi-flexors are frequently weaker than other limb muscles.

Pathophysiology of myasthenia gravis

Myasthenia is a familial, but not Mendelian disease. The evidence suggests that an autoimmune attack on the postsynaptic muscle membrane is the basis of acquired MG. Several autoantibodies are associated with acquired MG.

Autoantibodies in MG

Increased titers of antiacetylcholine receptor (AChR) antibodies are found in 80% of patients with generalized MG, and in 50% of patients with ocular myasthenia. Unfortunately, the role of these antibodies in the pathophysiology of MG is incompletely understood. Severity of symptoms does not correlate with the serum AChR concentration. Striational antibodies (StrAb) that react with contractile elements of skeletal muscle are found in more than 90% of MG patients who also have a thymoma, a tumor of the thymus gland. The serum concentration of StrAb does not correlate with disease severity. The main value of StrAb is in predicting thymoma. A new antibody, anti-MUSC has recently been found in AChR negative myasthenia patients.

The thymus in myasthenia gravis

Thymic abnormalities are associated with MG. Ten percent of patients have thymic tumors, and 70% have hyperplastic germinal centers. Most thymic tumors are benign and can be removed completely at surgery. (See under Thymectomy).

Diagnosis

The diagnosis of myasthenia is accomplished mainly by the clinical features. Intravenous administration of edrophonium chloride (Tensilon) is widely used as a diagnostic test. Tensilon is a rapidly acting anticholinesterase which provides brief improvement in myasthenic symptoms, especially ptosis, after intravenous administration. However, improved strength after edrophonium is not unique to MG. A specific, objective endpoint must be chosen, such as the interpalpebral distance in a patient with ptosis. Subjective improvement should not be the endpoint. In addition, the test must be carried out cautiously, since some patients may develop respiratory distress following injection. An ambu bag and a syringe containing atropine should always be on hand when a Tensilon test is performed.

Eighty percent of our patients with acquired generalized myasthenia and 55% with ocular myasthenia have serum antibodies that bind human AChR. While the AChR antibody concentration does not predict the severity of disease, elevated concentrations of antibodies in patients with a compatible clinical syndrome are confirmatory.

Repetitive nerve stimulation (RNS) can be carried out as part of a diagnostic electromyogram (EMG) study. RNS of a nerve supplying a symptomatic muscle produces a 10% decrement in amplitude, when one compares the first stimulus to the fourth or fifth. This fatiguing of the muscle is one of the few objective tests for a neuromuscular junction disorder. Single fiber EMG is a specialized technique that provides confirmatory diagnostic evidence. It is the most sensitive clinical test of neuromuscular transmission and confirms the diagnosis in almost all patients with MG.

Treatment of myasthenia gravis (MG)

Few controlled clinical trials for medical or surgical treatment of MG exist. There is a long experience, however, with clinical therapies for this disease, and the name *gravis* is no longer appropriate, since the disease is so treatable.

CHOLINESTERASE (CHE) INHIBITORS

ChE inhibitors allow greater acetylcholine (Ach) accumulation at the neuromuscular junction and prolong its effect. ChE inhibitors alone provide adequate chronic treatment in some patients with ocular myasthenia. Pyridostigmine bromide (Mestinon) is the most widely used ChE inhibitor. A typical adult oral dosage is 30–60 mg every 4–8 hours. The main dose related adverse effect is intestinal cramps and diarrhea. The dosage varies from day to day and during the same day.

THYMECTOMY

Thymectomy is widely used as a treatment for autoimmune MG but has never been proved effective by a double-blind, randomized clinical trial. The American Academy of Neurology recommends its use in patients with non-thymomatous autoimmune MG, to increase the probability of remission or improvement. It is also the recommended procedure for all patients with thymoma.

CORTICOSTEROIDS

Most patients experience marked improvement or complete relief of symptoms when treated with prednisone. Initial treatment is approximately 100 mg/day. When sustained improvement occurs, the regiman changes to every other day and is then tapered on a monthly schedule to a maintenance dose of 15–20 mg/kg/day. Weakness often recurs if the drug is stopped. Some patients become weaker at the onset of therapy but then respond. The main disadvantages of chronic corticosteroid therapy are the side effects.

IMMUNOSUPPRESSIVE DRUGS

Several immunosuppressive drugs are useful in managing patients with MG. The ones most widely used are azathioprine (Imuran), cyclosporine (Neoral or Gengraf), and mycophenolate mofetil (CellCept). Azathioprine is the oldest and least expensive. Symptoms respond, but usually only after a 6-month delay. The usual dose is 150 mg/day in three divided doses. A severe allergic flu-like syndrome occurs within 2 weeks in as many as 20% of patients and requires stopping the drug. Therefore, we maintain the initial dose of 50 mg daily for 2 weeks before increasing further. Improvement continues as long as the drug is used. Leukopenia and pancytopenia are possible adverse reactions requiring monitoring of blood counts.

The maintenance dose of mycophenolate mofetil is usually 2 g each day in two divided doses. Like azathioprine, monitoring is required for adverse reactions to bone marrow and liver.

Cyclosporine provides improvement in most patients. The initial dose is 5–6 mg/kg, given in two divided doses 12 hours apart. After 1 month, we adjust the dose to produce a trough serum CYA concentration of 75–150 ng/mL. We measure serum creatinine monthly and adjust the dose to maintain a creatinine level of less than 150% of pretreatment values. Renal toxicity and hypertension are the main adverse reactions.

PLASMA EXCHANGE AND INTRAVENOUS IMMUNOGLOBULIN

Plasma exchange (PE) and intravenous immunoglobulin (IVIG) are acute interventions to produce short-term improvement. Their use is mainly for patients with sudden worsening of myasthenic symptoms. Both are used as needed for patients with impending respiratory distress and always concomitantly with chronic therapy such as corticosteroids. A typical protocol of plasma exchange is to remove 2–3 L of plasma three times a week until improvement plateaus, usually after five–six exchanges. Intravenous immunoglobulin (IVIG) is usually provided as 2 g/kg of body weight divided into five portions given daily for 5 days.

Transitory neonatal myasthenia

A transitory MG affects 15% of newborns whose mothers have immune-mediated MG. The serum antibody concentration of the newborn and the mother are the same, but this level does not correlate with the severity of symptoms in the newborn or the mother. Once an affected mother delivers a newborn with transitory neonatal myasthenia, subsequent newborns are likely to be affected. The clinical syndrome includes hypotonia and feeding difficulty. Onset is from birth to 3 days postpartum. Passive transfer of maternal antibodies to the newborn does not explain the syndrome. The diagnosis is established by edrophonium (Tensilon) testing. Affected newborns require treatment with ChE inhibitors if feeding is impaired. Plasma exchange is a consideration in newborns with respiratory insufficiency.

Genetic myasthenic syndromes

Genetic forms of myasthenia are a heterogeneous group of disorders caused by abnormalities of neuromuscular transmission. Symptom onset is usually at birth or during infancy, though some do not present until young adult life. All genetic forms of myasthenia are transmitted by autosomal recessive inheritance, except the *slow-channel syndrome,* which is transmitted by autosomal dominant inheritance.

Congenital myasthenia

Congenital myasthenia is a clinical syndrome that encompasses several genetic neuromuscular defects. Male gender predominance is 2-to-1. Affected children develop ophthalmoparesis and ptosis during infancy. Mild facial paresis may be present as well. Ophthalmoplegia is often incomplete at onset but progresses to complete paralysis during infancy or childhood. Limb weakness is usually mild compared to ophthalmoplegia. Respiratory distress is unusual.

Familial infantile myasthenia

In familial infantile myasthenia, generalized hypotonia is present at birth, and the neonatal course is complicated by repeated episodes of life-threatening apnea and feeding difficulty. Assisted ventilation is often required. Arthrogryposis (congenital contractures at joints) may be present. Ocular muscle function is usually normal. Within weeks after birth, the child becomes stronger and ultimately breathes unassisted. However, episodes of life-threatening apnea occur repeatedly throughout infancy and childhood, even into adult life.

Slow-channel congenital myasthenic syndrome (SCCMS)

SCCMS is transmitted by autosomal dominant inheritance. The onset of symptoms always occurs after infancy, and the disease may present as late as the third decade. Weakness is slowly progressive, and atrophy is expected. Quinidine sulfate and fluoxetine may improve strength.

Lambert-Eaton myasthenic syndrome (LEMS)

Lambert-Eaton myasthenic syndrome is a presynaptic abnormality of ACh release. This is a relatively uncommon disorder, associated with malignancy in half of cases, usually small cell lung cancer (SCLC). The mechanism is an immune-mediated process directed against the voltage-gated calcium channels (VGCC) on nerve terminals.

CLINICAL FEATURES OF LEMS

The age at onset of Lambert-Eaton myasthenic syndrome is usually after 40 years. Both genders are equally affected. Weakness and pain of proximal leg muscles are the main symptoms. Weakness of the oropharyngeal and ocular muscles is mild. Strength first improves after exercise and then weakens. Tendon reflexes are reduced or absent, or they may enhance after repeated muscle contraction. Associated autonomic dysfunction includes dry mouth and postural hypotension. Unlike MG, the weakness in LEMS is not life-threatening.

Diagnosis of LEMS

The diagnosis of LEMS is predominantly clinical. The EMG is diagnostic, provided that the electromyographer is alerted to suspect the disease and performs repetitive stimulation studies at rapid rates. The amplitude of the compound motor action potential is small and further reduces in size following repetitive nerve stimulation at frequencies between 1 Hz and 5 Hz. The action potential size doubles in response to repetitive stimulation at 20–50 Hz. The diagnosis of LEMS requires an extensive search for an underlying malignancy, especially SCLC.

Treatment of LEMS

The initial treatment of LEMS is directed at the underlying malignancy, if one is found. Weakness may improve when cancer therapy is effective. ChE inhibitors are of little benefit. However, drugs that help release acetylcholine increase strength. Such drugs are diaminopyridine and guanidine. Neither is available on a commerical basis, but they are available on research protocols.

Both plasma exchange and IVIG provide transitory improvement in some patients with LEMS. Some patients respond to repeated courses of plasma exchange or IVIG. Prolonged use of prednisone and/or azathioprine is required. The long-term prognosis is variable and depends on the response of the underlying malignancy to treatment.

Botulism

The bacterium *Clostridium botulinum* produces a toxin that blocks the release of ACh from the motor nerve terminal. Most intoxications follow ingestion of contaminated food, but other forms follow wound infection or inhalation by infants.

Clinical features of botulism

Nausea and vomiting are the first symptoms of food-borne botulism. Home canning is often the source in adult cases. Newborns can ingest the live bacteria in honey and develop the disease. Neuromuscular symptoms begin 12–36 hours after exposure. Blurred vision, dysphagia, and dysarthria are the main symptoms of food-borne exposure. Pupillary responses to light are sluggish. Limb weakness is progressive, proximal more than distal, but tendon reflex responses, although diminished, are not absent. Autonomic dysfunction is common, especially in the newborn form. Symptoms consist of dry mouth, constipation, and urinary retention.

Diagnosis of botulism

The diagnosis of botulism requires culturing the organism from the wound or from the gastrointestinal tract of infants. Serum assays for botulinum toxin are available. The electromyographic findings in botulism include reduced amplitude of muscle action potentials and facilitation of action potential amplitudes by tetanic stimulation.

TREATMENT OF BOTULISM

Wound and food-borne infection is treated with antitoxin. Infantile botulism rarely requires treatment.

KEY REFERENCES

Andrews PI, Sanders DB. Myasthenia gravis in childhood. In: Jones RH, DeVivo DC, Darras BT, eds. *Neuromuscular Disorders of Infancy and Childhood*. Boston, MA: Butterworth-Heinemann; 2002:575–597.

Bedlack RS, Sanders DB. Steroid treatment for myasthenia gravis. *Muscle Nerve* 2002;55: 117–121.

Cherington M. Botulism: update and review. *Semin Neurol* 2004;24:155–163.

De Feo LG, Schottlender J, Martelli NA, et al. Use of intravenous pulsed cyclophosphamide in severe, generalized myasthenia gravis. *Muscle Nerve* 2002;26:31–36.

Engel AG. Congenital myasthenic syndromes. In: B Katirji, et al., eds. *Neuromuscular Disorders in Clinical Practice*. Boston, MA: Butterworth-Heinemann; 2002:953–963.

Fox CK, Keet CA, Strober JB. Recent advances in infant botulism. *Pediatr Neurol* 2005;32:149–154.

Gronseth GS, Barohn RB. Practice parameter: thymectomy for autoimmune myasthenia gravis (an evidence-based review). *Neurology* 2000;55:7–15.

Jones HR. Infantile botulism and other acquired neuromuscular junction disorders of infancy and childhood. In: Brown WF, Bolton CF, Aminoff MJ, eds. *Neuromuscular Function and Disease*. Philadelphia, PA: W.B. Saunders; 2002:1697–1702.

Mareska M, Gutmann L. Lambert-Eaton myasthenic syndrome. *Semin Neurol* 2004;24: 149–153.

Newsom-Davis J. Therapy in myasthenia gravis and Lambert-Eaton myasthenic syndrome. *Semin Neurol* 2003;23:191–198.

Sanders DB. Lambert-Eaton myasthenic syndrome: diagnosis and treatment. *Ann NY Acad Sci* 2003;998:500–508.

Scherer K, Bedlack RS, Simel DL. Does this patient have myasthenia gravis? *JAMA* 2005;293:1906–1914.

Shapiro RL, Hatheway C, Swerdlow DL. Botulism in the United States: a clinical and epidemiologic review. *Ann Intern Med* 1998;129:221–228.

Zaja F, Russo D, Fuga G, et al. Rituximab for myasthenia gravis developing after bone marrow transplant. *Neurology* 2000;55:1062–1063.

BRAIN TUMORS

Paul L. Moots, MD
and Michael L. Edgeworth, MD

INTRODUCTION

Brain tumors represent a significant cause of morbidity and mortality within the spectrum of diseases affecting the central nervous system (CNS). Primary brain tumors can vary greatly in terms of malignancy but even so-called benign tumors can become life-threatening by virtue of their infiltrative nature, making total resection impossible, and their ability to undergo malignant transformation. Brain tumors are a heterogeneous group of disorders with regard to their histology and cell of origin. Figure 36-1 shows the distribution of primary brain tumors by histology for all age groups. The majority of primary brain tumors are gliomas, arising from glial cells. Gliomas account for 40% of all primary brain tumors and 78% of primary malignant brain tumors. Metastatic tumors to the brain, principally from primary lung and breast carcinomas, are the most common neoplasms overall found in the brain. Although the etiology of most primary brain tumors remains unclear, a few genetic syndromes play a role in tumor formation, including neurofibromatosis, tuberous sclerosis complex, von Hippel-Lindau syndrome, Li-Fraumeni syndrome, basal cell nevus (Gorlin's) syndrome, Turcot syndrome, and ataxia telangiectasia.

The incidence of all primary benign and malignant brain tumors in the United States is 14.8 cases per 100,000 person-years, with a slight male predominance. An estimated 43,800 new cases of primary brain tumors are diagnosed each year. Eighteen thousand five hundred of these new cases are malignant tumors, representing about 1.35% of all cancers. The exact incidence of metastatic brain tumors is unknown but is estimated to be more than three to five times the incidence of primary brain tumors. Metastatic brain tumors are increasing in frequency, as patients with systemic cancers are surviving longer with improved therapies. The incidence rate of childhood (age < 20 years) primary nonmalignant and malignant brain and CNS

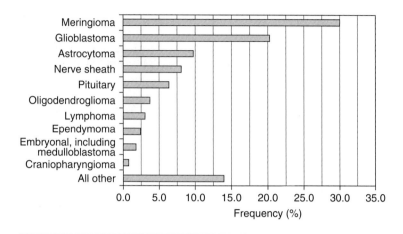

Figure 36-1 **Distribution of all primary brain and CNS tumors by histology.**

tumors is 4.3 cases per 100,000 person-years, with a slight male predominance. Between 2000 and 3000 children are diagnosed with a primary brain tumor each year. In the pediatric population, brain tumors are the most common nonhematologic malignancies, and malignant brain tumors represent the second leading cause of cancer death, after leukemias.

SIGNS AND SYMPTOMS

The symptoms and signs of CNS neoplasms represent a combination of localized, focal CNS dysfunction, such as focal seizures, aphasia, or hemiparesis, and superimposed, diffuse cerebral dysfunction, resulting from mass effect, hydrocephalus, and elevated intracranial pressure. Since the majority of adult gliomas are frontal, temporal, or parietal in origin, focal cerebral hemispheric symptoms predominate with these neoplasms. Metastases also have a predilection for the cerebral hemispheres, often arising at the gray-white junction, a distribution thought to reflect the path of greatest blood flow. Metastatic involvement of the cerebellum is considerably less common, whereas brainstem and intraparenchymal spinal cord metastases are rare.

The severity of symptoms due to brain tumors often reflects other factors in addition to location. Lesions involving homologous cerebral regions bilaterally, or disconnecting homologous areas, produce substantially greater functional disability than unilateral lesions. These principles hold true, regardless of the nature of the disease process, such as direct involvement by tumor, hydrocephalus, treatment-related toxicity, or coincidental CNS pathology unrelated to the neoplasm.

As with most types of CNS pathology, the rate of evolution of a CNS neoplasm has a significant impact on the severity of symptoms. Very slow-growing, noninfiltrative tumors such as meningiomas may become very large before any symptoms arise, and even then symptoms often develop slowly. Slowly growing neoplasms that infiltrate rather than compress brain tissue, such as low-grade gliomas, often present with partial seizures, without any other evidence of neurological deficit. More rapidly growing intra-parenchymal neoplasms such as high-grade gliomas and metastases tend to present with a subacute course of progressive focal symptoms over weeks to a few months. A 4 cm glioblastoma with surrounding edema may produce a life-threatening brain herniation, while a 4 cm low-grade astrocytoma in the same region may produce only focal seizures and otherwise remain asymptomatic.

Fulminant presentations of CNS neoplasms are not uncommon, and these can represent a life-threatening situation requiring emergency management. Generally, this type of presentation is related either to seizures or to a sudden rise in intracranial pressure, sometimes associated with bleeding into the tumor or acute hydrocephalus. The more common problem is seizures; these are sudden, often partial at onset, but they sometimes secondarily generalize, resulting in major convulsions. Once the seizure and postictal period are over, these patients often recover to baseline.

Even considering patients with aggressive intracerebral neoplasms, many present when neurological symptoms have not evolved to the point of being incapacitating. For example, among high-grade glioma patients, 60% present with a Karnofsky performance status of 70% or more, indicating largely independent functioning. The rate of symptom progression, over weeks to months for high-grade gliomas and metastases, and over a year or two for most low-grade gliomas, is slower than cerebrovascular syndromes and faster than neurodegenerative diseases such as Alzheimer's disease. These temporal profiles of symptom onset trigger clinical suspicions of a neoplasm. Neuroimaging, however, is even more useful in the diagnosis of brain tumors.

Seizures are a common symptom of brain tumors. Seizures are more common as a presenting feature in low-grade (70–80%) than in high-grade gliomas (20–30%), but even in high-grade tumors they represent a major, persistent cause of morbidity in about 25% of patients. Seizures are a presenting symptom in about 20% of metastatic brain tumors. Most seizures secondary to brain tumors are clinically localized, representing focal cerebral cortical dysfunction, but secondary generalization is common. If the patient is amnestic regarding the onset of the event and no one observed the event, the focal onset of the seizure is easily missed. Patients with seizures arising from underlying brain tumors have a greater likelihood of being refractory to anticonvulsant medications than those with idiopathic seizure disorders. Prophylactic anticonvulsant therapy is not recommended for brain tumor patients who have not had seizures.

Headaches are not as common in brain tumor patients as might be expected. In the absence of elevated intracranial pressure, only 36% of patients with supratentorial gliomas complain of headache. Headaches are more common among patients with brain metastases, occurring as a prominent symptom in about 50%. Tumor-associated headaches tend to be relatively modest and nondescript, except for their recurring, persistent, or progressive nature. There is a tendency for the pain to worsen with bending or straining. More severe headaches occur when substantial mass effect and elevated intracranial pressure develop. Severe headaches that accompany transient marked increases in intracranial pressure (*pressure waves*) are often accompanied by and sometimes relieved by vomiting. The classical early morning headache ascribed to elevated intracranial pressure related to brain tumors is seen infrequently.

Given the anatomic distribution of gliomas, personality and cognitive changes are often part of the presenting symptomatology and are among the most disabling symptoms associated with CNS neoplasms. Apathy and blunted or labile effect may be subtle but are strikingly common, and a large number of people are incorrectly treated for depression for months prior to the diagnosis of a CNS neoplasm. These neurocognitive deficits may arise from localized cerebral dysfunction. Common examples of focal cognitive abnormalities include apathy from frontal lobe dysfunction, aphasia from dominant temporal/frontal dysfunction, and neglect or denial of illness from nondominant parietal dysfunction. Progressive dementia-like presentations may be seen with high-grade gliomas invading the corpus callosum or deep frontal and midline structures, such as the thalamus. Multiple cerebral parenchymal metastases sometimes present with a progressive encephalopathy, often with subtle focal symptoms or signs. Metastatic involvement of the meninges and cerebrospinal fluid (CSF) (*carcinomatous meningitis*) often presents with encephalopathy as one component of a highly varied clinical picture. Cognitive impairment may also occur due to elevated intracranial pressure, with early or chronic herniation syndromes, or hydrocephalus. Families often give a history of personality change in patients with cognitive impairment; particularly in patients with frontal lobe tumors, this history is often more sensitive than the neurological examination. For most adults with primary CNS neoplasms such as gliomas, the decision-making process regarding medical care will at some point become the responsibility of caregivers, as the patient's capacity to comprehend, analyze, judge, and make decisions is progressively impaired. Particularly in regard to end-of-life issues, the need for early discussion is highlighted in this patient population.

Symptom management

The presence of severe or rapidly progressive symptoms from a brain tumor usually requires immediate efforts to stabilize the patient. The initial goal is to reduce mass effect and intracranial pressure, prior to undertaking definitive therapies. Attempting emergency surgical decompression or instituting radiation therapy without preliminary efforts to control edema and mass effect can result in dramatic deterioration.

Brain tumor edema is primarily vasogenic, or related to "leaky blood-brain barrier", and it responds to corticosteroid therapy. The synthetic corticosteroid, dexamethasone, has traditionally been used by neuro-oncologists because it has less mineralocorticoid activity than other corticosteroids, giving a better side effect profile. However, the same antiedema effect, and similar side effects, can be achieved with any of the commonly used corticosteroids. A typical dosing regimen for dexamethasone would be 10–40 mg IV once, followed by 4–16 mg IV every 6 hours. Improvement is often noted by 12 hours, maximal at 48–72 hours. Tapering to the lowest effective dose is recommended once definitive therapy for the tumor has been accomplished. Rapid tapering and abrupt discontinuation should be avoided in patients who have been on high-dose corticosteroids for longer than 10 days, because of the risk of adrenal insufficiency and the potential for rapid reaccumulation of cerebral edema, with neurological deterioration.

Other measures for stabilizing patients with fulminant presentations include hyperventilation and mannitol (see Chap. 23), or surgical intervention. Surgical intervention might include ventriculostomy for hydrocephalus or acute intracranial pressure elevation, or ultimately craniotomy for a decompressive resection.

DIFFERENTIAL DIAGNOSIS OF CNS MASS LESIONS

The major diagnostic considerations for most CNS mass lesions are various tumor types. Abscess, hematoma, infarction, contusion, acute inflammatory/demyelinating lesions, and others are sometimes difficult to distinguish from a tumor. Radiographic features, however, often allow the more likely diagnosis of a neoplasm. The distinction between various types of primary and metastatic tumors is often difficult by neuroimaging. As a rule of thumb, solitary mass lesions are primary, whereas multiple lesions are metastatic. In actuality, about 30–50% of metastatic brain tumors are solitary, and 5–10% of gliomas and 50% of CNS lymphomas are multiple.

Despite the tremendous advances in neuroimaging, biopsy remains the gold standard for the diagnosis of intracranial mass lesions, and establishing a tissue diagnosis is a guiding principle, the cornerstone of cancer treatment. Only in very select instances does the invasiveness and risk entailed in a neurosurgical procedure override the critical need of establishing a pathologic diagnosis. As more molecular markers for the diagnosis and treatment planning of cancers are discovered, the need to establish a specific diagnosis by tissue biopsy will only increase.

The most common exception to the need for a tissue diagnosis relates to meningiomas. These slow growing tumors have a very characteristic appearance and are almost always dural-based. Monitoring by repeated scanning can confirm the slow course. When a lesion suspected to be a meningioma arises under unusual circumstances, for example in a young person, biopsy confirmation is important. Some other, extra-axial mass lesions, such as acoustic nerve schwannomas and suprasellar craniopharyngiomas, have such characteristic appearances and locations on magnetic resonance imaging (MRI) that the diagnosis can be established to a high level of certainty.

Intrinsic brainstem masses are another exception to the rule requiring the establishment of a tissue diagnosis. When a brainstem mass is found in a child with progressive symptoms over months, the diagnosis is an infiltrating astrocytoma, usually high grade, in 95% of cases. Given the high risk of further dramatic neurological compromise in attempting to biopsy lesions in the brainstem, treatment is usually instituted empirically. A mass in the same location in an adult cannot be diagnosed as reliably by neuroimaging, but the risks of a biopsy may still be unacceptable.

The patient with a known systemic cancer and a newly discovered CNS mass may also not need a biopsy, as long as the systemic cancer is active and the neuroimaging is typical of a metastatic lesion. If the systemic cancer is part of the patient's past history but is inactive, then the documentation of a tissue diagnosis is essential. In this situation, a workup for active systemic cancer (blood work, chest x-ray, body computed tomography [CT], or even whole body positron emission tomography [PET] scanning) should be performed before undertaking an invasive neurosurgical procedure. The workup is based upon the predicted patterns of recurrence of the primary neoplasm and the presence or absence of specific systemic symptoms or signs, such as pain, cough, dyspnea, adenopathy, or hematuria. Extensive testing for an occult primary malignancy is warranted only if there is a metastasis, and no known primary neoplasm.

Nonneoplastic diagnoses are also important to consider in the workup of a suspected CNS neoplasm. These often represent disease processes that resemble tumors on MRI. Infection, especially a bacterial or fungal abscess, may look identical to a high-grade glioma and should be strongly considered in a patient with fever, meningismus, or a risk factor such as bacterial endocarditis. Stroke is often an initial diagnosis or concern in brain tumor patients who have presented with a rapid symptomatic decline or with seizure activity. An intraparenchymal hemorrhage is often considered a stroke but may arise from and mask an underlying neoplastic process; repeat imaging after the blood has cleared is essential for diagnosis. Neoplasms that frequently hemorrhage include metastatic melanoma, breast cancer, lung cancer, glioblastoma multiforme, and oligodendroglioma. Multiple sclerosis may also present with discrete, enhancing lesions similar in appearance to brain tumors, and a history of neurological sequelae separated by time and space would favor this diagnosis over a neoplasm. Other demyelinating or inflammatory processes, such as CNS vasculitis or sarcoidosis, may be considered as well. Lastly, trauma may leave permanent scarring in the brain parenchyma, which may look similar to a low-grade glioma. Posttraumatic lesions are often discovered incidentally, years after a significant head injury.

NEUROIMAGING

Imaging is a vital component to the management of patients with brain tumors. The advent of modern neuroimaging, with CT scanning in the mid-1970s and MRI scanning in the mid-1980s, dramatically improved the ability to diagnose brain lesions of many types, including tumors. Not only is imaging useful in treatment planning such as stereotactic biopsy, resection, and radiation therapy, but it is also critical in follow-up of patients to determine response to treatment or tumor progression. Contrast-enhanced CT and MRI provide the best anatomical detail of the tumor and surrounding brain. MR spectroscopy and PET give information about the molecular and metabolic nature of the tumors, respectively, which may aid in diagnostic dilemmas. Functional MRI and functional PET are being used to map critical neuronal components relative to the tumor location, to help prevent injury from neurosurgical intervention.

MRI with and without contrast is the most commonly used technique in brain tumor evaluation, because of its superior anatomical detail. Location of the tumor on MRI is often helpful in narrowing the differential diagnosis. For example, an extraparenchymal, dural-based tumor with homogenous contrast enhancement is most likely to be a meningioma (Fig. 36-2).

Primary CNS neoplasms tend to be hypointense on T1-weighted images and hyperintense on fluid-attenuated inversion recovery (FLAIR) and T2-weighted images (Fig. 36-3). Contrast enhancement of intraparenchymal tumors is reflective of breakdown of the blood-brain barrier and usually coincides with a more aggressive tumor subtype. High-grade gliomas, such as glioblastoma multiforme (Fig. 36-4), readily show enhancement with contrast, whereas low-grade gliomas (Fig. 36-3) do not. The number of lesions is also informative, as primary CNS neoplasms tend to be unifocal, whereas secondary (metastatic) CNS neoplasms are often multifocal and located at the border of the gray-white junction.

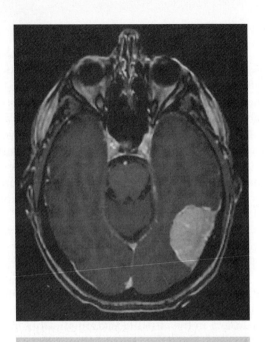

Figure 36-2. **T1-weighted contrast-enhanced MRI image of a left temporo-parietal meningioma.**

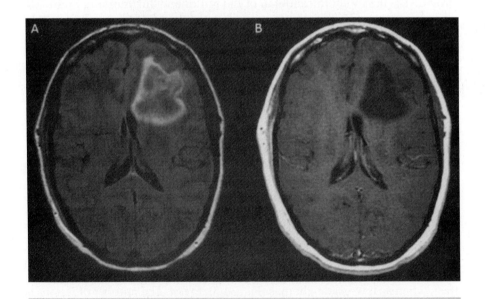

Figure 36-3. **MRI axial images of a patient with a low-grade oligodendroglioma.** Note that (A) shows the lesion is hyperintense on the fluid-attenuated inversion recovery (FLAIR) sequence and (B) reveals a hypointense lesion without enhancement on the contrast-enhanced T1-weighted sequence.

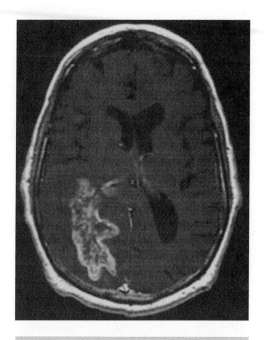

Figure 36-4. **T1-weighted contrast-enhanced MRI image of a right parieto-occipital glioblastoma multiforme.**

SPECIFIC CNS TUMORS

Gliomas

ASTROCYTOMA

Astrocytomas account for nearly 75% of all gliomas. Grading of the various subtypes of astrocytomas is based on the histologic appearance of the tumor. Most clinicians use the World Health Organization (WHO) grading system, which separates astrocytomas into grades I–IV based on cellularity, nuclear atypia, mitotic activity, microvascular proliferation, and tumor necrosis. Grade I astrocytoma, also known as juvenile pilocytic astrocytoma (JPA), is a childhood tumor with no tendency to progress to a higher grade, often curable with complete resection. Conversely, WHO grades II–IV astrocytomas are highly infiltrative by nature, making them essentially impossible to remove completely, despite what might appear to be a complete surgical resection by MRI. WHO grade II astrocytomas are also referred to as low-grade astrocytomas (LGA). Histologic subtypes of LGA include fibrillary, protoplasmic, and gemistocytic astrocytomas. Grades III and IV are considered high-grade tumors and referred to as anaplastic astrocytoma (AA) and glioblastoma multiforme (GBM), respectively.

Low-grade astrocytomas occur more frequently in young adults, with peak onset between 30 and 40 years of age. They have a tendency to progress to higher grades over time. Anaplastic astrocytomas (AAs) also tend to progress to a higher grade (i.e., glioblastoma multiforme, GBM), but GBMs commonly develop de novo, without any prior history of a lower grade neoplasm. Genetic abnormalities are known to play a role in the formation, proliferation, and progression of astrocytomas. They are hereditary in less than 5% of cases. Acquired mutations leading to glioma formation have been associated with previous radiation therapy and with exposure to chemicals such as nitroso- compounds and aliphatic hydrocarbons, but in most instances the cause of these abnormalities is unknown.

The clinical course of patients with an astrocytoma, especially LGA, is best predicted by the tumor grade. Genetic abnormalities in the tissue also correlate with the grade of the tumor. Several clinical features are also useful in predicting outcome. Good prognostic factors include lower grade histology, age < 40 years, good performance status, radiographically complete resection, and presentation with seizures. LGA patients often have remissions lasting several years after treatment. Astrocytomas occur most commonly in the frontal, temporal, and insular regions. A rare variant called *gliomatosis cerebri* is characterized by infiltration of a glioma into more than two lobes of the brain. AA and GBM patients progress much more rapidly, despite therapeutic interventions. Astrocytomas, with the exception of WHO grade I tumors, are considered incurable despite surgical, radiation and chemotherapeutic options. The 5-year survival rates for JPA, LGA, AA, and GBM are approximately 91%, 47%, 29%, and 3%, respectively.

Treatment options generally include surgery, radiation therapy, and chemotherapy. If amenable, a gross total resection (GTR) by MRI is the initial treatment of choice for all astrocytomas. Radiation therapy is known to be effective in decreasing mass effect and tumor burden and in improving neurological symptoms in astrocytoma patients, but it is often reserved for AA and GBM patients or in older LGA patients not amenable to GTR. LGA following GTR may be followed conservatively until evidence of tumor progression, as one large study showed no difference in progression-free survival or overall survival with early versus delayed radiation therapy. There is no clearly proved role for chemotherapy in LGA patients. Treatment for AA and GBM usually includes postoperative, fractionated radiation therapy delivered daily over 5–6 weeks. This is given focally to the tumor bed and a surrounding margin in order to spare normal brain from potential radiation-induced injury. Recent evidence has shown that concomitant chemotherapy, using temozolomide (Temodar, an alkylating agent), and radiation therapy prolongs overall survival in GBM patients, the first chemotherapy agent proved to extend life in these patients. Temozolomide is also given to AA patients, though strong clinical evidence for this practice is lacking. Other chemotherapeutic options and experimental agents are available and widely used, but their efficacy remains unproved.

OLIGODENDROGLIOMA

Oligodendrogliomas account for 9% of all gliomas. The WHO grading scale for oligodendrogliomas includes only two grades, low-grade oligodendroglioma (LGO) and anaplastic oligodendroglioma (AO). The peak age of onset of LGO is about 40, whereas that for AO is 50 to 60. Histologically, these tumors demonstrate a "honeycomb" or "fried egg" pattern with clear cytoplasm forming perinuclear haloes that represent a fixation artifact. Calcifications are more frequent than in astrocytomas and can be present in the tumor itself or surrounding cortex. There is often a pronounced capillary network giving a "chicken wire" appearance. AO are characterized by increased cell density, with nuclear anaplasia, increased mitotic activity, and necrosis. The term oligoastrocytoma is sometimes used when distinct areas of astrocytoma and oligodendroglioma occur in the same tumor.

Surgical and radiation therapy options are similar to those addressed above with astrocytomas. Oligodendrogliomas tend to be more sensitive to chemotherapy than astrocytomas and usually carry a better prognosis. Chemosensitivity was first noted in the late 1980s with a regimen of procarbazine, CCNU, and vincristine (PCV). Later, chemosensitivity was noted to be associated with specific genetic abnormalities, specifically loss of heterozygosity at chromosomes 1p and 19q. Temozolomide has also been shown to be effective in LGO and AO patients with loss of heterozygosity at 1p and 19q and is commonly used as the first-line chemotherapeutic agent, because of the hematological toxicities associated with the PCV regimen. Prognostic factors are also similar to those noted above with astrocytomas. The 5-year survival rates for LGO and AO are 70% and 40%, respectively.

EPENDYMOMA

In children, ependymomas are relatively common CNS neoplasms. They tend to arise in the lateral (40%) or fourth ventricle (60%). Not all have an obvious connection to the ventricular system. They are better circumscribed than most other gliomas but do not have a true capsule separating the tumor from adjacent brain tissue. Still, careful resection alone can be curative. More often, postoperative radiation is given to the local area, particularly if obvious residual tumor is identified on postoperative MRI scanning. MRI scanning of the entire neuraxis and evaluation of CSF cytology is also recommended because of a slightly higher tendency for CSF dissemination than other gliomas (10%). Chemotherapy has been used in very young children and occasionally is effective enough to allow radiation to be deferred, but in general these neoplasms are not highly chemosensitive. They have a high rate of local recurrence and a high mortality, with 5-year survival approximately 40%.

Ependymomas in adults are substantially different from the childhood tumors. A few young adults have neoplasms that are the equivalent of the childhood form. More often, ependymomas in adults are very well circumscribed nodules in the cerebellopontine angle, cervical spinal cord, or lumbosacral spinal canal. Resection is often the only treatment needed. Local recurrence is not rare, but long-term survival is very high. The 5-year survival for intraspinal ependymomas in adults is 85%. The combination of multiple meningiomas, multiple ependymomas, and bilateral acoustic schwannomas is characteristic of neurofibromatosis type II. This disorder is due to a mutation on chromosome 22.

Medulloblastoma/primitive neuroectodermal tumor

Medulloblastoma is a common childhood brain tumor that arises from the embryonal precursors of the granule cells of the cerebellar cortex. Abnormalities in the genetic program for granule cell proliferation and differentiation underlie the development of this tumor. Histologically similar neoplasms arising in the supratentorial region or pineal region are referred to as primitive neuroectodermal tumors. They are so rare that the tendency to lump them together with medulloblastoma has had practical benefits in clinical trials, but increasingly molecular and clinical features that distinguish them are being established. For example, the pineal region pineoblastoma sometimes arises in patients with the hereditary retinoblastoma syndrome, an inherited mutation in the retinoblastoma tumor suppressor gene.

Medulloblastoma is often a rapidly growing tumor. The tendency for CSF dissemination is high (10–30%) compared with other primary neuroepithelial tumors. Staging the neuraxis with complete MRI scanning of the spine and CSF cytology is required. Systemic metastases occur in about 5%, most often involving the bone marrow. About 25–50% have hydrocephalus. Resection of the primary tumor will reestablish adequate CSF flow dynamics; only 25% require ventriculoperitoneal shunt placement. Definitive therapy includes surgical resection and craniospinal radiation with a boost to the tumor bed. *Standard risk* patients, those with little residual tumor on postoperative MRI and no evidence of metastases, have a good prognosis with radiation only, with 5-year survival 70–80%. *High-risk* patients, who have a large residual tumor or metastases, have a 5-year survival of 0% when treated with radiation alone. The addition of chemotherapy increases survival to 40–60%. In recent years, trials have looked at the merit of adding chemotherapy for standard risk patients and lowering the craniospinal radiation dose in order to reduce the delayed toxicities of radiation. The treatment of very young children (< 3 years) and of adults with medulloblastoma requires substantial modifications due to age-related, differing toxicities.

Primary CNS lymphoma

Primary CNS lymphoma is the most common of a small group of malignant neoplasms that arise in the brain but are not of neuroepithelial origin. There is no lymphatic drainage of the brain proper, yet a small population of migrating lymphocytes is present in the brain at any time and is presumed to be the source of CNS lymphomas. Until the 1970s, CNS lymphoma was a rare tumor of mid-to-late adult life. The advent of effective immunosuppression in the management of renal and other transplants was associated with the first reports of CNS lymphoma in immunocompromised patients. Soon thereafter, a high incidence of CNS lymphoma was observed in patients with human immunodeficiency virus/acquired immunodeficiency syndrome (HIV/AIDS), as that epidemic began. The development of aggressive antiretroviral therapy for HIV has decreased the incidence of CNS lymphoma in AIDS patients. Epidemiologic studies, however, have suggested that CNS lymphomas in immunocompetent individuals are increasing in incidence.

CNS lymphoma is almost always a high-grade B-cell non-Hodgkin's lymphoma (NHL). It presents with subacute, progressive symptoms over weeks or months. The MRI typically shows an enhancing mass, although multiple lesions are common and infiltration beyond the lesion seen on MRI is typical. CSF involvement is present in 10–30%. Ocular involvement is present in 5–10%. Systemic sites are involved at diagnosis in less than 5%. Conversely, most instances of systemic NHL metastasizing to the CNS produce neoplastic meningitis rather than parenchymal metastases. One important exception is testicular NHL which often involves the brain parenchyma. When the diagnosis of CNS lymphoma is strongly suspected, corticosteroids should be avoided prior to the time of biopsy, if possible. Corticosteroids can cause rapid lysis of tumor cells, resulting in an inconclusive biopsy. The steroid response is rarely sustained for more than a few weeks or months.

The treatment of immunocompetent patients centers on chemotherapy and radiation. Surgical resection is not beneficial because of the infiltrative nature of the tumor and the high likelihood of response to other modalities. Chemotherapy agents that are active against lymphoma and also have good blood-brain barrier penetrance are the first choice for most patients. High-dose methotrexate is most commonly used. Standard chemotherapy regimens used for systemic NHL, such as cyclophosphamide, doxorubicin (Adriamycin), vincristine (Oncovin), and prednisone (CHOP), are not effective. Many CNS lymphomas are CD20 positive, and the use of the monoclonal antibody, rituximab is being tested currently.

If radiation is used, the treatment needs to include the whole brain. Dementia is common after this treatment, occurring in about 50% of long-term survivors. If a complete or near complete response is achieved with chemotherapy, radiation can be deferred until tumor progression. Current reports indicate a 3–4-year median survival for patients receiving both chemotherapy and radiation. Radiation therapy alone provides a 10–12-month median survival.

METASTATIC CANCER INVOLVING THE CNS

Parenchymal brain metastases

Brain metastases appear to be increasing in frequency, owing in part to improved treatments for systemic cancers. Unfortunately, treatments aimed at the underlying tumor and systemic metastases are rarely effective in controlling brain metastases. Once a tumor has metastasized to the brain, survival is short; median survival is 4–6 months, with 2-year survival of less than 10%. About half of brain metastases encountered at autopsy are single lesions. Clinical studies estimate development of brain metastases from systemic cancers at 8.5%, with the majority occurring late in the course of the disease. The five most common primary sites for brain metastases are lung, breast, colorectal, kidney, and melanoma. Spread to the CNS occurs most commonly through hematologic seeding of molecularly altered tumor cells, via arterial circulation. Implantation often occurs at the gray-white junction, and watershed areas of arterial circulation in the brain tend to be a classic location.

Management of brain metastases depends on the primary site of origin, stage of systemic disease, number of brain metastases, and patient performance status. Routine brain imaging for systemic cancer patients without neurological symptoms is usually not recommended. Lung cancer is the main exception to this rule, as 3–10% of newly diagnosed non-small cell lung cancer and 15% of small cell lung cancer patients have identifiable brain metastases. Once melanoma has become metastatic to any organ, the occurrence of brain metastases is markedly increased (about 40% in one autopsy series) and may justify routine surveillance in this patient population as well. Presenting signs and symptoms of metastatic brain tumors are commonly headache, focal neurological deficits, and seizures.

Treatment is aimed at controlling the disease while maintaining quality of life. Although survival is short, a subgroup of patients with good prognostic factors warrant vigorous treatment strategies aimed at prolonging overall survival. The strongest prognostic factors are age < 65 years, good performance status, a solitary brain metastasis, and a controlled primary tumor with absence of systemic disease. Whole brain radiotherapy (WBRT) was the treatment of choice in the past but is now reserved for patients with unfavorable prognostic factors or widespread disease. A typical dose is 30 Gy delivered over 10 fractions. Newer modalities of delivering radiation have led to better treatment options for some patients. Stereotactic radiosurgery (SRS) delivers a one-time, small, well-defined beam of radiation to a specific target, sparing surrounding brain. Surgical resection or SRS is now the favored treatment for patients with good prognostic factors and limited intracranial disease. The results of SRS are similar to those of surgical resection, but SRS often worsens adjacent cerebral edema for a few months. Tumors larger than 3 cm in diameter are poor SRS targets, because of difficulty producing a sharply contoured beam, essential for limiting radiation to the surrounding brain. Large tumors also develop worse post-treatment edema. An advantage of SRS over surgery is that multiple lesions can be treated in one procedure. If more than three lesions are present, standard fractionated whole brain radiation is usually chosen. The role of chemotherapy is debated, but certain tumor types are amenable to chemotherapy, including lung cancer, breast cancer, germ cell tumors, and choriocarcinoma.

Epidural metastases with spinal cord compression

Spinal cord injury from cancer almost always results from a tumor growing in the epidural space. Eighty percent reach the epidural space by extension from the vertebral body, a late complication of bone metastases. Breast, prostate and lung cancers lead the list of primary types, each having a high likelihood of dissemination to bone. Most of the remaining 20% of cases result from extension of paraspinal tumors through the neural foramen. Lymphomas are the most common type epidural, spinal tumors. Intradural nodules large enough to compress the spinal cord are an occasional feature of carcinomatous meningitis (see below). Metastasis directly to spinal cord is rare.

Back pain is the initial symptom in 60–90% of patients with epidural spinal cord compression. Pain precedes the neurological symptoms by weeks to months. For this reason, every cancer patient should be repeatedly asked about new back pain, and every positive report should be evaluated in detail. This often means imaging the spine, usually with MRI. The thoracic region is most often affected, followed by lumbar, then cervical. By comparison, degenerative joint and disc disease of the spine more commonly involves the lumbar and cervical regions. Pain due to vertebral metastasis is usually near the level of bone involvement and is aggravated by local percussion of the spine. Unlike disc disease, lying down tends to worsen the pain, presumably because of venous engorgement and edema. Excruciating pain with movement suggests mechanical instability of the spine and may reflect a pathologic collapse of the vertebrae. Patients with cervical cord compression sometimes report Lhermittes's phenomenon (paresthesias shooting downward with neck flexion).

The most common symptoms after pain are weakness and sensory disturbance below the level of the lesion. Patients often report a belt- or band-like sensation around the trunk at or just below the level of the lesion, indicating radicular symptoms in addition to myelopathy. Autonomic symptoms, especially bladder incontinence or retention, and gait disturbance are prominent features. The classical examination findings include bilateral corticospinal tract signs and a truncal sensory level to pain, temperature, and light touch a segment or two below the actual level of cord impingement. Compression below the T12 or L1 vertebral body produces a cauda equina syndrome rather than a myelopathic picture. The Brown-Séquard syndrome is uncommon with external compression, being more typical of intrinsic cord lesions. About 10% of patients will have a gait ataxia without classical myelopathic signs. These patients are difficult to diagnose.

MRI scanning usually shows abnormal signal from the vertebral body marrow plus an irregular, enhancing lesion that distorts and compresses the spinal cord and obliterates the surrounding CSF. These masses do not follow anatomic boundaries and may be difficult to visualize. Multiple vertebral levels may be involved. Remarkably, the epidural neoplasm almost never transgresses the dura. CSF leakage, neoplastic meningitis, and direct extension into the spinal cord proper are extremely rare.

Emergency measures for neurological stabilization rely heavily on corticosteroids. Dexamethasone 100 mg IV once followed by 24 mg every 6 hours is a common regimen. Pain control often is greatly aided by the corticosteroid, but most patients also require narcotics. Surgical resection of the tumor and the vertebral body followed by radiation for 10–14 fractions is the best treatment but can be undertaken in only a very select group of patients. Most patients receive radiation alone. Surgical decompression by dorsal laminectomy followed by radiation is not more effective than radiation alone.

Leptomeningeal metastases (neoplastic meningitis)

Neoplastic meningitis can result from metastatic spread through the blood stream, by perineural spread along cranial or spinal nerve roots, or from metastatic deposits in the brain or choroid plexus. Although the term *carcinomatous meningitis* is often used interchangeably with *neoplastic meningitis*, there are important differences in the incidence, treatment, and long-term control of neoplastic meningitis caused by different tumor types.

For many acute leukemias and some high-grade lymphomas, involvement of the meninges is so common that even in the absence of symptoms or CSF abnormalities therapy to the CNS (*CNS prophylaxis*) is routinely advised. Among nonhematologic cancers in adults, none involve the meninges or CSF frequently enough to recommend routine prophylaxis. The most common causes are breast cancer, lung cancer, and melanoma, although essentially any cancer can on rare occasion seed the meninges.

The presenting symptoms are widely varied but include combinations of cranial nerve, spinal nerve root, and cognitive dysfunction. They may be fulminant or subacute, but almost never chronic. Headache is common (40%), as is hydrocephalus. Meningeal enhancement on MRI is seen in > 85% of patient with solid tumors, but less often in lymphoma and leukemia. The enhancement may be subtle or patchy or include obvious nodules. Meningeal enhancement, however, is very nonspecific, and confirmation by CSF analysis is strongly recommended. CSF abnormalities are present in every patient. Typically the protein is elevated (80–90%), the glucose is low (30–40%), and there is a lymphocyte predominant pleocytosis (60–70%). Cytology is positive in 60–90% if multiple taps are performed. Tumor markers such as carcinoembryonic antigen (CEA) can be helpful for solid tumors.

Flow cytometry can be helpful for leukemias and lymphomas when cytology is negative. Meningeal biopsy is rarely used, and usually not helpful.

CSF flow patterns are often disturbed due to impairment of reabsorption at the arachnoid villi or accumulation of tumor cells and fibrosis in the basilar cisterns or other subarachnoid sites. This is a poor prognostic feature and also impedes delivery of chemotherapies that are administered directly into the CSF. Many authors suggest assessment of CSF dynamics by nuclear cisternography, the injection of a radionucleotide into the CSF with nuclear imaging at various times over 12–24 hours to assess the distribution of the marker. Ventriculoperitoneal shunting may be very helpful as a symptomatic treatment if hydrocephalus is present.

Radiation to symptomatic regions is the best therapy for most solid tumors involving the leptomeninges. Progression of symptoms is often halted. Focal radiation to areas of CSF block is also recommended. In practice, both objectives often require whole brain radiation. Cranial spinal radiation would seem to be advantageous, but is generally too morbid.

Intrathecal chemotherapy is used in selected cases; the neoplasms that respond the best are breast cancer, small cell lung cancer, and lymphoma. Chemotherapy can be administered via a lumbar puncture, but better distribution is achieved when administered through a reservoir/catheter system into the lateral ventricle (Ommaya reservoir). Agents that are routinely available for intrathecal treatment include methotrexate, ARA-C, and thiotepa. A slow-release form of ARA-C, Depocyt, has demonstrated good activity against lymphoma and some solid tumors. A few other cytoxic agents, some monoclonal antibodies, and interferons have been used by this route. Systemic chemotherapy such as high-dose methotrexate is also used in selected patients.

The median survival for patients with carcinomatous meningitis from solid tumors is about 4 months. Symptom control can be achieved in many patients, but long-term tumor control is not common, and only 10% survive more than a year. Carcinomatous meningitis is a late occurring complication, and for patients who have widely disseminated cancers or poor performance status simple palliative care is commonly chosen.

Meningioma

Meningiomas are the most common extraparenchymal CNS tumors. They are usually present as a solitary mass compressing the brain from the lateral convexity (20%) or parasagittal region (17%), as a skull base mass compressing cranial nerves particularly in the sphenoid wing or parasellar region (28%), subfrontally in the olfactory groove (10%), posterior fossa (14%), or in the spine or other locations (10%). Many are asymptomatic, and it is common to find a small meningioma as a coincidental finding on a CT or MRI obtained for unrelated symptoms. There is a wide variety of histologic patterns, although 95% are histologically low grade. A small number, termed atypical meningiomas, display mitotic figures. Less common still are anaplastic, invasive tumors termed malignant meningiomas.

The majority of meningiomas occur in women (female:male—3:1), and many have estrogen and progesterone receptors. The peak incidence is in the fifth through seventh decades. They can occur as part of hereditary cancer syndromes, most notably neurofibromatosis type II. They are also known to arise as treatment-related second tumors years after radiation for tumors of the head and neck region.

Complete resection is curative for most patients. The survival in this group at 5, 10, and 15 years is 93%, 80%, and 68%. However, incomplete resection is common for lesions that encase cranial nerves, arterial structures such as the carotid artery, or venous structures such as the sagittal sinus. After subtotal resection the 5-, 10- and 15-year survival rates are 63%, 45%, and 9%. Some authors have favored radiation for incompletely resected meningiomas. More often, the residual tumor is monitored by MRI every 6–12 months. Reresection, fractionated radiation, or stereotactic radio-surgery are used for subsequent progression. Radiation is used as part of the initial treatment plan after resection in patients with malignant melanomas. Chemotherapy and hormonal therapy have been attempted for recurrent meningiomas, but with very little success.

KEY REFERENCES

Baldwin RT, Preston-Martin S. Epidemiology of brain tumors in childhood—a review. *Toxicol Appl Pharmacol* 2004;199(2):118–131.

Behin A, Hoang-Xuan K, Carpentier AF, et al. Primary brain tumours in adults. *Lancet* 2003;361:323–331.

CBTRUS. Statistical report: Primary Brain Tumors in the United States. Central Brain Tumor Registry of the United States 1998–2002, 2005.

Cairncross JG, Macdonald DR. Successful chemotherapy for recurrent malignant oligodendroglioma. *Ann Neurol* 1988;23:360–364.

Cairncross JG, Ueki K, Zlatescu MC, et al. Specific genetic predictors of chemotherapeutic response and survival in patients with anaplastic oligodendrogliomas. *J Natl Cancer Inst* 1998;90:1473–1479.

Chamberlain MC. Neoplastic meningitis. *J Clin Oncol* 2005;23:3605–3613.

Delattre JY, Krol G, Thaler HT, et al. Distribution of brain metastases. *Arch Neurol* 1988;45:741–744.

Forsyth PA, Posner JB. Headaches in patients with brain tumors: a study of 111 patients. *Neurology* 1993;43:1678–1683.

Gavrilovic IT, Posner JB. Brain metastases: epidemiology and pathophysiology. *J Neurooncol* 2005;75:5–14.

Glantz MJ, Cole BF, Forsyth PA, et al. Practice parameter: anticonvulsant prophylaxis in patients with newly diagnosed brain tumors. Report of the Quality Standards

Subcommittee of the American Academy of Neurology. *Neurology* 2000;54: 1886–1893.

Karim AB, Maat B, Hatlevoll R, et al. A randomized trial on dose-response in radiation therapy of low-grade cerebral glioma: European Organization for Research and Treatment of Cancer (EORTC) Study 22844. *Int J Radiat Oncol Biol Phys* 1996;36:549–556.

Mirimanoff RE, Dosoretz DE, Linggood RM, et al. Meningioma: analysis of recurrence and progression following neurosurgical resection. *J Neurosurg* 1985;62:18–24.

Moots PL, Maciunas RJ, Eisert DR, et al. The course of seizure disorders in patients with malignant gliomas. *Arch Neurol* 1995;52:717–724.

Moots PL. Pitfalls in the management of patients with malignant gliomas. *Semin Neurol* 1998;18:257–265.

Patchell RA, Tibbs PA, Regine WF, et al. Direct decompressive surgical resection in the treatment of spinal cord compression caused by metastatic cancer: a randomised trial. *Lancet* 2005;366:643–648.

Posner JB, Chernik NL. Intracranial metastases from systemic cancer. *Adv Neurol* 1978;19:579–592.

Shapiro WR, Green SB, Strike TA, et al. Randomized trial of three chemotherapy regimens and two radiotherapy regimens and two radiotherapy regimens in postoperative treatment of malignant glioma. Brain Tumor Cooperative Group Trial 8001. *J Neurosurg* 1989;71:1–9.

Soffietti R, Costanza A, Lasuzzi E, et al. Radiotherapy and chemotherapy of brain metastases. *J Neurooncol* 2005;75:31–42.

Stupp R, Mason WP, van den Bent MJ, et al. Radiotherapy plus concomitant and adjuvant temozolomide for glioblastoma. *N Engl J Med* 2005;352:987–996.

Walker MD, Alexander E Jr, Hunt WE, et al. Evaluation of BCNU and/or radiotherapy in the treatment of anaplastic gliomas. A cooperative clinical trial. *J Neurosurg* 1978;49:333–343.

CHAPTER 37

BRAIN DEATH, PERSISTENT VEGETATIVE STATE, AND MINIMALLY CONSCIOUS STATE

INTRODUCTION

One of the most difficult tasks a neurologist faces in clinical practice is the request to prognosticate on the likelihood of recovery of a patient in coma after severe brain injuries. The easiest case is that of brain death, and we shall consider that first. Only a small minority of comatose patients, however, reach a state of brain death. The vast majority remain in states in which some brain function remains. Especially problematic, as anyone who has followed the news of Terri Schiavo and other legal cases knows, is medical decision making in patients with persistent vegetative or minimally conscious states.

BRAIN DEATH

The criteria for brain death are relatively straightforward. The criteria were created by a Presidential Commission in 1981, and most states and hospitals have more or less accepted them, with varying degrees of legal certitude. Death in the past meant cardiac death, or loss of heart rhythm and pumping. With traumatic brain injury, massive stroke or cerebral hemorrhage with herniation, or cardiac arrest with hypoxic encephalopathy, the brain can be irretrievably damaged, yet the heart can beat on, with maintenance of blood pressure and function of the other organs.

By the Presidential Commission criteria, brain death really means loss of brainstem functions. The criteria are shown in Table 37-1. The first criterion

Table 37-1 **Criteria for Brain Death**

Coma
Absent respirations, including apnea testing with pCO_2 >60
Absent pupillary light reflexes
Absent corneal reflexes
Absent eye movements, including oculocephalic and oculovestibular reflexes
Absent gag and cough reflexes
Absent motor responses other than spinal reflexes
Absent withdrawal from sensory stimuli

Source: American Academy of Neurology. Practice parameters: assessment and management of patients in the persistent vegetative state. Report of the Quality Standards Subcommittee of the American Academy of Neurology. Copyright AAN, 1994.

of brain death is coma, complete unresponsiveness. The second is complete apnea. Apnea should be confirmed by a formal apnea test, in which the patient's ventilator is temporarily turned off, and 100% oxygen is given via a cannula placed into the endotracheal tube. The goal is to have the patient off mechanical ventilation for 10 minutes; at the end of this period, blood gases are taken to make sure that the pCO_2 is elevated above 60 mm Hg. Since both hypoxia and hypercapnea are stimulants of ventilation, both hypoxia and hypercarbia must be achieved to ensure that complete apnea is present. Simply disconnecting the ventilator for 2–3 minutes, which will usually achieve hypoxemia, is not sufficient for apnea determination. It takes much longer to achieve hypercarbia, particularly in an intensive care patient on a ventilator, in whom hyperventilation and hypocarbia are often part of the treatment plan (see Chap. 23).

Brain death implies loss of all brainstem reflexes and functions. The pupils should be completely unreactive, and the eyes should be fixed in midposition, with no movement either spontaneously, with movement of the head (oculocephalic maneuver), or with ice water calorics (oculovestibular maneuver). The corneal reflexes must be absent. Stimulation of the face or nostrils with a noxious stimulus such as a sharp Q-tip produces no response whatever. There must be no gag reflex, even during endotracheal suctioning. There should be no spontaneous movement of the limbs, nor a clear response to noxious stimuli such as sternal rub or pinch on the limbs. Muscle stretch (deep tendon) reflexes can be present, since these are mediated at spinal cord level. Two additional criteria require that the patient must not have sedative drugs on board which could depress brainstem reflexes, and the patient should not be hypothermic. Caution was also advised in children below 5 years of age.

Loss of all brainstem function prevents the cerebral cortex from being awake or responsive. We often do not know if the cortex itself is damaged, but the available experience confirms that complete loss of brainstem function augurs the permanent loss of all brain functions. No patient with complete loss of brainstem function, including all of the above criteria, has ever recovered.

The original Presidential Commission criteria for brain death required a waiting period. If the cause was hypoxia or unknown, two examinations of the type described above had to be performed at 24-hour intervals. If the cause was known, as with a massive stroke or cerebral hemorrhage, the waiting period was only 12 hours. This could be reduced to 6 hours with a confirmatory laboratory test. The Commission did not advocate a specific laboratory test, listing cerebral angiography, radioisotope cerebral blood flow study, electroencephalogram (EEG), brainstem auditory evoked response (BAER), and somatosensory evoked response (SER) as alternative tests.

LABORATORY TESTS TO CONFIRM BRAIN DEATH

The traditional test used to confirm brain death is the EEG, which should be "flat" or isoelectric in brain death. This test has technical difficulties, in that patients in intensive care units are likely to show various electrical artifacts on EEG from all of the equipment operating around them. In recent years, other tests have been developed to get around the limitations of the EEG. Evoked responses, either auditory or somatosensory, can document an absence of response, equally predictive as the EEG in terms of no prognosis for recovery. Various techniques have been used to measure cerebral blood flow; as the brain swells, perfusion of the brain usually ceases. This can be measured by arteriography, by an isotope cerebral blood flow study, or by transcranial Doppler ultrasonography. If any of these tests confirms brain death, the waiting period before final determination of brain death can be reduced to 6 hours.

MANAGEMENT OF BRAIN DEATH

The Presidential Commission criteria for brain death have been widely accepted nationally, though not specifically backed up by national law. A patient who is brain dead can, in practice, be declared dead and removed from the ventilator and other life support. In practice, this is usually not done without the family's agreement. Occasionally, families disagree among themselves or refuse to grant permission to remove life support, and hospital ethics committees and even legal authorities must become involved. The other practical repercussion of a brain death declaration is that organs can potentially be harvested for transplant procedures. In many states, representatives of organ donor organizations are the ones empowered to discuss the issue of organ donation with the families. If the brain dead patient is to be an organ donor, life support apparatus must be maintained until the organs are harvested.

PERSISTENT VEGETATIVE STATE

Persistent vegetative state (PVS) is a condition in which the patient has intact brainstem functions, but no evidence of function of the cerebral cortex. The term was coined by Jennett and Plum in 1972. Physicians have sought to develop a set of criteria that would provide certainty, similar to that of brain death, that the patient in this state will have no meaningful recovery. PVS is distinguished from several other states of reduced consciousness, which may be more common.

The American Academy of Neurology, along with representatives of the American Neurological Association, Child Neurology Society, American Association of Neurological Surgeons, and American Academy of Pediatrics set up a Multi-Society Task Force to establish criteria for the PVS. The guidelines, published in 1994, have also been adopted as a practice guideline by the American Academy of Neurology. At least 10,000–25,000 adults and 6000–10,000 children in the United States were estimated in 1995 to have PVS. The criteria for diagnosis of PVS, shown in Table 37-2, must be made at least 1 year after traumatic brain injury in young patients, and at least 3 months after nontraumatic illnesses.

The Task Force reviewed case series from the literature including 434 adults and 106 children with traumatic brain injury, and 169 adults

Table 37-2 **Requirements for the Examination of a PVS**

(1) No evidence of awareness of self or environment, no interaction with others
(2) No meaningful response to stimuli
(3) No receptive or expressive language
(4) Return of sleep-wake cycles, arousal, even smiling, frowning, and yawning
(5) Preserved brainstem/hypothalamic autonomic functions to permit survival
(6) Bowel and bladder incontinence
(7) Variably preserved CN and spinal reflexes

Source: Multi-Society Task Force on PVS. Medical aspects of the persistent vegetative state (second of two parts). *N Engl J Med* 1994;330:1572–1579.

and 45 children with nontraumatic injuries, mostly related to hypoxia. Of patients in PVS for more than 3 months after nontraumatic injuries, the probability of moderate disability or good recovery was less than 1% (99% confidence intervals 0–4%). In those patients who were still in PVS at 6 months, the probability of any reasonable recovery was 0%. No patient has been reported to recover after a full year of PVS, not even patients with traumatic brain injury. Patients in well publicized legal cases, such as Karen Ann Quinlan, Nancy Cruzan, and Terri Schiavo, have remained in this state for years, and no such cases have recovered.

The criteria for PVS make clear that the patient can have periods of sleep alternating with periods of an awake-like state, in which the eyes are open and may move about, and the patient may breathe, yawn, open the mouth, chew, perhaps even briefly turn towards stimuli, but not interact meaningfully with others. There is always the possibility that family members will see such movements as "meaningful" responses. It is true that patients who are minimally responsive may respond more to family members than to the many nurses and physicians who enter the patient's room each day and night. On the other hand, the criteria for PVS are well substantiated by abundant patient experience; as long as all of the criteria are fulfilled, including the time period, the prognosis can be confidently predicted as nil for meaningful recovery.

Many specific etiologies of brain injury can result in PVS. After acute traumatic and nontraumatic brain injury, PVS evolves out of an initial coma. In degenerative and metabolic disorders of the nervous system, the patient gradually sinks into PVS from a more responsive state. Severe developmental malformations of the central nervous system can produce PVS, but only in anencephaly can PVS be diagnosed before 3 months of observation. In all cases, PVS is a diagnosis based on observation over time.

A semantic debate surrounds the distinction between persistent and permanent vegetative states. In general, a vegetative state can be suspected at 1 month after an acute brain injury or hypoxia. Permanent vegetative state can be diagnosed after 3 months in nontraumatic and after 12 months in traumatic brain injuries. Note that this definition of permanent vegetative state is equivalent to the definition of persistent vegetative state given earlier. The guideline also states: "A PVS patient becomes permanently vegetative when the diagnosis of irreversibility can be established with a high degree of clinical certainty, i.e., when the chance of regaining consciousness is exceedingly rare."

Laboratory tests in PVS

Diagnostic tests such as computerized tomography (CT) or magnetic resonance imaging (MRI) scans can confirm that much of the cerebral cortex has been damaged. Functional brain imaging modalities such as functional magnetic resonance imaging (fMRI), single photon emission computed tomography (SPECT), and positron emission tomography (PET) scanning may be used to document the lack of arousal of the cortex to stimuli. These tests, however, remain investigational and have been validated only in small case series. The Multi-Society Task Force stated that diagnostic tests "may support the diagnosis of PVS, but none adds to the diagnostic specificity with certainty." This recommendation has not changed in the years since the Task Force publication.

Management of the PVS patient

Once a diagnosis of PVS has been made with certainty, a prognosis of no possibility of meaningful recovery can be given. Most patients in PVS are no longer dependent on ventilators, and life support in this situation may mean a feeding tube to provide hydration and nutrition. Removal of such simple, supportive care is the cause of great moral, philosophical, and legal debate, as was seen in the recent Terri Schiavo case. A final provision of the American Academy of Neurology practice guideline discusses the decision to withhold fluids and nutrition via a feeding tube (see Table 37-3). In practice, many families decide well before the time criteria for PVS have been satisfied that they do not want to see their loved one kept "alive" on life support without meaningful interaction with other people. Decisions to withdraw life support are often made before the full PVS criteria are met. Most states recognize the right of patients to refuse medical care, and this refusal is equally valid if provided before the event, in the form of an advanced directive. The spectacular legal cases, such as that of Terri Schiavo, develop in cases where no advanced directive exists, and the family members cannot agree on what the patient would have wanted.

Table 37-3 **Policy on Nutrition and Hydration**

(1) "The decision to discontinue fluid and nutrition should be made in the same manner as other medical treatment decisions";
(2) "Artificial provision of nutrition and hydration is analogous to other forms of life-sustaining treatment, such as . . . a respirator";
(3) "Administration of fluids and nutrition by medical means, such as a G-tube, is a medical procedure"; and
(4) "Treatments which provide no benefit to the patient or the family may be discontinued . . . Medical treatment provides no benefit to patients in a PVS, once the diagnosis is established."

Source: American Academy of Neurology. Practice parameters: assessment and management of patients in the persistent vegetative state. Report of the Quality Standards Subcommittee of the American Academy of Neurology. Copyright AAN, 1994.

MINIMALLY CONSCIOUS STATE

A more recent category of patients who have some, but very limited consciousness, is called the *minimally conscious state* (MCS). This designation was adopted at a conference in 2002. MCS may be as much as 10 times more common than PVS. Unlike PVS, the prognosis of individual patients in MCS has not been well defined by clinical studies, and the ethical implications are more questionable. These patients have some minimal evidence of conscious awareness and interaction with other people and with the environment. Table 37-4 lists the proposed criteria for MCS.

Management of the MCS patient

The implications of a diagnosis of MCS are not well defined. There is no time criterion for diagnosis; presumably, patients in MCS soon after an injury or cardiac arrest may improve progressively, whereas those who have taken months to reach this state would be unlikely to make a qualitatively good recovery. Much of the debate in the Terri Schiavo case rested on whether she truly had PVS, or whether she might have MCS. The Florida courts, based

Table 37-4 **Criteria for Minimally Conscious State**

To diagnose MCS, limited but clearly discernible evidence of self- or environmental awareness must be demonstrated on a reproducible or sustained basis by one or more of the following behaviors:
(1) Follows simple commands
(2) Gestural or verbal yes/no responses (regardless of accuracy)
(3) Intelligible verbalization
(4) Purposeful behavior, including movements or effective behaviors that occur in contingent relationship to relevant environmental stimuli and are not due to reflexive activity. Some examples of qualifying purposeful behavior are
  Appropriate smiling or crying in response to the linguistic or visual content of emotional but not to neutral topics or stimuli
  Vocalizations or gestures that occur in direct response to the linguistic content of questions
  Reaching for objects that demonstrates a clear relationship between object location and direction of reach
  Touching or holding objects in a manner that accommodates the size and shape of the object
  Pursuit eye movement of sustained fixation that occurs in direct response to moving or salient stimuli

Source: Giacino JT, Ashwal S, Childs N, et al. The minimally conscious state: definition and diagnostic criteria. *Neurology* 2002;58:349–353.

on review of expert testimony, found that criteria for PVS were satisfied, and the higher courts did not reverse this finding. The application of an advanced directive would still be ethically appropriate in patients with longstanding MCS, but the legal implications have not been decided.

KEY REFERENCES

American Academy of Neurology. Practice parameters: assessment and management of patients in the persistent vegetative state. Report of the Quality Standards Subcommittee of the American Academy of Neurology. Copyright AAN, 1994.

Beuthien-Baumann B, Handrick W, Schmidt T, et al. Persistent vegetative state: evaluation of brain metabolism and brain perfusion with PET and SPECT. *Nucl Med Commun* 2003;24:643–649.

Els T, Kassubek J, Kubalek R, et al. Diffusion-weighted MRI during early global cerebral hypoxia: a predictor for clinical outcome? *Acta Neurol Scand* 2004;110:361–367.

Giacino JT, Ashwal S, Childs N, et al. The minimally conscious state: definition and diagnostic criteria. *Neurology* 2002;58:349–353.

Gostin LO. Ethics, the Constitution, and the dying process. The case of Theresa Marie Schiavo. *JAMA* 2005;293:2403–2407.

Jennett B, Plum F. Persistent vegetative state after brain damage: a syndrome in search of a name. *Lancet* 1972;1:734–737.

Kampfl A, Schmutzhard E, Franz G, et al. Prediction of recovery from post-traumatic vegetative state with cerebral magnetic-resonance imaging. *Lancet* 1998;352: 1763–1767.

Laureys S, Faymonville ME, Peigneux P, et al. Cortical processing of noxious somatosensory stimuli in the persistent vegetative state. *Neuroimage* 2002;17: 732–741.

Multi-Society Task Force on PVS. Medical aspects of the persistent vegetative state (first of two parts). *N Engl J Med* 1994;330:1499–1508.

Multi-Society Task Force on PVS. Medical aspects of the persistent vegetative state (second of two parts). *N Engl J Med* 1994;330:1572–1579.

Perry JE, Churchill LR, Kirshner HS. The Terri Schiavo case: legal, ethical, and medical perspectives. *Ann Intern Med* 2005;143:744–748.

President's Commission for the Study of Ethical Problems in Medicine and Biomedical Research, Defining Death. Guidelines for the determination of brain death. *JAMA* 1981;246:2184–2186.

Quality Standards Subcommittee of the American Academy of Neurology. Practice parameters for determining brain death in adults (summary statement). *Neurology* 1995;45:1012–1014.

Wijdicks EFM, Cranford RE. Clinical diagnosis of prolonged states of impaired consciousness in adults. *Mayo Clin Proc* 2005;80:1037–1046.

Wijdicks EFM. The diagnosis of brain death. *N Engl J Med* 2001;344:1215–1221.

NEURODIAGNOSTIC TESTS

Karl E. Misulis, MD, PhD

INTRODUCTION: SELECTION OF TESTS

This chapter will review common neurodiagnostic tests ordered by and often performed and/or interpreted by neurologists. We shall also briefly review neuroimaging tests such as computed tomography (CT) and magnetic resonance imaging (MRI), which are usually performed by radiology facilities. Specific tests are indicated for defined indications. There are two somewhat opposing points of view regarding neurodiagnostic and radiologic tests. On the one hand, the clinician is in the best position to determine what tests are needed; by this criterion, the test should be performed without other justification than it is needed, in the clinician's judgment. The opposing point of view is that mere opinion is not a justification for expensive testing. Reimbursement usually depends on justification to the payor that the procedure is needed and justified. The neurophysiologist or radiologist who directs, performs, and interprets the tests is not a mere technician, but a diagnostic consultant who is in a position to determine when certain tests and procedures are clinically indicated. For example, electroencephalography (EEG) is not indicated for evaluation of patients for headache.

Before ordering any test, whether a chemical test on the blood, an X-ray or imaging procedure, or a neurophysiological study, the physician should determine the purpose of the test. A test ordered without a clear purpose, or knowledge of what is being looked for with the test, is likely to be confusing rather than helpful. The neurologist should always go as far toward diagnosis as possible with the tools of the history and physical examination, with laboratory tests used mainly for confirmation.

Electroencephalography

EEG is the recording of cerebral potentials from the brain. The main purpose of the EEG is for the assessment of patients with suspected seizures, although the test may also be done for assessment of coma, brain death, and other indications.

EEG THEORY

All neurons conduct electricity, but the magnitude of the charge movements is not large enough that the activity of a single neuron can be detected by scalp electrodes. Only synchronous activity in many neurons can be detected by scalp recordings. EEG rhythms detected at the scalp, including the normal background rhythms of the brain, sleep patterns, and alerting responses, represent the simultaneous activation of many neurons. Epilepsy can produce abnormally synchronous activation of neurons, which can often be detected by scalp electrodes.

EEG METHODS

EEG electrodes are cup-shaped, metal discs, which are placed onto the scalp. A conducting gel acts as a maleable extension of the electrode and is placed inside the cup to help reduce impedance between the scalp and electrode.

An array of electrodes covers the scalp. The electrodes then pass to the EEG machine, which amplifies the signal from each electrode. The potentials emanating from the specific electrodes are compared to display the electrical activity of the surface of the brain. The electrodes are compared in various combinations, termed *montages*. The individual montages have strengths and weakness, and there is a degree of personal preference among neurophysiologists in the use of montages, within some general guidelines. Recordings are of varying duration, from 20 minutes to days. Long-term recordings are used to try to capture seizures on EEG (Fig. 38-1).

EEG RESULTS

EEG recordings are very complex and must be interpreted in light of a number of factors including state (awake, drowsy, sleep, lethargy, coma), age (premature to elderly), and activation during the recording (photic, tactile, auditory). For this reason, computerized interpretation of EEG will likely never be adequate, although computer analyses are helpful for power spectral analyses and spike detection. Visual examination by the neurophysiologist will likely remain the gold standard.

The EEG is analysed for (1) background activity, (2) transients, and (3) response to activation.

Background activity consists of a combination of EEG rhythms for which normal patterns have been established for awake, drowsy, and sleep states for patients from about 29 weeks conceptional age to patients in their eighties.

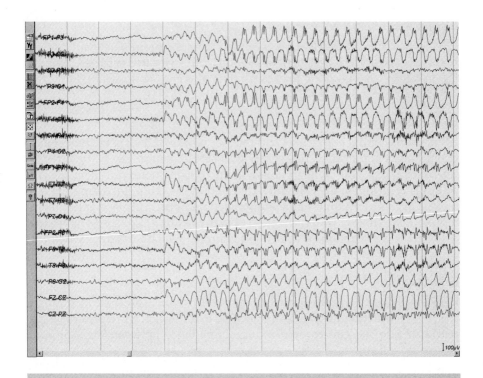

Figure 38-1 ***EEG showing absence seizure.*** EEG of a patient with absence epilepsy, showing the spike-wave pattern which begins about 4 seconds into the recording. The EEG up to that point is normal.

Recordings of patients outside these bounds have to be interpreted with caution and with disclaimers.

Transients are brief potential changes on EEG. They may include normal potentials due to partial arousal, movement, or other physiologic potentials, or pathologic transients such as seizure activity.

Response to activation refers to changes in the EEG during photic stimulation, hyperventilation, or simply auditory or tactile stimulation. Photic stimulation and hyperventilation are performed to enhance the detection of seizure activity in awake patients. Auditory and tactile stimulation are used to try to evoke a response in patients with severe encephalopathy.

INTERPRETATION

The most common interpretation of EEG in the outpatient setting is "normal." This means that the background was normal for the clinical states, there were no seizure discharges with activation procedures, and there were no pathologic transients.

The most common interpretation of EEG of hospitalized patients is "abnormal, consistent with encephalopathy." The most common reason for neurologic evaluation in the hospital is confusion, which produces slowing and disorganization of the background of the EEG. *Paroxysmal* or *epileptiform discharges*, referred to in medical slang as "seizure discharges" are also common, and may be the most common finding in some hospitals, particularly those with epilepsy monitoring units. The word *seizure* should always refer to a clinical spell, not just an EEG discharge, and not all patients with paroxysmal discharges have epilepsy. Table 38-1 lists common EEG findings and their interpretations.

Table 38-1 **EEG Findings**

Finding	Interpretation	Clinical correlate
Normal background	Normal	Normal patients. Patients with seizures and some other disorders may have normal EEGs despite their disorder.
Diffuse slowing of the background	Abnormal, consistent with a diffuse encephalopathy	Many possible causes, including metabolic, toxic, infectious, vascular, degenerative, and neoplastic.
Focal slowing of the background	Abnormal, consistent with a focal structural lesion	Many possible causes of focal slowing, including tumors, stroke, injury, infection.
Generalized epileptic transients	Abnormal, consistent with seizure disorder of the generalized type	Seen in patients with absence of epilepsy, juvenile myoclonic epilepsy, and other types, although the appearance differs between these.
Focal epileptic transients	Abnormal, consistent with a seizure disorder of the focal type	Usually seen in patients with focal seizures. May also be seen with or without seizures in patients with focal structural lesions.
Periodic discharges over one or both hemispheres	Abnormal, indicative of disturbance of cortical function	Seen in patients with destructive lesions such as HSV encephalitis, some prion diseases, and anoxia.

Figure 38-1 shows an EEG montage of 18 channels. This EEG happened to record a 3/second, generalized, spike/wave, epileptiform discharge, very typical of what is seen in *absence* (formerly called "petit-mal") epilepsy.

Neuromuscular electrophysiology

Neuromuscular electrophysiological testing consists of two main parts: nerve conduction studies (NCS) and electromyography (EMG). The two are usually used together. The EMG/NCS, as it is commonly called, must be focused on the specific problem at hand; as such, it is best performed under the direct supervision of a trained neurophysiologist. An untrained technician or physician cannot give consistent, high quality studies. In addition, accurate clinical information of the patient's symptoms and signs must be available, in order for the appropriate tests to be selected. If this information is lacking, the neurophysiologist must perform a clinical neurology consultation before beginning electrical studies.

NERVE CONDUCTION STUDY

NCS use nerve stimulation with recording from the peripheral nerves and muscles. The NCS is divided into the following: (1) sensory NCS, (2) motor NCS, (3) F-wave study, (4) H-reflex study, and (5) repetitive nerve stimulation (RNS) study.

Sensory NCS is performed by stimulating a pure sensory portion of a nerve while recording proximal to this. The proximal portion may be a mixed nerve, but the motor component is not activated because only sensory fibers are stimulated. The sensory nerve conduction velocity (NCV) is determined by dividing the distance between the stimulating and recording electrodes, by the latency of the sensory nerve action potential (SNAP). The NCV is expressed in meters/second. Tables must be consulted to know the normal values, though in general NCVs above 40 m/second are usually normal.

Motor NCS is performed by recording from a muscle while stimulating the peripheral nerve proximal to the muscle. The nerve may be motor or mixed; stimulation of the sensory nerve has no significant direct effect on the muscle. If you calculate the conduction velocity from the stimulation site to the recording site on the muscle, an artificially low velocity will be recorded since there is a delay in neuromuscular transmission and because the conduction velocity of the muscle is different from that of the motor nerves. Therefore, two stimulation points are used on the innervating nerve. The distance between the two stimulating sites is divided by the difference in the latencies of the compound motor action potential (CMAP) after stimulation at the two sites. This is the motor NCV. For motor conduction between the most distal stimulating point on the nerve and the muscle, the latency in milliseconds is simply expressed as a *distal latency*. Again, normal values for these latencies must be looked up.

F-wave, H-reflex, and RNS (repetitive nerve stimulation) studies are specialized studies using electrical stimulation. The F-wave detects conduction of the proximal portion of peripheral nerves, from the limb to the spine. The H-reflex is essentially the electrophysiologic correlate of the achilles reflex. RNS is used to look for neuromuscular transmission disorders such as myasthenia gravis, Lambert-Eaton myasthenic syndrome, and botulism (Chap. 35).

ELECTROMYOGRAPHY

EMG is performed by inserting a needle electrode into a muscle and recording muscle fiber action potentials at rest and with voluntary contraction. There is no electrical stimulation. Normal muscles are electrically silent at rest, so discharges are usually abnormal unless the patient is not truly relaxing the muscle. With voluntary contraction, the EMG shows a compound action potential for each motor unit, or group of muscle fibers activated by a single motor axon. Acute denervation of the muscle results in reduced numbers of motor unit potentials. Chronic denervation results not only in fewer units, but the remaining units have a polyphasic appearance and are often larger in amplitude than normal motor unit potentials (MUPs). The large amplitude, polyphasic potentials reflect reinnervation of denervated muscle fibers by surviving axons, leading to larger-than-normal motor units. In contrast to denervating disorders, myopathies do not reduce the number of motor units. Instead, each unit is smaller, and the reduced synchrony of firing of the muscle fibers produces a brief, polyphasic appearance.

By the rationale explained above, the EMG can usually differentiate the following disorders: (1) acute denervation, (2) chronic denervation, and (3) myopathy. In an acute neuropathy or nerve injury, only acute denervation changes should be present. In a chronic neuropathy, both acute and chronic denervation changes may coexist. After full recovery from a nerve injury, only chronic changes should remain.

USE OF NEUROMUSCULAR ELECTROPHYSIOLOGIC TESTS FOR DIAGNOSIS

NCS and EMG are of tremendous value in narrowing the differential diagnosis of patients with possible neuromuscular disorders. The selection of tests is often a combination of what is requested by the clinician and the neurophysiologist's planning as findings become available. For example, if the clinical question is weakness and the NCS shows severe demyelination, the approach of the neurophysiologist to the EMG will be different from that if the NCS had been normal. Table 38-2 summarizes the typical findings on EMG/NCS in common patterns of peripheral neuropathy and motor neuron disorders. Table 38-3 summarizes the use of neuromuscular electrophysiology in the diagnosis of a few, specific neuropathies. Clinical information on these disorders is found in Chap. 33.

Table 38-2 **Implications of Neurophysiologic Findings on EMG/NCS**

NCS	EMG	Physiology	Disorder
Slow	Normal	Demyelination	Acute or chronic inflammatory demyelinating neuropathies (AIDP or CIDP)
Normal	Widespread distal denervation	Axonal neuropathy	Many neuropathies including toxic, metabolic, and some inherited
Normal	Widespread proximal and distal denervation	Motor neuron degeneration	Amyotrophic lateral sclerosis (ALS)
Slow	Distal denervation	Mixed axonal/demyelinating polyneuropathy	Many metabolic, toxic, and inherited neuropathies

Table 38-3 **Electrophysiological Findings in a Few Specific Neuromuscular Disorders**

Disorder	Pathology	NCS	EMG
Diabetic neuropathy: mononeuropathy multiplex	Damage to multiple single nerves, noncompressive	Slowing of selected nerve conductions	Chronic denervation in the distributions of the neuropathy
Diabetic neuropathy: polyneuropathy	Polyneuropathy with distal and mainly axonal predominance	Mild slowing of motor and sensory NCS	Widespread distal chronic denervation, sometimes with active denervation
Acute inflammatory demyelinating polyradiculoneuropathy (AIDP)	Autoimmune demyelination	Slowing of motor and sensory NCS	Normal
Chronic inflammatory demyelinating polyradiculoneuropathy (CIDP)	Autoimmune demyelination	Slowing of motor and sensory NCS	Usually normal, although denervation can be seen
Amyotrophic lateral sclerosis (ALS)	Degeneration of upper and lower motor neurons	Normal	Acute and chronic denervation

Evoked potentials

Evoked potentials (EP) are used much less than they were a few years ago. Neurologists continue to use EPs for evaluation of patients with suspected multiple sclerosis (MS) and for patients who are undergoing intraoperative monitoring during surgery. There are three commonly used modalities: (1) brainstem auditory evoked potential (BAEP), (2) somatosensory evoked potential (SSEP), and (3) visual evoked potential (VEP).

BAEP evaluates conduction from the inner ear to the brainstem and through the brainstem. Before the days of MRI, this was the most sensitive test for acoustic neuroma and could also give evidence for a brainstem lesion, which would be difficult to see on CT. BAEP is still used in the neonatal intensive care unit (ICU) for evaluation of neonates for brainstem maturity. BAEP is performed by using specialized headphones to deliver sounds into the ears and recording from the scalp. Thousands of stimuli are given and the responses are averaged by computer, so that the consistent, evoked potential lifts out of the random, electrical noise.

SSEP evaluates conduction of sensory nerve axons ascending in the posterior columns of the spinal cord to the brainstem and cerebrum. In the past, this was useful for looking for spinal cord lesions, but MRI has proved superior for this purpose. SSEP is still used for intraoperative monitoring during spinal surgery. Absence of the SSEP has also been found to predict a poor prognosis in patients with traumatic brain injury. SSEP is performed by electrically stimulating peripheral nerves and recording from the skin overlying the spinal cord, brainstem, and brain.

VEP is used for evaluating conduction of the optic nerve to the chiasm and the optic tract and radiations. With MRI, the retrochiasmal areas can be directly imaged, and hence VEP is not used much for diagnosing hemisphere lesions. The VEP is very sensitive to demyelination of the optic nerve, a lesion that is difficult to see on MRI, so VEP still has a function in this arena. VEP is performed by having the patient look at a visual stimulus, often two changing checkerboard patterns, though in less responsive patients a bright flash can be used. Potentials from the brain are recorded, which are interpreted to determine whether one or both optic nerves are affected by demyelination or other lesion.

Computed tomographic imaging and CT angiography

Computerized tomography (CT) uses X-rays to image the body in two dimensions. Three-dimensional reconstructions can be created by computer software but are not immediately available. Neurologic uses of CT imaging include the brain, spine, and vasculature. Although some of the functions of the CT have been eclipsed by MRI, CT remains a valuable diagnostic tool.

The CT is composed of an X-ray emitter and a series of detectors. The patient moves through this array, and the output of the detectors is recorded for multiple slices through the body. The slices can be from 1 to 10 mm apart.

The data from the detectors is used for calculations, which indicate bone and tissue density through each slice. This is a two-dimensional representation of the body at this slice.

Data from adjacent slices can be used to reconstruct three-dimensional images of selected areas. Since the CT imaging gives average densities over a vertical slice, and there may be gaps between slices, the three-dimensional reconstruction is imperfect.

Iodinated contrast agents (often referred to as "dye") are sometimes used to visualize blood vessels or areas of increased vascular permeability. This is particularly helpful for visualization of tumors, vascular malformations, and infections.

Brain CT

CT of the brain is most commonly used for screening patients in the emergency department (ED) with stroke, head injury, or other cause of neurologic deficit. Although indications are individualized, as with all tests, the main indications for CT are (1) significant traumatic brain injury; (2) focal neurological deficit; (3) unexplained, severe headache; (4) altered mental status (confusion, lethargy, or coma); and (5) seizures.

Brain CT is typically performed in the ED for these reasons, but it is performed less often for elective evaluation of neurologic conditions. MRI is often chosen over CT because of superior anatomic resolution and other advantages. CT is performed when MRI cannot be undertaken because a patient is claustrophobic, uncooperative, or has an implanted electronic or mechanical device such as a cardiac pacemaker or deep brain stimulation electrode.

Traumatic brain injury can produce lucency (hypodensity) in the brain due to edema or tissue damage. If there is hemorrhage, the density will be increased. A mixture of lucency and increased density is common, indicating a hemorrhagic component of a traumatic contusion. Hemorrhage has increased density; as discussed in Chap. 24, hemorrhage can arise within the brain substance (intraparenchymal), within the spinal fluid (subarachnoid hemorrhage), under the dura (subdural hematoma), or overlying the dura (epidural hematoma). Edema from a contusion is often not evident immediately on CT, so a patient with significant head injury may have a normal emergent CT.

Strokes can be ischemic or hemorrhagic. An ischemic stroke is hypodense on CT, but the CT may be negative for as long as 2–3 days. In addition, the areas of infarction and edema are both hypodense and may be difficult to distinguish from each other. Also, patients with small vessel infarctions may have such small areas of damage that the CT remains negative even after 3 days. Hemorrhages are of increased density, regardless of the specific intracranial location. Blood decreases in density over a period of a few weeks, going through an isodense phase, and finally a hypodense phase. Strokes sometimes have a mixed appearance, with some hemorrhage into the area of infarction. In addition, hemorrhages often produce surrounding edema after 1–2 days. Without the initial CT, hemorrhage with edema can be difficult to differentiate from hemorrhage into an infarction. Figure 38-2 shows a CT scan of a patient who developed an acute right middle cerebral artery territory stroke a few hours before the scan.

Brain abscesses produce an area of variable lucency, but usually the wall of the abscess enhances with contrast administration. This results in a *ring-enhancing* appearance, with less enhancement in the relatively avascular center of the abscess. Ring enhancing lesions can be abscesses, tumors, or even strokes or cerebral hemorrhages a few days to 2–3 weeks after onset.

Brain tumors have a variable appearance. Benign or low-grade tumors (see Chap. 36) can have any density from lucent to isodense to hyperdense,

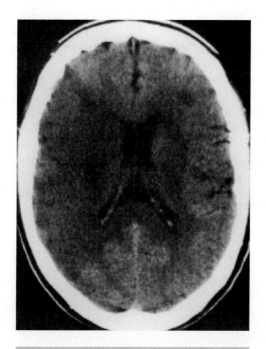

Figure 38-2 **CT scan of a patient with acute ischemic stroke.** CT of the brain showing a normal left hemisphere (right side of the figure) and loss of the normal architecture of the right hemisphere (left side of the figure). There is obliteration of the cortical sulci, mass effect pressing on the right ventricle, and diffuse hypodensity of the tissue within the right middle cerebral artery territory. This patient had an acute ischemic stroke.

though not to the extent of hemorrhage. Benign tumors do not usually enhance much with contrast administration. Malignant tumors such as metastases and high-grade primary brain neoplasms are often of decreased or variegated density, and they strongly enhance with contrast administration. The enhancement can be homogenous, heterogenous, or ring-like.

Differentiation of an abscess from a malignant tumor can be impossible on CT, since both can produce a ring-enhancing lesion. Multiple lesions are more likely to be metastases than abscesses, although subacute bacterial endocarditis can be associated with multiple cerebral abscesses.

Differentiation of malignant primary from metastatic tumor can also be difficult on CT. Multiple enhancing lesions are usually metastatic. The history of a known systemic malignancy also favors metastases.

SPINE CT

Spine CT is usually performed for trauma patients with suspected spinal fracture. CT is often more readily available than MRI, and studies of patients in spinal support devices can be scanned more easily by CT than MRI. Reconstructions can provide a three-dimensional image of the spine, indicating integrity, fracture, and/or instability of the spine.

A compression fracture of the spine is typically of the vertebral body and is generally a stable lesion. The CT can show if there is retropulsion of fragments into the spinal canal. A burst fracture destroys the vertebra, so that the fragments can impinge on surrounding tissues, most importantly the spinal canal. Odontoid fracture is a serious injury with high-cervical instability, which can result in paralysis or death.

CT angiography

CT angiography (CTA) has recently reduced the use of conventional catheter angiography for patients with suspected cerebrovascular disease. CTA is performed by administering iodinated dye intravenously and performing high-resolution, high-speed CT scanning of the brain. Complex calculations produce three-dimensional reconstructions of the arteries, which can show normal vessels, arterial plaques, stenoses, dissections, and embolic occlusions. The cerebral veins can also be imaged, helping in the diagnosis of venous sinus or cerebral vein thrombosis or occlusion.

CTA cannot be performed on patients with severe allergies to iodinated dye or in patients with any degree of renal failure. In these patients, MRA or selective catheter angiography is preferable.

Magnetic resonance imaging (MRI, MRA, and MRV)

MRI is the gold standard for structural imaging in the brain and spine. Specific imaging sequences can reveal abnormalities such as infarct, hemorrhage, tumor, developmental defect, trauma, inflammatory disorder, multiple sclerosis, and some degenerative conditions.

MRI involves placing the patient in a strong magnetic field. The field is perturbed by a radiofrequency pulse, and detectors measure the response of the atoms to the pertubation. Through complicated calculations, two-dimensional and three-dimensional images are created. MRI has greater spatial resolution than CT, and it avoids the problem of bone artifacts in the skull. It thus shows the brain to greater advantage. Specific imaging sequences are helpful in revealing acute or remote infarction (stroke), acute or remote traumatic brain injury, acute or remote hemorrhage, demyelinating plaques suggestive of MS, brain tumors; brain abscesses, developmental disorders, and meningitis.

MRI has been particularly useful in acute stroke (Chap. 24). Diffusion weighted imaging (DWI) reflects stagnation in the extracellular space and detects ischemic infarction within an hour or two of onset, remaining positive for 2–4 weeks. Perfusion weighted imaging (PWI, an image of blood flow with contrast infusion) can also show hypoperfused areas in the brain in acute stroke. The difference between DWI and PWI is thought to delineate the *ischemic penumbra* of tissue that is ischemic but not yet necrotic, perhaps identifying patients who can still be helped by thrombolytic therapy. Figure 38-3 shows a DWI in a patient with an acute ischemic stroke in the

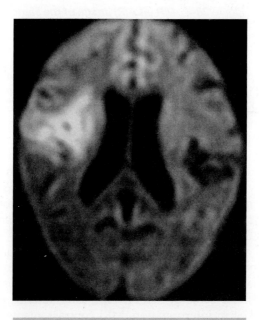

Figure 38-3 **MRI of a patient with an acute right middle cerebral artery territory stroke.** Diffusion-weighted imaging shows brightness in the right hemisphere (left side of the image) indicating a region of acute ischemia.

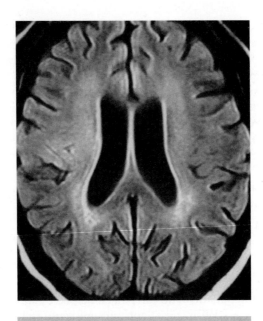

Figure 38-4 **MR (FLAIR) image of the same
patient as Fig. 38-3.**

right middle cerebral artery territory; this lesion was not detectable on a
FLAIR image (Fig. 38-4). A picture of a perfusion-weighted MR image was
shown in Fig. 24-4. Cerebral hemorrhage can also be imaged on MRI via the
T2* or *gradient echo* sequence, in which both acute and chronic blood products
produce a dark signal. The time course of changes in the standard T1- and T2-
weighted sequences with hemorrhage are more complex than those of CT.

In MS, plaques are bright on T2 and FLAIR images, an appearance that
can be shared by small infarcts, or even tumors or abscesses. Plaques of MS
tend to line up along the ventricles and are especially prominent in white
matter pathways such as the corpus callosum. Enhancement of a T2-bright
lesion indicates that it is acute or subacute.

Tumors and abscesses may vary in their appearance on MRI. As in CT
scanning, enhancement with contrast agents is helpful in detecting high-
grade or malignant lesions. As was discussed under CT, abscesses, and even
subacute strokes and cerebral hemorrhages can enhance with contrast, so
care must be taken in interpretation. MRI contrast agents are *paramagnetic*
rather than iodinated and rarely produce allergic reactions or renal changes;
this is another advantage of MR imaging over CT.

Magnetic resonance angiography (MRA) refers to MR imaging of the arteries
of the brain and neck. Flowing blood makes a magnetic image, and MRA is

actually imaging blood flow rather than the anatomy of the vessels. Accurate views of the carotid and vertebral vasculature can be obtained, however, especially with use of paramagnetic contrast agents and with a very cooperative patient. MRA is ordered especially in patients with stroke, transient ischemic attack (TIA), or those in whom there is consideration of aneurysm.

Magnetic resonance venography (MRV) refers to MR imaging of the cerebral veins and venous sinuses. MRV is used mainly for patients with suspected venous thrombosis, including patients with headache and signs of increased intracranial pressure, pregnant patients with headache and focal symptoms or signs, and some patients with seizures.

MRI, MRA, and MRV cannot be performed on patients with implanted devices including permanent pacemakers, implanted defibrillators, and depth electrodes for deep brain stimulation. Also, some clinicians feel that recently-inserted coronary or cerebrovascular stents and aneurysm clips pose a risk to a patient during MRI. As mentioned in the CT section, MR is also problematic in patients who are claustrophobic or uncooperative, though MR can be performed under sedation.

Angiography

Conventional catheter angiography is often considered the gold standard for evaluation of cerebrovascular disease. Ultrasound, CTA, and MRA have reduced the number of angiograms performed, but this technique is far from obsolete. The noninvasive studies can overestimate the level of stenosis; operative decisions without an angiogram should always be made with full understanding of the limitations of noninvasive studies.

Catheter angiography is performed by passing a catheter usually via the femoral artery, entering near the groin. The catheter is threaded rostrally, and selective injections into the carotid and vertebral arteries show the extracranial and intracranial vessels.

Angiography is usually performed when the diagnostic considerations include stroke, TIA, vasculitis, aneurysm, or vascular malformation. Angiography is also necessary for intra-arterial thrombolytic therapy in acute stroke, or to permit extraction of an embolus via a clot-extraction device (see Chap. 24). Other advantages of angiography over MRA or CTA include the detection of small vessel changes such as vasculitis or small aneurysms or arteriovenous malformations (AVMs). Interventional procedures to coil aneurysms, embolize AVMs, or perform angioplasty and stenting for arterial stenosis must be done via catheter angiography.

The angiogram may show the following changes: arterial occlusion, arterial stenosis, arterial plaque, aneurysm, arteriovenous malformation (AVM), vasculitis, or venous occlusion. Arteriograms also show the patterns of collateral blood flow in cerebrovascular occlusive disease, and they are necessary for the Wada test (see Chap. 25) used to document cerebral dominance

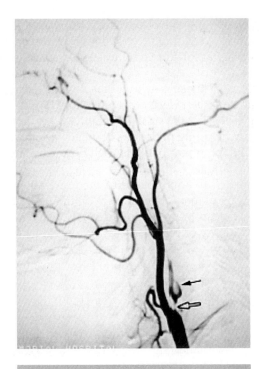

Figure 38-5 **Cerebral arteriogram showing internal carotid artery stenosis.** Catheter angiography of the carotid artery. The open arrow shows an area of marked narrowing at the origin of the internal artery as it separates from the external carotid artery (the ECA always has multiple branches). The dark arrow shows a small amount of contrast distal to the stenosis with an irregular appearance, suggesting clot or plaque in the bulb of the internal carotid artery.

in patients in whom surgical ablation is planned for epilepsy or for AVMs or brain tumors. Figure 38-5 shows a cerebral arteriogram in a patient with severe stenosis of the internal carotid artery.

Performance of cerebral angiography should normally be planned after evaluation by or consultation with neurology, neurosurgery, or vascular surgery. In many instances, adequate vascular assessment can be made from noninvasive studies. Catheter angiography has a small but significant risk of ischemic stroke, local hemorrhage, and renal insufficiency.

KEY REFERENCES

Abou-Khalil BE, Misulis KE. *Atlas of EEG and Seizure Semiology*. Philadelphia, PA: Elsevier; 2006.

Biola H, Crowell K, Grover F Jr. Clinical inquiries. Which imaging modality is best for suspected stroke? *J Fam Pract* 2005;54:538–539.

Chemali KR, Tsao B. Electrodiagnostic testing of nerves and muscles: when, why, and how to order. *Cleve Clin J Med* 2005;72:37–48.

Cueva RA. Auditory brainstem response versus magnetic resonance imaging for the evaluation of asymmetric sensorineural hearing loss. *Laryngoscope* 2004;114: 1686–1692.

Gandhi D. Computed tomography and magnetic resonance angiography in cervic-ocranial vascular disease. *J Neuroophthalmol* 2004;24:306–314.

Misulis KE, Head TC. *Essentials of Clinical Neurophysiology*. 3rd ed. Boston, MA: Butterworth Heinemann; 2003.

Smith SJ. EEG in the diagnosis, classification, and management of patients with epilepsy. *J Neurol Neurosurg Psychiatry* 2005;76(ii Suppl. 2):2–7.

Tsushima Y, Endo K. MR imaging in the evaluation of chronic or recurrent headache. *Radiology* 2005;235:575–579.

van Baalen B, Odding E, Maas AI, et al. Traumatic brain injury: classification of initial severity and determination of functional outcome. *Disabil Rehabil* 2003;7;25: 9–18.

Walsh P, Kane N, Butler S. The clinical role of evoked potentials. *J Neurol Neurosurg Psychiatry* 2005;76(ii Suppl.2):16–22.

Weinstock-Guttman B, Baier M, Stockton R, et al. Pattern reversal visual evoked potentials as a measure of visual pathway pathology in multiple sclerosis. *Mult Scler* 2003;9:529–534.

Young RJ, Destian S. Imaging of traumatic intracranial hemorrhage. *Neuroimaging Clin N Am* 2002;12:189–204.

NOTE: Page numbers followed by *f* or *t* indicate figures or tables, respectively.